SECOND EDITION

BASIC CLINICAL REHABILITATION MEDICINE

SECOND EDITION

Basic Clinical
Rehabilitation Medicine

Mehrsheed Sinaki, M.D., M.S.

Professor of Physical Medicine and Rehabilitation
Mayo Medical School
Consultant
Department of Physical Medicine and Rehabilitation
Mayo Clinic and Mayo Foundation
Rochester, Minnesota

With Contributors

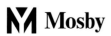 Mosby

St. Louis Baltimore Boston Chicago London Madrid Philadelphia Sydney Toronto

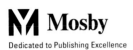
Mosby
Dedicated to Publishing Excellence

Publisher: George Stamathis
Editor: Robert Hurley
Developmental Editor: Joyce-Rachel John
Project Supervisor: Carol A. Reynolds
Project Supervisors: Deborah Thorp, Frances Perveiler
Proofroom Manager: Barbara M. Kelly
Manufacturing Supervisor: Betty Richmond
Designer: Carol A. Reynolds

Printed in the United States of America.
Composition by Clarinda.
Printing/binding by Maple Vail.

1 2 3 4 5 6 7 8 9 0 97 96 95 94 93

Library of Congress Cataloging-in Publication Data
Basic clinical rehabilitation medicine / [edited by] Mehrsheed Sinaki.
  —2nd ed.
     p.   cm.
  Includes bibliographical references and index.
  ISBN 0-8016-7991-5
  1. Medicine, Physical.   2. Medical rehabilitation.   I. Sinaki,
Mehrsheed.
  [DNLM: 1. Rehabilitation.   WB 320 B311 1993]
RM700.B315   1993
617'.03—dc20   93-4035
DNLM/DLC   CIP
for Library of Congress

CONTRIBUTORS

Karen L. Andrews, M.D.
Senior Associate Consultant,
  Department of Physical Medicine
  and Rehabilitation, Mayo Clinic and
  Mayo Foundation; Assistant Professor
  of Physical Medicine and
  Rehabilitation, Mayo Medical
  School; Rochester, Minnesota

Richard Paul Bonfiglio, M.D.
Vice President, Medical Affairs, and
  Medical Director, Bryn Mawr Rehab,
  Malvern, Pennsylvania

Stephen W. Carmichael, Ph.D., D.Sc.
Chair, Department of Anatomy, Mayo
  Clinic and Mayo Foundation;
  Professor of Anatomy, Mayo Medical
  School; Rochester, Minnesota

Carl W. Chan, M.D.
Consultant, Department of Physical
  Medicine and Rehabilitation, Mayo
  Clinic and Mayo Foundation;
  Assistant Professor of Physical
  Medicine and Rehabilitation, Mayo
  Medical School; Rochester,
  Minnesota

Jon B. Closson, M.D.
Consultant, Department of Physical
  Medicine and Rehabilitation, Mayo
  Clinic and Mayo Foundation;
  Instructor in Physical Medicine and
  Rehabilitation, Mayo Medical
  School; Rochester, Minnesota

Janet M. Cogoli, M.D.
Formerly, Senior Resident Associate in
  Physical Medicine and
  Rehabilitation, Mayo Graduate
  School of Medicine, Rochester,
  Minnesota. Currently, Fairlawn
  Rehabilitation Hospital, Worcester,
  Massachusetts

Robert W. DePompolo, M.D.
Chair, Department of Physical
  Medicine and Rehabilitation, Mayo
  Clinic and Mayo Foundation;
  Assistant Professor of Physical
  Medicine and Rehabilitation, Mayo
  Medical School; Rochester,
  Minnesota

Peter T. Dorsher, M.D.
Formerly, Senior Associate Consultant,
  Department of Physical Medicine
  and Rehabilitation, Mayo Clinic and
  Mayo Foundation; Instructor in
  Physical Medicine and
  Rehabilitation, Mayo Medical
  School; Rochester, Minnesota.
  Currently, Associate Medical
  Director, Rehabilitation Hospital of
  Baton Rouge, Baton Rouge,
  Louisiana

Rolland P. Erickson, M.D.
Consultant, Department of Physical
  Medicine and Rehabilitation, Mayo
  Clinic Scottsdale, Scottsdale,
  Arizona; Assistant Professor of
  Physical Medicine and
  Rehabilitation, Mayo Medical
  School; Rochester, Minnesota

Steven V. Fisher, M.D.
Chairperson, Department of Physical
  Medicine and Rehabilitation,
  Hennepin County Medical Center;
  Associate Professor, University of
  Minnesota; Minneapolis, Minnesota

Gail L. Gamble, M.D.
Consultant, Department of Physical
  Medicine and Rehabilitation, Mayo
  Clinic and Mayo Foundation;
  Assistant Professor of Physical
  Medicine and Rehabilitation, Mayo
  Medical School; Rochester,
  Minnesota

v

Sherwin Goldman, M.D.
Consultant, Impairment Evaluation Center, Mayo Clinic and Mayo Foundation; Assistant Professor of Orthopedics, Mayo Medical School; Rochester, Minnesota

Toni J. Hanson, M.D.
Consultant, Department of Physical Medicine and Rehabilitation, Mayo Clinic and Mayo Foundation; Assistant Professor of Physical Medicine and Rehabilitation, Mayo Medical School; Rochester, Minnesota

David G. Hurrell, M.D.
Fellow in Cardiovascular Diseases, Mayo Graduate School of Medicine, Rochester, Minnesota

Mary L. Jurisson, M.D.
Consultant, Department of Physical Medicine and Rehabilitation, Mayo Clinic and Mayo Foundation; Instructor in Physical Medicine and Rehabilitation, Mayo Medical School; Rochester, Minnesota

Edward R. Laskowski, M.D.
Consultant, Department of Physical Medicine and Rehabilitation, and Co-Chair, Sports Medicine Center, Mayo Clinic and Mayo Foundation; Assistant Professor of Physical Medicine and Rehabilitation, Mayo Medical School; Rochester, Minnesota

James F. Malec, Ph.D.
Consultant, Department of Psychiatry and Psychology, Mayo Clinic and Mayo Foundation; Associate Professor of Psychology, Mayo Medical School; Rochester, Minnesota

Joseph Y. Matsumoto, M.D.
Consultant, Department of Neurology, Mayo Clinic and Mayo Foundation; Assistant Professor of Neurology, Mayo Medical School; Rochester, Minnesota

Dennis J. Matthews, M.D.
Chairman and Medical Director, Rehabilitation Center, The Children's Hospital; Clinical Assistant Professor, Department of Rehabilitation Medicine, University of Colorado, Health Sciences Center; Denver, Colorado

John C. McMichan, M.B.,B.S., Ph.D.
Consultant, Department of Anesthesiology, Mayo Clinic Scottsdale, Scottsdale, Arizona; Associate Professor of Anesthesiology, Mayo Medical School, Rochester, Minnesota

Malcolm C. McPhee, M.D.
Chair, Department of Physical Medicine and Rehabilitation, Mayo Clinic Scottsdale, Scottsdale, Arizona; Associate Professor of Physical Medicine and Rehabilitation, Mayo Medical School; Rochester, Minnesota

John L. Merritt, M.D.
Formerly, Consultant, Department of Physical Medicine and Rehabilitation, Mayo Clinic and Mayo Foundation; Professor of Physical Medicine and Rehabilitation, Mayo Medical School; Rochester, Minnesota. Currently, Medical Director, Tustin Rehabilitation Hospital and in private practice, Tustin, California

Neil E Miller, P.T.
Physical Therapist, Department of Physical Medicine and Rehabilitation, Mayo Clinic and Mayo Foundation, Rochester, Minnesota

Bahram Mokri, M.D.
Vice Chair, Department of Neurology, Mayo Clinic and Mayo Foundation; Associate Professor of Neurology, Mayo Medical School; Rochester, Minnesota

Donald W. Mulder, M.D.
*Emeritus member, Department of
Neurology, Mayo Clinic and Mayo
Foundation; Emeritus Professor of
Neurology, Mayo Medical School;
Rochester, Minnesota*

Kevin P. Murphy, M.D.
*Formerly, Resident in Physical
Medicine and Rehabilitation, Mayo
Graduate School of Medicine;
Instructor in Physical Medicine and
Rehabilitation, Mayo Medical
School; Rochester, Minnesota.
Currently, Associate Medical
Director, Polinsky Medical
Rehabilitation Center, Associate
Professor, University of Minnesota
School of Medicine, Duluth,
Minnesota, and Attending Staff
Consultant, The Duluth Clinic Ltd.,
Duluth, Minnesota*

David L. Nash, M.D.
*Consultant, Department of Physical
Medicine and Rehabilitation, Mayo
Clinic and Mayo Foundation;
Assistant Professor of Physical
Medicine and Rehabilitation, Mayo
Medical School; Rochester,
Minnesota*

Stephen F. Noll, M.D.
*Consultant, Department of Physical
Medicine and Rehabilitation, Mayo
Clinic and Mayo Foundation;
Assistant Professor of Physical
Medicine and Rehabilitation, Mayo
Medical School; Rochester,
Minnesota*

**John H. Noseworthy, M.D.,
F.R.C.P.(C)**
*Head of a Section of Neurology, Mayo
Clinic and Mayo Foundation;
Associate Professor of Neurology,
Mayo Medical School; Rochester,
Minnesota*

Terry H. Oh, M.D.
*Consultant, Department of Physical
Medicine and Rehabilitation, Mayo
Clinic and Mayo Foundation;
Assistant Professor of Physical
Medicine and Rehabilitation, Mayo
Medical School; Rochester,
Minnesota*

Joachim L. Opitz, M.D.
*Consultant, Department of Physical
Medicine and Rehabilitation, Mayo
Clinic and Mayo Foundation;
Professor of Physical Medicine and
Rehabilitation, Mayo Medical
School; Rochester, Minnesota*

Jane L. Reiman, M.D.
*Formerly, Consultant, Department of
Physical Medicine and
Rehabilitation, Mayo Clinic and
Mayo Foundation; Assistant Professor
of Physical Medicine and
Rehabilitation, Mayo Medical
School; Rochester, Minnesota.
Currently, Physiatrist, Lutheran
General Health Systems, Park Ridge,
Illinois*

Elizabeth A. Rivers, O.T.R., R.N.
*Burn Rehabilitation Specialist, St. Paul
Ramsey Medical Center, St. Paul,
Minnesota; Part-Time Clinical
Instructor, University of Minnesota;
Minneapolis, Minnesota*

Daniel E. Rohe, Ph.D
*Consultant, Department of Psychiatry
and Psychology, Mayo Clinic and
Mayo Foundation; Assistant Professor
of Psychology, Mayo Medical
School; Rochester, Minnesota*

Ann H. Schutt, M.D.
*Consultant, Department of Physical
Medicine and Rehabilitation, Mayo
Clinic and Mayo Foundation;
Associate Professor of Physical
Medicine and Rehabilitation, Mayo
Medical School; Rochester,
Minnesota*

Lee D. Shibley, P.T.
*Formerly, Physical Therapist,
Department of Physical Medicine
and Rehabilitation, Mayo Clinic and
Mayo Foundation, Rochester,
Minnesota. Currently, Captain, USAF
Biomedical Science Corps, Staff
Physical Therapist at Wilford Hall
Medical Center, Lackland AFB, Texas*

Ray W. Squires, Ph.D.
*Director, Cardiovascular Health Clinic,
and Director, Exercise
Electrocardiography Laboratory,
Mayo Clinic and Mayo Foundation;
Assistant Professor of Medicine,
Mayo Medical School; Rochester,
Minnesota*

Lynne M. Stempien, M.D.
*Assistant Medical Director,
Rehabilitation Center, The Children's
Hospital; Clinical Assistant Professor,
Department of Rehabilitation
Medicine, University of Colorado,
Health Sciences Center; Denver,
Colorado*

G. Keith Stillwell, M.D., Ph.D.
*Emeritus member, Department of
Physical Medicine and
Rehabilitation, Mayo Clinic and
Mayo Foundation; Emeritus Professor
of Physical Medicine and
Rehabilitation, Mayo Medical
School; Rochester, Minnesota*

Jeffrey M. Thompson, M.D.
*Consultant, Department of Physical
Medicine and Rehabilitation, Mayo
Clinic and Mayo Foundation;
Assistant Professor of Physical
Medicine and Rehabilitation, Mayo
Medical School; Rochester,
Minnesota*

Gudni Thorsteinsson, M.D.
*Chair, Department of Physical
Medicine and Rehabilitation, Mayo
Clinic Jacksonville, Jacksonville,
Florida; Assistant Professor of
Physical Medicine and
Rehabilitation, Mayo Medical
School; Rochester, Minnesota*

David C. Weber, M.D.
*Senior Associate Consultant,
Department of Physical Medicine
and Rehabilitation, Mayo Clinic and
Mayo Foundation; Instructor in
Physical Medicine and
Rehabilitation, Mayo Medical
School; Rochester, Minnesota*

PREFACE TO THE SECOND EDITION

The purpose of this book, as in the previous edition, is to provide the reader with a basic knowledge of most of the areas in rehabilitation medicine and with specific details about the practical management of the conditions that are most common in the daily practice of physical medicine and rehabilitation.

The prevalence of detailed, informative books on physical medicine and rehabilitation during the past 8 years has necessitated a book that provides easier access to some of the rehabilitative measures without extensive reading.

To fulfill readers' needs in additional areas of rehabilitation medicine, we have extensively revised several of the original chapters and added new tables and figures. In addition, several new chapters are added. Several new contributors have participated in this edition. This book is the overall effort of the contributors and editor to provide basic scientific knowledge in various areas of rehabilitation medicine in a condensed manner.

I am especially grateful to my dear friend and editor, Mrs. LeAnn Stee, for her editorial efforts. I also thank other members of the Section of Publications for their excellent editorial assistance, especially Mrs. Mary Jane Badker, Mrs. Virginia Dunt, Mrs. Dorothy Tienter, Mrs. Jen Schlotthauer, Miss Mary Schwager, and Miss Renée Van Vleet. Very special thanks and appreciation are expressed to Mrs. Sandy Fitzgerald for her superb secretarial assistance and dedication.

Mehrsheed Sinaki, M.D., M.S.

PREFACE TO THE FIRST EDITION (1987)

The first class of Mayo Medical School, composed of 40 students, began its studies in September 1972. These young men and women of high enthusiasm and intellect are carefully selected from many applicants. It was not until the academic year of 1974–1975 that those students began their rotation through the Department of Physical Medicine and Rehabilitation. Since then, our Department has not been the same. Their remarkable desire to learn and their inquisitiveness have enhanced our staff members' enthusiasm for educating and have enriched our academic lives. Some of these students have joined us as residents and colleagues and have furthered our cause for practice, education, and research. The original lecture series for the medical students was developed by Gordon M. Martin, M.D., chairman of the Department at that time. During the subsequent few years, the course was further strengthened through the efforts of Gudni Thorsteinsson, M.D., then chairman of the undergraduate committee for the Department of Physical Medicine and Rehabilitation, before he passed his responsibilities to me in 1980. Several members of our Department taught various topics. Gradually, the lectures and handouts were revised and a syllabus was developed. G. Keith Stillwell, M.D., and Malcolm C. McPhee, M.D., succeeding department chairmen, provided much encouragement.

The idea of preparing this book was crystallized after repeatedly being told by many of our students that we should write a book that they could use for the course. The material presented in the lecture series formed the basis of this book. It is aimed at medical students. Because excellent extensive books are available that contain detailed information on various subjects of rehabilitation, lengthy discussions have been avoided to enable the reader to grasp the concepts for rehabilitation of commonly encountered problems without elaborate reading. In addition to medical students, this book will be useful to junior residents in the field of physical medicine and rehabilitation and to physicians and residents in other fields.

I thank my colleagues in the Department of Physical Medicine and Rehabilitation for their support, for their enthusiastic teaching of the medical students, and for making the preparation of this book possible. My special gratitude goes to Roy S. Rogers III, M.D., Associate Dean for Academic Affairs of the Mayo Medical School, for his contagious enthusiasm, encouragement, and support over the years and to Mr. Jack E. Uhlenhopp, Administrative Assistant of the Mayo Medical School, for his many efforts and help. My thanks go also to members of the Section of Publications. I am deeply indebted to the efforts of LeAnn Stee for her skillful editorial work and her constructive advice. I particularly thank Roberta J. Flood for her assistance in meeting deadlines and facilitating production of the book, and my appreciation goes to Mary Jane Badker, editorial assistant, and to Dorothy Tienter, proofreader, for their efforts. I gratefully acknowledge the interest and advice of Mr. Brian C. Decker, publisher.

Mehrsheed Sinaki, M.D., M.S.

CONTENTS

PART I

Introduction to Physical Medicine and Rehabilitation

1 | Current Concepts and Practical Aspects of Physical Medicine and Rehabilitation

Mehrsheed Sinaki

G. Keith Stillwell

The primary goal of rehabilitation medicine is the achievement of maximal independence for handicapped persons by using the organized efforts of knowledgeable personnel in the health sciences and social service areas.

DEFINITIONS

The scope and aims of rehabilitation have been conveyed by investigators in the field. Krusen[1] defined the field as follows.

> Physical medicine and rehabilitation involves the medical examination and evaluation of the disabilities of handicapped patients, the prescription and medical supervision of physical and occupational therapy and other forms of therapy, the training of the handicapped person in ambulation and self-care and medical supervision and coordination of other rehabilitation procedures.

Krusen[1] described rehabilitation as follows.

> Rehabilitation involves treatment and training of the patient to the end that he may attain his maximal potential for normal living physically, psychologically, socially, and vocationally.
>
> Rehabilitation is a creative procedure which includes the cooperative efforts of various medical specialists and their associates in other health fields to improve the physical, mental, social, and vocational aptitudes of persons who are handicapped, with the objective of preserving their ability to live happily and productively on the same level and with the same opportunities as their neighbors.

3

The goal of rehabilitation is to decrease the dependence of the handicapped or disabled person by developing, to the greatest extent possible, the abilities needed for adequate functioning in the individual's situation.

In rehabilitation medicine, a patient's abilities rather than disabilities are stressed. "Rehabilitation medicine is the use of all methods of diagnosis and treatment which will restore the disabled individual to as nearly normal as possible."[2]

Rehabilitation should involve the progressive transition from the rehabilitation facility to home, to work, and into the community; this transition should be smooth and planned and engineered with care, foresight, and knowledgeable effort.

During recent years, medical schools have increasingly recognized the importance of physical medicine and rehabilitation, and free-standing rehabilitation centers and hospital-based rehabilitation facilities and programs have proliferated. Also, increases in the aging population and serious disabling injuries have enhanced the need for physical medicine and rehabilitation.

The team approach used in the field of physical medicine and rehabilitation involves all medical specialties. Resources of available, cooperating, trained personnel are more important than the facility. Each team is based on the individual patient's requirements. Desirable rehabilitation-oriented personnel include internists, physiatrists, neurologists, orthopedists, pediatricians, psychiatrists, speech pathologists and therapists, rehabilitation nursing personnel, physical therapists, occupational therapists, social service workers, psychologists, the patient's family, clergy, insurance carriers, vocational counselors, vocational placement services, and specialized personnel for deficits such as blindness, deafness, and mental retardation.

In the United States, associations of physicians interested in physical therapeutics date as far back as 1890 and have as their surviving descendant the American Congress of Rehabilitation Medicine. Its membership is not limited to physicians. The other principal professional organization, whose membership is limited to physiatrists, is the American Academy of Physical Medicine and Rehabilitation, founded in 1938. A smaller group, the Association of Academic Physiatrists, provides, among other functions, liaison with the Association of American Medical Colleges.

Historically, Frank H. Krusen, M.D., is regarded as the father of physical medicine, and Howard A. Rusk, M.D., was the foremost leader in the expansion of medical rehabilitation during and after World War II. The American Board of Physical Medicine was established in 1947; "rehabilitation" was added to the name in 1949.

Several disease-oriented organizations have rehabilitation as a major concern, such as the American Academy for Cerebral Palsy and Developmental Medicine, the American Spinal Injury Association, and the Muscular Dystrophy Association. The National Rehabilitation Association is principally concerned with state and federal vocational rehabilitation programs.

REFERENCES

1. Krusen FH. The scope of physical medicine and rehabilitation. In: *Handbook of physical medicine and rehabilitation*. 2nd ed. Philadelphia: WB Saunders, 1971:1–13.
2. Gullickson G Jr, Licht S. Definition and philosophy of rehabilitation medicine. In: Licht S, ed. *Rehabilitation and medicine*. Baltimore, Maryland: Waverly Press, 1968:1–14.

PART II

Evaluation of the Patient in Rehabilitation Medicine

2

History Taking and Evaluation of Patients

Rolland P. Erickson

Toni J. Hanson

Malcolm C. McPhee

As with other facets of medicine, the cornerstone of rehabilitation medicine is a thorough and useful evaluation[1] of the patient. For patients who are hospitalized in a rehabilitation unit for comprehensive care, a complete general medical workup is necessary to manage the common medical problems that will need to be managed by the physiatrist serving as primary physician. The disability cannot be isolated from preexisting and concurrent general medical problems.

In addition, certain aspects of the rehabilitation evaluation go beyond the traditional medical workup.[2] Activities of daily living are those endeavors that are accomplished on a daily basis in order to maintain personal independence. The abilities to eat, bathe, groom, toilet, turn in bed, rise, sit, lie, transfer (from bed to chair, chair to toilet, or chair to car), accomplish mobility (walk with or without gait aids or operate a wheelchair), speak, hear, see, and think have an impact on the ability to live independently. Disability occurs when these and other skills of independent living are impaired. These functional skills must be assessed to identify the most appropriate rehabilitation intervention. For example, consider a patient with recent hemiparesis and aphasia. The neurologist evaluates the patient to determine cause (cerebral thrombosis, hemorrhage, embolism, or tumor), proper acute management, and prevention of progression of the impairment (hemiparesis and aphasia). The physiatrist evaluates the patient not only to identify strategies for reduction of impairment (muscle reeducation and strengthening) but also to decipher maneuvers that minimize the disability (inability to dress, bathe, or ambulate) that has resulted from the impairment.

One soon realizes that the rehabilitation evaluation is not limited to a specific organ system. Instead, a truly comprehensive quality to the assessment emerges. In that the goal of rehabilitation is to maximize an individual's mental, social, vocational, and physical usefulness, the influence of the individual's impairment on work, play, family life, and sexuality must also be assessed and appropriate strategies identified.

Following is an outline of a clinical evaluation applicable to rehabilitation. In its complete form it should be useful for the comprehensive assessment of a patient admitted to a rehabilitation unit. For patients evaluated as outpatients or in consultation with a non-rehabilitation physician, parts of it may be used.

OUTLINE OF CLINICAL EVALUATION

History

Chief complaint
History of present illness, including medications and dosages
Functional abilities (Table 2–1)

Review of Systems

Constitution: fever, chills, sweats, fatigue, weight change
HEENT
Head: headaches
Eyes: scotoma, pain, dryness
Ears: earache, drainage
Nose: epistaxis, drainage, congestion
Throat and mouth: teeth, gums, tongue, eating, sores, masses, voice
Respiratory: cough, sputum, hemoptysis, wheezing, dyspnea, pleuritic chest pain
Cardiovascular: chest pain, dyspnea, orthopnea, paroxysmal nocturnal dyspnea, palpitations, claudication, murmur, exercise tolerance
Gastrointestinal: pain, nausea, vomiting, stool consistency, blood from mouth or rectum, jaundice, change in bowel habits

TABLE 2–1
Assessment of Functional Abilities

Function	Independent	Independent With Aids	Needs Some Assistance	Totally Dependent
Feeding				
Dressing				
Hygiene				
Toileting				
Bed activities				
Transfers				
Mobility/wheelchair				
Mobility/gait				
Driving				

Genitourinary: dysuria, pyuria, hematuria, retention, incontinence, sensation, stones, urinary tract infection

Females: menses and bleeding, pain, pregnancies, miscarriages, live births, menopause

Males: erection, ejaculation, progeny, pain

Neurologic

Cranial nerves

I: altered sense of smell

II, III, IV, VI: diplopia, blurring, field cuts, glasses

V: weakness of masticating muscles

VII: facial weakness, dysarthria, loss of taste

VIII: deafness, imbalance, dizziness, tinnitus

Motor: weakness, tremors, clumsiness

Gait: stability, falls, endurance

Sensory: loss or change, pain

Cognitive, perceptual: changes in memory or thinking

Personality: changes

Muscles: pain, weakness, hypertrophy, atrophy

Skeleton: fracture, deformity

Joints: stiffness, limited motion, pain, swelling

Past Medical History

Allergies

Blood transfusions and reactions

Childhood illness

Surgical procedures

Hospitalizations not involving surgical procedures

Injuries

Immunizations: include pneumococcal and flu vaccines

Illnesses: diabetes, hypertension, pneumonia, coronary artery disease, hepatitis, bronchitis, chronic obstructive pulmonary disease, scarlet fever, rheumatic fever, cancer

Travel

Family History

Family members and their health

History of hereditary disease, hypertension, cancer, diabetes, heart disease

Patient Profile

Social history

Habits

Diet: for secondary prevention of risk factors

Drugs, alcohol, smoking

Family: members, others at home, marital status
Architectural accessibility of home
Vocational history
Avocational interests
Psychologic history
Previous life-style
Past and current responses to stress

Physical Examination

Vital signs: blood pressure, pulse, temperature, respiration
Skin and lymphatics
HEENT
Head: signs of trauma, surgical wounds
Eyes: nystagmus, conjunctivae, sclerae, funduscopic examination
Ears: otoscopic examination
Nose: inspection
Throat and mouth: inspection and palpation, gums and teeth, swallowing
Neck: quality of jugular and carotid pulsations, bruits, nodes, thyroid
Chest: structure, respiratory rhythm, clubbing, inspection, palpation, percussion, auscultation, diaphragm
Cardiovascular: heart sounds, peripheral pulses (grading)
Abdomen: bowel sounds, tenderness, organomegaly, masses
Genitourinary: flank tenderness, external genitalia, pelvic examination
Rectal: sphincter tone, masses, prostate, stool
Neurologic
Mental status
Level of consciousness: coma, stupor, somnolence, confusion, reaction to verbal, visual, tactile, and painful stimuli
Intellect: orientation, calculation, retention, recent and past memory, general information, similarities, abstractions
Personality: description of cooperation, behavior and affect
Thought: fears, preoccupations, insight, fixed ideas, delusions, illusions, hallucinations
Complex sensory functions: agnosias, body scheme, concepts of time, space, configuration
Performance of complex acts: apraxia, perseveration
Language: listening (single- and multiple-step commands), reading, speaking, writing
Speech: respiration, phonation, articulation, resonance, prosody
Handedness
Handwriting sample
Cranial nerves
I: smell
II: visual acuity and fields
III, IV, VI: pupillary responses, extraocular muscles, nystagmus
V: masseter, pterygoids

VII: corneal reflex, facial muscles
VIII: hearing (watch), Weber, Rinne, Romberg tests
IX, X, XI: sternocleidomastoid, taste, gag
XII: tongue
Reflexes
   Muscle stretch reflexes: jaw (nerve V), biceps (C5–C6), brachiora-
      dialis (C5–C6), triceps (C6–C8), quadriceps (L2–L4), internal
      hamstring (L4–L5, S1–S2), external hamstring (L5, S1–S2), gas-
      trocnemius-soleus (L5, S1–S2)
   Superficial reflexes: corneal (nerves V–VIII), gag (nerves IX–X),
      epigastric (T6–T9), hypogastric (T11–L1), cremasteric (L1–L2),
      anal (S3–S5), bulbocavernous (S2–S4)
   Pathologic reflexes: Babinski, Chaddock
Sensation
   Test extremities, thorax, abdomen, genitalia, perineum
   Superficial touch and pain, deep pain, position sense, vibration,
      stereognosis, temperature (hot and cold), extinction to bilateral
      confrontation
Coordination/rapid alternating movements
   Sitting and standing balance
   Rapid alternating movements
   Finger-nose-finger test
   Heel-toe test
Musculoskeletal
Inspection: atrophy, swelling, skin changes
Palpation: swelling, spasm, tenderness
Range of motion
   Passive
   Active
Joint stability: tests, subluxations, dislocations
Manual muscle testing (see below)
Gait (see below)

Manual Muscle Testing

Manual muscle testing is helpful for ascertaining the degree and extent
of muscle weakness. Grading muscle strength involves assigning a specific value (by adjective or number) to the strength of muscles (Table
2–2). Manual muscle testing is of benefit clinically for diagnosing neuromuscular diseases, designing effective therapy programs, evaluating
the need for assistive devices, and following the course of a disease and
its response to treatment (through periodic reevaluations); it can also be
of benefit for determining subsequent physical, medical, and surgical
management of neuromuscular diseases. Various factors influence manual muscle testing, including the presence or absence of pain, spasticity, fatigue, age and sex of a patient, upper motor neuron disorders,
communication problems, conversion reactions, other psychologic fac-

TABLE 2–2.
Systems Used to Grade Muscle Strength

Strength	Criteria	Grading System[3]					
		Mayo Clinic PM & R* (No.)	Mayo Clinic Neuro* (No.)	Kendall (%)	National Foundation for Infant Paralysis (%)	Wright and Lovett (Word & Letter)	Aids to Investigation of Peripheral Nerve Injury (No.)
Normal	Muscle has the ability to move the body part through the available arc of motion and hold against gravity and maximal resistance	0	0	90%–100%	100%	Normal N	5
Good	Muscle moves the part through the available arc of motion against gravity but accepts less than maximal resistance	1	−1	70%–90%	75%	Good G	4
Fair	Muscle moves the part through the available arc of motion against gravity but cannot accept any additional resistance	2	−2	40%–60%	50%	Fair F	3
Poor	Muscle can complete the arc of motion but only with elimination of the effects of gravity	3	−3	10%–30%	25%	Poor P	2
Trace	A feeble visible or palpable contraction of muscle (or prominence of a tendon) without production of motion	3+†	−3, −4	5%		Trace T	1
Total paralysis	No contraction of muscle	4	−4	0%	0%	Zero 0	0

*Neuro, neurology; PM & R, physical medicine and rehabilitation.
†In the Mayo Clinic PM & R system (following the numerical value): + = weaker than designated grade; − = stronger than designated grade.

tors (for example, low motivation or fear), and the expectations of the examiner.

When manual muscle testing is performed,[3] joint motion should be assessed, preferably with the patient moving the part actively through the available range of motion. Evaluation of the presence of cocontraction and substitution patterns is important. Positioning should be checked. The muscle should be tested in an antigravity position, and stabilization proximal to the segment tested should be ensured. The examiner applies resistance proximal to the next distal joint and in the direction opposite to the movement produced by the muscle contraction. Assessment of posture as a clue to muscle weakness, as well as ambulation patterns, is recommended. Also, strong antigravity muscles such as the dorsiflexors and plantar flexors of the ankle should be evaluated by heel and toe gait, respectively.

Gait

Numerous factors cause deviations in the normal pattern of walking, including (1) restriction of joint motion (including contractures), (2) pain with movement or weight bearing, (3) muscle weakness, (4) changes in sensation, (5) lack of coordinated movement, and (6) amputations or other changes in the status of soft tissues. Careful observation of the patient during standing and walking with identification of deviations is a valuable component of the physical evaluation process.

DIAGNOSES

A logical listing of a patient's diagnoses based on the history and physical examination summarizes the clinical findings. Both medical and rehabilitation diagnoses are stated, along with a succinct comment on the prognosis and the expected duration of treatment. It is increasingly important to document the diagnoses in order of rehabilitation significance because third-party payers (Medicare, Workmen's Compensation, and private insurance carriers) review them to determine payment based on the appropriateness of admission.

GOALS

Rehabilitation goals should continue to be refined at patient care conferences; however, at the time of the initial evaluation, general statements are made relating to short- and long-term goals. Plans for impairment reduction and improvement in functional status are clearly stated, as is the expected placement after dismissal. Medical goals are determined, including diagnostic studies and medications needed and problems requiring close scrutiny.

COMMENT

The requirements of a clinical evaluation can vary from evaluation of a specific joint to a comprehensive examination for admission to a rehabilitation unit. The detail needed and the time available will guide the examiner in determining the items to be selected for the clinical evaluation.

Presenting the results of the history and physical examination to an experienced clinician can help the medical student develop skills for problem identification and problem solving.

Clearly, the clinical evaluation remains a most important skill for the medical student to develop. Learning this skill never really ends.

REFERENCES

1. Mayo Clinic and Mayo Foundation. Clinical examinations in neurology. 5th ed. Philadelphia: WB Saunders, 1981.
2. Erickson RP, McPhee MC. Clinical evaluation. In: DeLisa JA, Currie DM, Gans BM, Gatens PF Jr, Leonard JA Jr, McPhee MC, eds. Rehabilitation medicine: principles and practice. Philadelphia: JB Lippincott, 1988:25−65.
3. Kendall FP, McCreary EK. Muscles testing and function. 3rd ed. Baltimore, Maryland: Williams & Wilkins, 1983.

3

Examination of Joints

John L. Merritt
Mehrsheed Sinaki

A prerequisite for the examination of any part or system of the human body is a thorough understanding of that part's anatomy and function for correct examination, recording, and interpretation. This chapter is not a review of joint anatomy or function because excellent texts on these subjects are already available; instead, this chapter is intended to present principles of joint examination that will assist the examiner in obtaining and interpreting the results.

An incomplete and inaccurate examination can result from the imposing number of human joints and the prodigious extent of joint landmarks, functions, and signs. All these factors may provide a setting for random and careless joint evaluation. The best guard against such is to develop a "routine" or system, whether the evaluation is of 1, 10, or 174 joints.

METHODICAL EXAMINATION

Adherence to a methodical evaluation is essential when a thorough examination of joints is needed.[1] Whether one begins with the upper extremities and then proceeds to the trunk and then the lower extremities or the reverse can often be determined by personal choice, patient position, or convenience, but variation in the order of examination should only rarely be the case. Deviations from one's established routine invite oversights and errors. The following sequence is suggested. With the patient standing, the lower back should be examined first, including the sacrum, coccyx, and sacroiliac and lumbar spine. The thoracic spine should be examined next; the patient will need to lie down to complete this part of the evaluation. Then the patient sits on the edge of the examination table or bed. The neck, skull, and temporomandibular joints are examined. The upper extremities are next approached, proceeding from proximal to distal joints. Finally, the lower extremities are examined, also from proximal to distal. Whether examining the back, neck, or upper or lower extremities, each joint pair should be symmetrically evaluated, first the right side and then the left (the "right first rule")—with one exception, which is described below. Measurements are recorded similarly: right/left (for example, knees [passive]: 5° to 110°/15° to 75°).

MOTION

Joint motion should be determined before the joints are palpated.[2, 3] Range of motion should include first active motion, then active assisted or passive motion. When the range is abnormal, goniometry (for peripheral joints) or skin distraction measurements (for the spine) should be added.[4, 5] Motions that cause pain and painful arcs of motion should be noted and recorded. After active and passive motions have been recorded, resistance to active motion (this may also serve as an evaluation of muscle strength) and any pain caused by isometric contractions are noted.[6] Although strength assessment includes appraisal of active, against-gravity movements, strength determination concludes with isometric resistance.

In patients with suspected or known arthritis, bursitis, or tendinitis, it is essential for the examiner to position himself or herself so as not to be overcome and not to allow movement during testing of resistance to motion.[7–9] Isometric resistance is usually tolerated, but painful isotonic movements are unwarranted and uncomfortable and may interfere with the remainder of the examination. Every effort should be made to ensure as little discomfort as possible.[1] If the examination is unnecessarily painful, patient trust and confidence in the examiner are undermined and assessment of relaxed, passive motions becomes impossible. This mistrust may even spill over into poor compliance to treatment recommendations and thus sabotage the very purpose of the joint examination.

In this light, whenever joint pain is reported to be asymmetric, relaxed passive examination of *the least painful side* should be performed first in order to enhance trust between patient and examiner and to allow the patient a better understanding of what motion or activity is to be attempted. This is the single exception to the "right first rule." A simple explanation to the patient before each step as to what is to be performed and what is to be examined aids the patient and examiner. Pain, muscle spasm, and splinting are thus minimized. When active assisted or passive movements are to be performed, a gentle, careful grip that supports the painful joint and avoids other tender areas is essential.

LIMITATION OF MOTION

When evaluating joint motion, one is, of course, already formulating a differential diagnosis. During this time, the four categories into which the causes of limitation of joint motion generally fall should be kept in mind.[10]

The first cause of limitation of joint motion is contractures. Contractures may be caused by the shortening of collagen fibers in muscle, tendon, ligaments, or, most frequently, the joint capsule itself. Capsular contractures (adhesive capsulitis) are a common consequence of infrequent or incomplete ranging of joints and often of surgical procedures, trauma, arthritis, tendinitis, bursitis, or neuromuscular disorders. Ligamentous contractures have similar broad causes but are more significant in the neck and back than in peripheral joints. Tendon and muscle contractures are often considered congruous, but careful studies have shown that these contractures are predominately intramuscular and that associated tendons themselves are not frequently contracted.

Motion limited by contractures has a special "feel" when the joint is passively moved.[6, 8] This has been called a soft "end-feel" and is a slow, gradual resilience at the end of an arc of passive motion. This is in contrast to the hard "end-feel" or "block" at the end of an arc of motion described below.

The second cause is capsular distention.[10] Joint capsules allow full arcs of joint motion only because of the existence of large, lax capsular redundancies (Fig. 3–1). These capsular redundancies may restrict motion not only when they are contracted (for example, adhesive capsulitis) but also when they are distended by fluid or synovial proliferation. This is the primary cause of loss of motion in inflammatory arthritis and after trauma. The capsular redundancies are already tense, and further movement of the joint is thus limited by the already taut, interlaced capsular collagen fibers. Further movement will thus only cause pain or tears of the joint capsule fibers.

The third cause is intra-articular loose bodies, which may limit joint motion by mechanically impinging on joint surfaces. Torn menisci, synovial plicae, loose cartilaginous fragments, and villonodular synovitis are some examples of intra-articular loose bodies.

The fourth cause is cartilaginous incongruity. Degenerative or inflammatory erosion of joint surface cartilage is the frequent cause. The resulting lack of a smooth surface for joint approximation may result in a sudden barrier to motion. Both intra-articular loose bodies and cartilaginous incongruity usually have a hard "end-feel"—the joint comes to an abrupt halt and does not move as further slow, gentle, unidirectional pressure is applied.[6]

Limitation of joint motion may, of course, and frequently does, result from combinations of these four causes. For example, traumatic hemarthrosis may restrict motion by capsular distention, but a torn meniscus may also be present. As the hemarthrosis resolves but motion continues to be restricted by cast, splint, pain, or inactivity, the joint capsule may contract as the joint fluid is absorbed.[10] An adhesive capsulitis may be the consequence.[9] Degenerative joint disease may limit motion by joint surface incongruity, but associated degenerative meniscal fragments may further limit motion. Pain and inactivity may concomitantly contribute to a superimposed joint capsule contracture. However, because the treatment strategies for each of the four categories of limitation of motion are divergent, understanding the contribution of each will promote a more logical and ef-

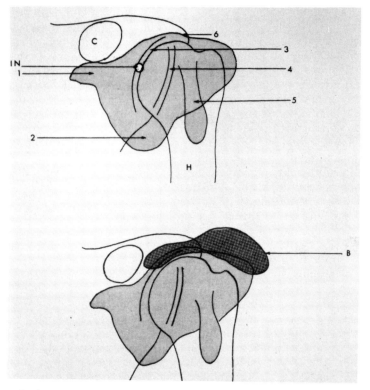

Figure 3–1

Arthrograms. Shaded area on shoulder joint depicts normal arthrogram. C, Coracoid process; H, humerus; IN, anterior site of injection into glenohumeral joint. (1) Subscapular bursa that normally communicates directly with shoulder joint and thus fills in normal arthrogram. As dye injection distends capsule, it hangs as dependent pouch under joint 2. (3) Superior medial surface of humerus. (4) Line of lesser density caused by underlying glenoid labrum. (5) Synovial lining that is pouch accompanying biceps tendon sheath in intertubercular groove a distance of some 2 inches. (6) Subacromial bursa and rotator cuff. Rotator cuff tear will permit dye to extend into subacromial bursa, superior to smooth line above humeral head, above and "around corner" of greater tuberosity, B. (From Cailliet R. Shoulder pain. Philadelphia: FA Davis, 1966:61. By permission.)

ficacious therapeutic plan. The physical examination of the joint is essential for development of such a therapeutic plan.

PALPATION

Palpation should be performed only after active, passive, and resistive joint motions have been assessed. Palpation should include joint margins, synovium, bursae, and accessible tendons. Palpation includes an appraisal of swelling, tenderness, stability, crepitation, deformities, and "joint play."[1, 8]

The synovium is the soft tissue of the joint proper. Normal synovium is not palpable because it is only a few cells in thickness. A swollen synovial membrane has a "boggy" feel, somewhat like the feel of modeling clay or fresh dough.[1, 7] An inflammatory arthritis is synonymous with synovitis. Synovitis is readily palpated. Therefore, learning to "feel" synovial thickening is a fundamental skill for the diagnosis of arthritis. A thickened, inflamed synovial membrane is readily palpable to the experienced examiner in all extremity joints from the elbow and knee distally. Practice is required to appreciate swollen, proliferative synovium, but this skill is not difficult to achieve with practice and frequent comparison with normal joints.

Synovial fluid is present in a normal joint in such minute quantities that it, like normal synovium, also is not palpable.[1] Palpation of fluid in a joint is abnormal and usually associated with synovitis. Joint fluid (effusion) may be obvious by visual or palpatory inspection. Fluid may be further identified by applying pressure over the joint and observing a readily reducible bulge at the margins of the joint.

Crepitations are grating vibrations that may be palpated or sometimes heard during motion. They result from cartilaginous roughening from degenerative or, less frequently, inflammatory processes. Inflammatory or degenerative changes in tendons and associated structures, however, may also produce crepitations. Of less significance is joint "snapping" due to tendon and ligament slipping over bony surfaces during motion. The stability of the supporting ligamentous structures should next be determined by passive joint manipulation. Specific techniques are available for each joint. Deformities of bony architecture, contractures, and articular subluxations should be noted and recorded.

"JOINT PLAY"

In addition to testing ligamentous stability by specific relaxed passive joint manipulation techniques, minor joint motions should also be estimated. A typical joint has major and minor motions.[5, 6, 8] Major motions may include flexion, extension, adduction, abduction, or rotation.[5] All joints also have minor motion, called "joint play."[8] This small motion is a passive gliding motion perpendicular to and along the axis of the articulating bones (Fig. 3–2). Restrictions of joint play motions are associated with tight joint capsules and intra-articular obstructions.[6] These minor joint motion restrictions, restrictions of joint play, are the basis for spinal and peripheral joint mobilization and manipulation techniques.[8]

THE RECORDING CHART

Collection of a large amount of data can lead to a record that is unwieldy and difficult to review.[2, 3] However, a permanent record of all joint

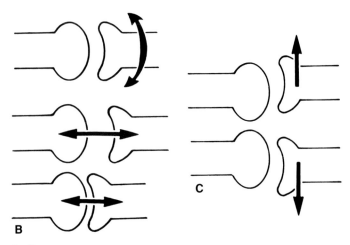

Figure 3–2
Joint play. *A*, Major motions: flexion, extension, and rotation. *B*, Longitudinal minor motion. *C*, Transitional, gliding, minor motion.

examinations is essential for prescribing and monitoring treatment. A convenient and useful charting system, the STL system, has been in use at the Mayo Clinic for many years (Fig. 3–3).[1] "S" indicates synovitis (objective and palpable synovial swelling or synovial effusion), "T" denotes joint tenderness, and "L" designates limitation of motion. "S," "T," and "L" can all be graded from 1 to 4: grade 1 is the slightest detectable involvement, grades 2 and 3 are moderate to severe abnormalities, and grade 4 is the most severe (rarely used) grade. Motions of the shoulder, elbow, wrist, fingers, knee, and ankle are often recorded more precisely by goniometry, when abnormal. Incomplete finger flexion can also be recorded in centimeters of flexion lag from the end of the nail bed to the transverse palmar crease. Thoracic and lumbar motions are best recorded with a motion diagram, onto which one can record grades of motion (0 to 4) and color in the arcs that are painful.[6] Traditional goniometry of thoracolumbar spine motion is an inaccurate and worthless effort. The skin distraction methods of Martin[1] (C7–S1 distraction during flexion) and of Schober (Fig. 3–4) and the inclinometer method of Loebl (Fig. 3–5) (lumbar spine) are the most convenient and reproducible objective clinical measurements of spine motion.[4]

TENDINITIS AND BURSITIS

The most common joint symptom is pain. Most joint pain is not from arthritis but from tendinitis and bursitis. Because the prognoses and therapies for arthritis, bursitis, and tendinitis are different, distinguishing these disorders is important. A regard to some simple observations, however, can help to differentiate them.[6] Pain is produced by active and passive motions in all planes in the presence of significant synovitis. In contrast, ten-

Name _____ Date _____

Joint	Right (Rt.) S	T	L	Comments	Left (Lt.) S	T	L	Comments
T-M	0	0	0		0	0	0	
S-C	0	0	0		0	0	0	
M-S	0	0	0					
A-C	0	0	0		0	0	0	
Sh	0	2		Abd. 60° (or grade 1+)	0	0	0	
				Ext. rot. 60° (or grade 1+)				
				Int. rot. 60° (or grade 1+)				
Elb	0	0	0		0	0	0	
Wr	1+	1-		Dorsiflexion 35° (or grade 2)	0	0	0	
MCP	0	0	0 ⎫		MCP$_2$ 1	1-	0 ⎫	
PIP	0	0	0 ⎬ Fist 100%		PIP$_2$ 1+	0	0 ⎬ Fist 100%	
DIP	0	0	0 ⎭		0	0	0 ⎭	
Hip	0	0	0		0	0	0	
Kn	1	1		Ext. 15° (or grade 1)	0	0	0	
				Flex. 115° (or grade 1)				
Ank	0	0	0		0	0	0	
S-T	0	0	0		0	0	0	
MTP	0	0	0		MTP$_2$ 1	1	0	
PIP	0	0	0		0	0	0	
DIP	0	0	0		0	0	0	

Spine
  Cervical
    Atlas (vertebrae 1 & 2) T$_0$ L$_0$
    Vertebrae 3-7 T$_0$ L$_0$
  Thoracic
    Costochondral T$_0$ L$_0$
    Chest expansion 12.5 cm
  Lumbar T$_0$ L$_0$
    Lumbosacral T$_0$ L$_0$
  Sacroiliac T$_0$
  Coccyx T$_0$
Posture—Mild upper thoracic rounding
Gait—Normal

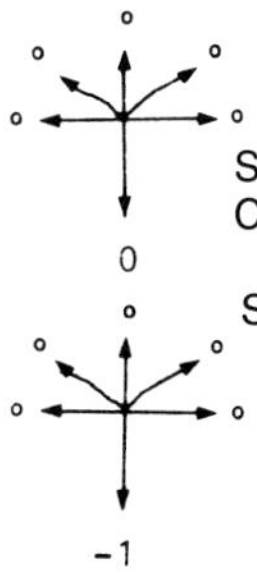

Spine flexion:
C7-S1 = 8.5 cm
Schober = 5.0 cm

Examiner _____

Figure 3–3

Example of chart used to record results of joint examination. Joints: T-M, temporomandibular; S-C, sternoclavicular; M-S, manubriosternal; A-C, acromioclavicular; Sh, shoulder; Elb, elbow; Wr, wrist; MCP, metacarpophalangeal; PIP, proximal interphalangeal; DIP, distal interphalangeal; Kn, knee; Ank, ankle; S-T, subtalar; MTP, metatarsophalangeal. Finding: S, swelling; T, tenderness; L, limitation of motion. (From Polley and Hunder.[1] By permission of the publisher.)

dinitis produces pain primarily with active and resistive motions but not with, or as intensely with, passive motion, and then only in planes where the tendon or its associated muscle is placed under tension. Pain can be elicited by isometric resistance in tendinitis (Fig. 3–6). Bursitis is associated with painful arcs of active and passive motion but not with isometric resistance. Thus, if one observes active and then passive movements and finally isometric resistance to that motion, the differentiation is clearer. Confirmation can then be established by direct palpation.

As an example, if one noted shoulder and arm pain with active shoul-

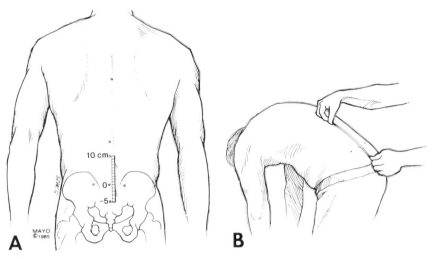

Figure 3-4

Modified Schober flexion test. *A,* With subject standing erect but relaxed, top of sacrum ("0") is identified by spinal intersection of horizontal line joining dimples of Venus (denoted by small circular marks to left and right of zero), and points 10 cm above and 5 cm below are marked. *B,* Subject bends forward maximally, and distance between the upper and lower marks is measured in centimeters. This value minus 15 is amount of lumbar flexion. (From Merritt et al.[4] By permission of Mayo Foundation.)

der abduction but not with passive abduction or active flexion, supraspinatus tendinitis would be suspected.[6] Shoulder arthritis and subacromial bursitis (both are causes of shoulder pain during active abduction) would be less likely diagnoses. Further confirmation of the diagnosis of supraspinatus tendinitis could (and should) be made by isometrically resisting abduction while the arm is in an abducted and internally rotated position. Finally, palpation of the supraspinatus tendon is performed with the shoulder in internal rotation, adduction, and extension. Subacromial bursitis would produce pain on active and passive abduction but not with isometric resistance to abduction and not with active or passive shoulder flexion.

Lateral epicondylitis ("tennis elbow," common extensor tendinitis) should, likewise, be established not only by direct palpation but also by reproduction of pain during active and resisted wrist extension and supination. Medial epicondylitis ("golfer's elbow") should similarly be confirmed by resisted wrist pronation and flexion.

SHOULDER IMPINGEMENT SYNDROME

The impingement syndrome is a common shoulder syndrome that results from the unique characteristics of the rotator cuff muscle groups.[9] The supraspinatus muscle is a major shoulder abductor, but it also, during active contraction, pulls the head of the humerus inferiorly into the inferior

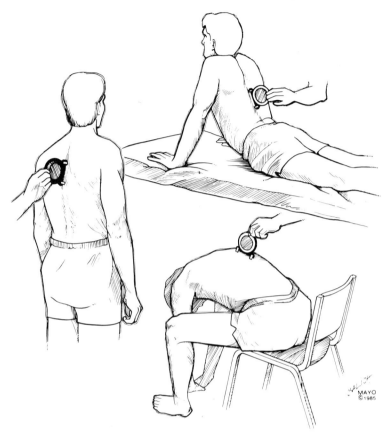

Figure 3–5
Loebl measurements. Spinal tangents are measured with an engineer's inclinometer. From these measurements, angles and degrees of movement are calculated. (From Merritt et al.[4] By permission of Mayo Foundation.)

portion of the glenoid. This active muscular contraction may, however, be disrupted in conditions of cuff degeneration, rupture, or tears. When this mechanism fails to pull the head downward and the humerus is rotated, the greater tuberosity impinges on the acromion, trapping the intervening supraspinatus tendon and subacromial bursa (Fig. 3–7). Repeated impingement results in trauma and further inflammatory changes in these structures, which in turn result in edema and swelling in these structures, which further increase impingement with less abduction.

PRINCIPLES OF GONIOMETRY

The method of measuring and recording joint motion as presented here is based on the principles of the neutral zero method described by

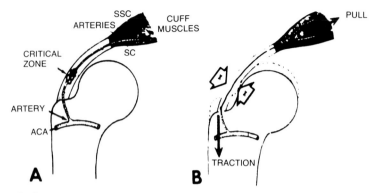

Figure 3-6

Blood circulation. *A*, Circulation to rotator cuff. Arterial branch from anterior circumflex artery (ACA) enters from bone. Suprascapular (SSC) and subscapular (SC) branches merge to enter from muscle. Critical zone of tendon is anastomosis that is patent when arm is supported and inactive. *B*, Traction on cuff from dependent arm or from pull of contracting cuff muscle elongates tendon and renders critical zone (arrows) relatively ischemic. (From Cailliet.[9] By permission of the publisher.)

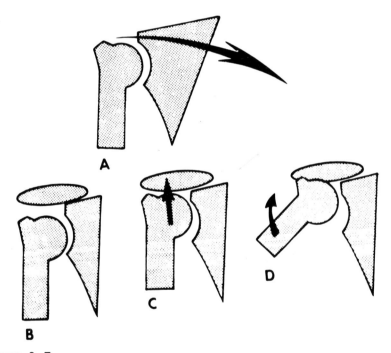

Figure 3-7

Impingement syndrome. *A*, Supraspinatus muscle and tendon abduct and set head of humerus inferiorly into glenoid. *B*, Normal, relaxed relationship. *C*, Defective rotator cuff results in superior gliding of humerus in glenoid. *D*, Impingement of greater tuberosity on inferior surface of acromion.

Cave and Roberts in 1936.[11] In this method, all motions of the joint are measured from a defined zero starting position. Thus, the degrees of motion of the joint are added in the direction of the joint motion from this position. The extended "anatomic position" of an extremity is, therefore, accepted as 0° rather than 180°.

GENERAL PRINCIPLES OF MEASUREMENT OF RANGE OF MOTION OF JOINTS

The instrument used is called a goniometer (Fig. 3−8). It consists of two rigid shafts that intersect at a hinged joint.[5] The protractor is fixed to the shafts so that motion can be read directly from the scale in degrees. The axis of the goniometer should coincide with the appropriate axis of motion in the joint being measured. This point can be determined by moving the joint through the range of motion and visually estimating the site of rotation. The shaft of the goniometer should be aligned parallel to the long axis of limb segments that are associated with the joint being measured. One of these segments must be stabilized for an accurate reading of the actual joint motion. The "starting position" in Figures 3−9 through 3−41 is defined as the point at which the movable segment is at 0°.[12] With minor exceptions, this is also the anatomic position. If the subject has a limitation of motion that prevents assuming the starting position, this is recorded as the number of degrees from zero. (Example: Normal flexion of the elbow is expressed as 150°. In the case of a flexion contracture, the reading might be 15° to 150°. If the subject has excessive mobility beyond the starting position, this reading is expressed as a negative value from the zero position by some authors and as a positive value by others. To avoid confusion, it is better to use the term "hyperextension" and the degree of hyperextension after it. "Hyperextension" can occur frequently in the elbow and the knee joints. The "measurement" is defined as the reading on the scale that reflects the maximal amount of motion available in a joint in a given plane of orientation. Two types of substitution that must be avoided in measurement are (1) deviation from the plane of motion and (2) movement of the limb segment designated as the baseline. When recording data, the motion should be indicated as passive or active.

BONY LANDMARKS

The following are fixed bony landmarks or guides for alignment of the goniometer for accurate measurements.[1]
Surface anatomy:

Scapula:
Spine
Acromial process

Axillary and vertebral borders
Inferior angle
Clavicle:
  Sternal (convex) or acromial (concave) extremity
  Suprasternal notch or jugular notch
Humerus:
  Greater tubercle
  Lesser tubercle
  Bicipital groove
  Lateral epicondyle
  Medial epicondyle
Ulna:
  Olecranon process
  Head of ulna
  Styloid process
  Medial border
Radius:
  Lateral surface
  Styloid process
Carpal bones
Metacarpal bones
Phalanges:
  Distal and proximal extremity
  Medial and lateral borders
Pelvis:
  Crest of the ilium
  Anterosuperior iliac spine
  Posterosuperior iliac spine
  Iliac tuberosity
  Pubic symphyses
Femur:
  Greater trochanter
  Adductor tubercle
  Lateral epicondyle
  Medial epicondyle
Tibia:
  Medial condyle
  Lateral condyle
  Tibial tuberosity
  Anterior border
  Medial surface
  Medial malleolus
Fibula:
  Styloid process
  Head
  Lateral malleolus
Tarsals
Metatarsals

Phalanges
Spine:
  Spinous processes (C−2 to L−5)
  Sacrum
  Coccyx

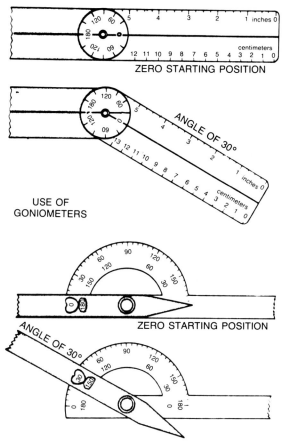

Figure 3−8
After the landmarks of a joint are defined, the goniometer is used to measure motion. (From Measuring and recording of joint motion.[12] By permission of the publisher.)

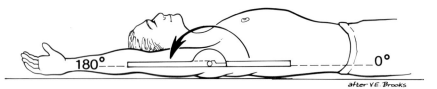

Figure 3–9
Shoulder flexion. (From Erickson et al.[13] By permission of the publisher.)

Starting position
Supine
Arm at side with hand pronated

Measurement
Sagittal plane
Substitution to avoid:
    Arching back
    Rotating trunk
Goniometer:
    Axis lateral to joint and just below acromion
    Shaft parallel to mid-axillary line of trunk
    Shaft parallel to midline of humerus

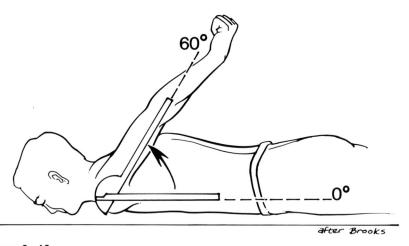

Figure 3–10
Shoulder hyperextension. (From Erickson et al.[13] By permission of the publisher.)

Starting position
Prone
Arm at side with hand pronated

Measurement
Sagittal plane
Substitution to avoid:
    Lifting shoulder from table
    Rotating trunk
Goniometer:
    Same as described for Figure 3–9

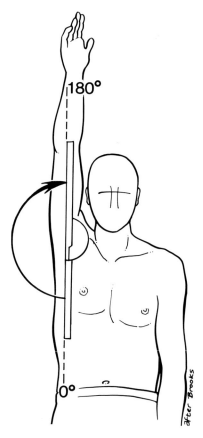

Figure 3–11

Shoulder abduction. (From Erickson et al.[13] By permission of the publisher.)

Starting position
Supine
Arm at side

Measurement
Frontal plane (must externally rotate shoulder to
    obtain maximum)
Substitution to avoid:
    Lateral motion of trunk
    Rotation of trunk
Goniometer:
    Axis anterior to joint and in line with acromion
    Shaft parallel to midline of trunk
    Shaft parallel to midline of humerus

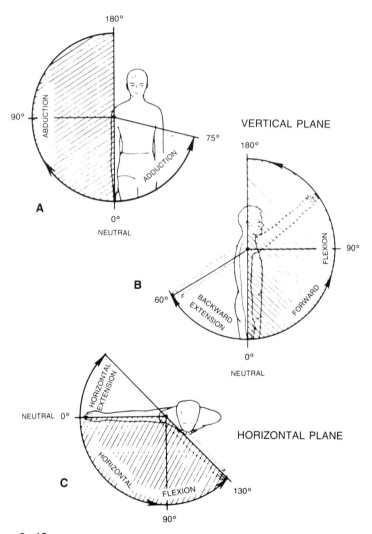

Figure 3–12

Shoulder. Zero starting position: patient standing erect, arm at side of body. *A* and *B*, Vertical or upward motion: abduction and adduction *(A)* and forward flexion and backward extension *(B)*. *C*, Horizontal motion: flexion and extension. (From Measuring and recording of joint motion.[12] By permission of the publisher.)

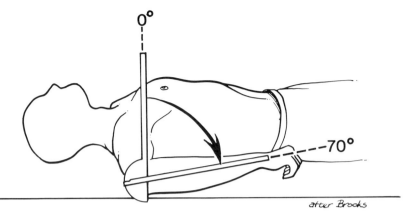

Figure 3–13

Shoulder internal rotation. (From Erickson et al.[13] By permission of the publisher.)

Starting position

Supine
Arm abducted to 90° and elbow off table
Elbow flexed to 90° and hand pronated
Forearm perpendicular to floor

Measurement

Transverse plane
Substitution to avoid:
   Protracting shoulder
   Rotating trunk
   Changing angle at shoulder or elbow
Goniometer:
   Axis through longitudinal axis of humerus
   Shaft perpendicular to floor
   Shaft parallel to midline of forearm

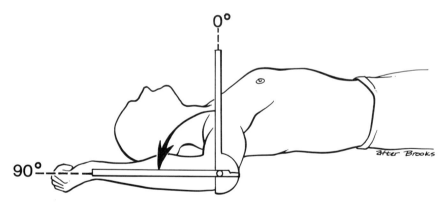

Figure 3–14

Shoulder external rotation. (From Erickson et al.[13] By permission of the publisher.)

Starting position

Same as described for Figure 3–13

Measurement

Transverse plane
Substitution to avoid:
   Arching back
   Rotating trunk
   Changing angle at shoulder or elbow
Goniometer:
   Same as described for Figure 3–13

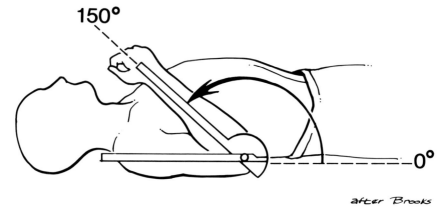

Figure 3-15
Elbow flexion. (From Erickson et al.[13] By permission of the publisher.)

Starting position
Supine
Arm at side with elbow straight
Hand supinated

Measurement
Sagittal plane
Goniometer:
    Axis lateral to joint and through epicondyles of
        humerus
    Shaft parallel to midline of humerus
    Shaft parallel to midline of forearm

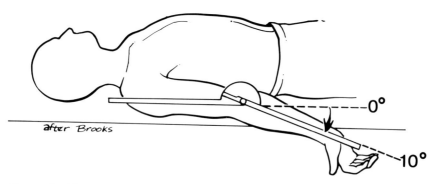

Figure 3-16
Elbow hyperextension. This illustration demonstrates the method of measuring excessive mobility past the "normal" starting position. (From Erickson et al.[13] By permission of the publisher.)

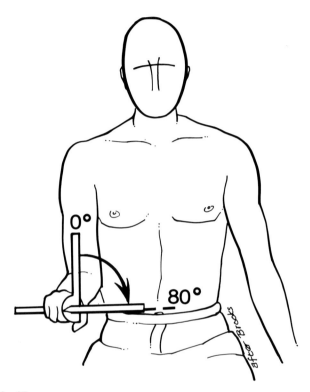

Figure 3–17
Forearm pronation. (From Erickson et al.[13] By permission of the publisher.)

Starting position	***Measurement***
Sitting (or standing)	Transverse plane
Arm at side with elbow held close to trunk	Substitution to avoid:
Elbow bent to 90°	Trunk rotation
Forearm in neutral position between pronation and supination	Moving arm
	Changing angle at elbow
Wrist in neutral position	Angulating wrist
Pencil held securely in mid-palmar crease	Goniometer:
	Axis through longitudinal axis of forearm
	Shaft parallel to midline of humerus
	Shaft parallel to pencil (on thumb side)

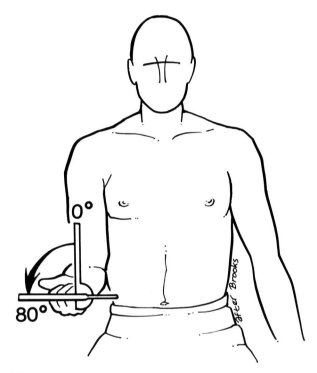

Figure 3–18
Forearm supination. (From Erickson et al.[13] By permission of the publisher.)

Starting position	***Measurement***
Same as described for Figure 3–17	Same as described for Figure 3–17

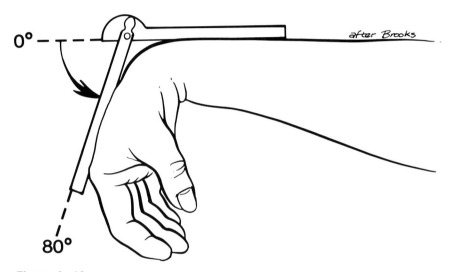

Figure 3–19
Wrist flexion. (From Erickson et al.[13] By permission of the publisher.)

Starting position
Elbow bent
Forearm and wrist in neutral position

Measurement
Sagittal plane
Goniometer:
    Axis over dorsum of wrist (in line with 3rd metacarpal bone)
    Shaft on mid-dorsum of forearm
    Shaft on mid-dorsum of hand

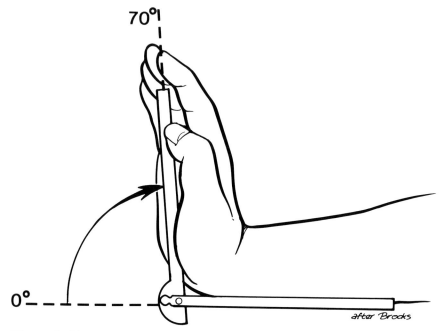

Figure 3–20
Wrist extension. (From Erickson et al.[13] By permission of the publisher.)

Starting position
Same as described for Figure 3–19

Measurement
Sagittal plane
Goniometer:
    Axis on ventral surface of wrist (in line with 3rd metacarpal bone)
    Shaft on mid-ventral surface of forearm
    Shaft on mid-palmer surface of hand

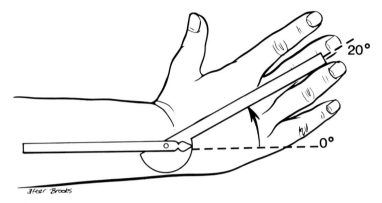

Figure 3–21
Wrist radial deviation. (From Erickson et al.[13] By permission of the publisher.)

Starting position
Forearm pronated
Wrist in neutral position

Measurement
Frontal plane
Goniometer:
    Axis over dorsum of wrist centered at
      mid-carpal bone
    Shaft on mid-dorsum of forearm
    Shaft on shaft of 3rd metacarpal

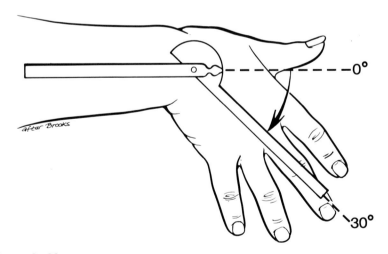

Figure 3–22
Wrist ulnar deviation. (From Erickson et al.[13] By permission of the publisher.)

Starting position
Same as described for Figure 3–21

Measurement
Same as described for Figure 3–21

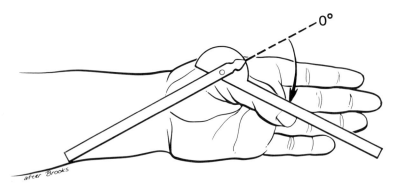

Figure 3–23

First metacarpophalangeal flexion. (From Erickson et al.[13] By permission of the publisher.)

Starting position
Elbow slightly flexed
Hand supinated
Fingers and thumb extended

Measurement
Frontal plane
Goniometer:
  Axis on lateral aspect of metacarpophalangeal joint
  Shaft parallel to midline of first metacarpal
  Shaft parallel to midline of proximal phalanx

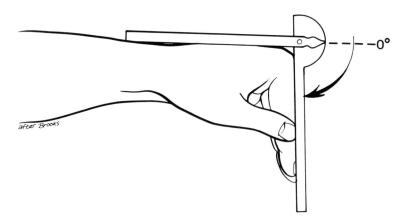

Figure 3–24

Second, third, and fourth metacarpophalangeal flexion. (From Erickson et al.[13] By permission of the publisher.)

Starting position
Elbow flexed
Hand pronated
Wrist in neutral position

Measurement
Sagittal plane
Goniometer:
  Axis on mid-dorsum of joint
  Shaft on mid-dorsum of metacarpal
  Shaft on mid-dorsum of proximal phalanx

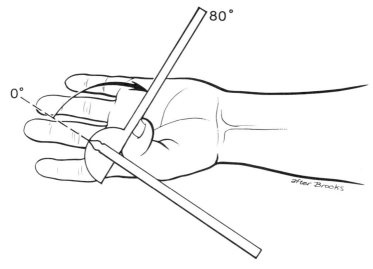

Figure 3–25

First interphalangeal flexion. (From Erickson et al.[13] By permission of the publisher.)

Starting position
Elbow flexed
Forearm supinated
Interphalangeal joint extended

Measurement
Frontal plane
Goniometer:
  Axis on lateral aspect of interphalangeal joint
  Shaft parallel to midline of proximal phalanx
  Shaft parallel to midline of distal phalanx

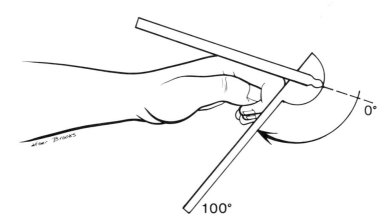

Figure 3–26

Second, third, and fourth interphalangeal flexion. (From Erickson et al.[13] By permission of the publisher.)

Starting position
Elbow flexed
Forearm pronated
Interphalangeal joint extended

Measurement
Sagittal plane
Goniometer:
  Axis over dorsal aspect of joint
  Shaft over mid-dorsum of proximal phalanx
  Shaft over mid-dorsum of more distal phalanx

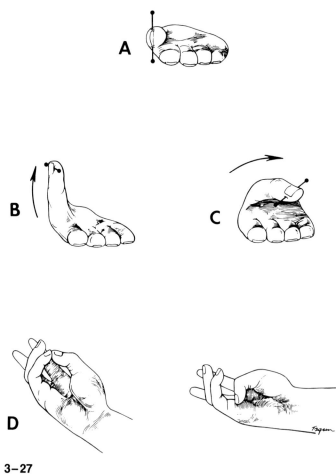

Figure 3–27

Thumb, opposition. *A,* Zero starting position. *B,* Abduction. *C,* Rotation. *D,* Flexion, two methods: tip, or pulp, of thumb touches tip of fifth finger (left) or tip of thumb touches base of fifth finger (right). (From Measuring and recording of joint motion.[12] By permission of the publisher.)

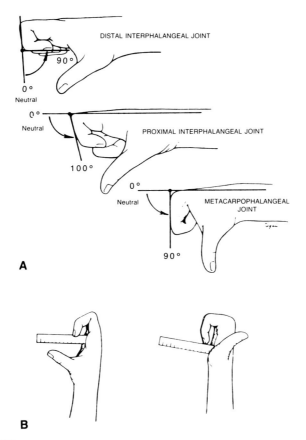

Figure 3–28

Fingers, flexion. Zero starting position: extended fingers parallel to each other, in line with plane of dorsum of hand and wrist. *A,* Flexion of joints of fingers. *B,* Composite motion of flexion, estimated with a ruler as distance from tip of finger to (1) distal palmar crease (left) and (2) proximal palmar crease (right). (From Measuring and recording of joint motion.[12] By permission of the publisher.)

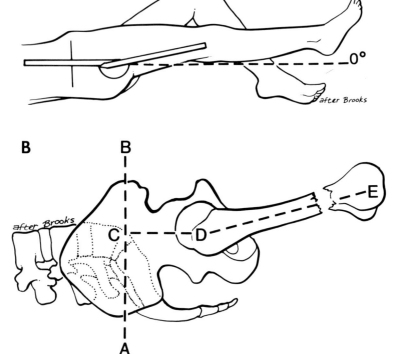

Figure 3–29
Hip extension. (From Erickson et al.[13] By permission of the publisher.)

Position	*Measurement*
Lying on side (or supine)	Sagittal plane
Lower leg bent for support	Draw line from anterior superior to posterior superior iliac spines (B-A)
	Drop a perpendicular to the greater trochanter (C-D)
	Center axis of goniometer at greater trochanter (D)
	Shaft along perpendicular (C-D)
	Shaft along shaft of femur (D-E)

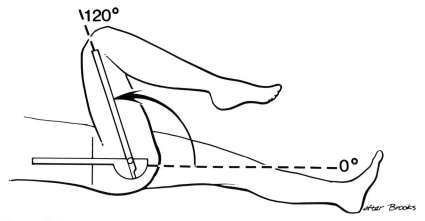

Figure 3-30

Hip flexion. (From Erickson et al.[13] By permission of the publisher.)

Position

Supine or lying on side (may flex lower knee
  slightly for support)

Measurement

Sagittal plane
Relocate greater trochanter and redraw
  C-D as described for Figure 3-29
Goniometer:
    Same as described for Figure 3-29

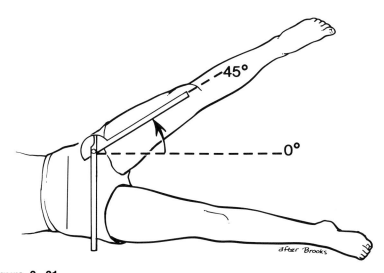

Figure 3-31

Hip abduction. (From Erickson et al.[13] By permission of the publisher.)

Position

Lying supine

Measurement

Frontal plane
Mark both anterior-superior iliac spines,
    and draw a line between them
Goniometer:
    Axis over hip joint
    Shaft parallel to line between spines
      of ilium
    Shaft along shaft of femur

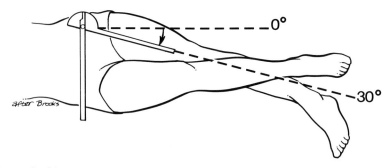

Figure 3-32

Hip adduction. (From Erickson et al.[13] By permission of the publisher.)

Position
Lying supine
Leg extended and in neutral position

Measurement
Frontal plane
Mark both anterior superior iliac spines, and
   draw a line between them
Goniometer:
   Axis over hip joint
   Shaft parallel to line between spines of ilium
   Shaft along shaft of femur

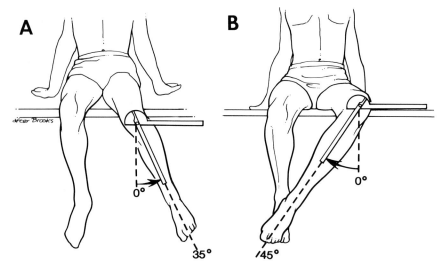

Figure 3-33

A, Hip internal rotation. B, Hip external rotation. (From Erickson et al.[13] By permission of
the publisher.)

Position
Sitting; can also be measured in
   prone or supine position
   (indicate on record which position
Knee flexed to 90°

Measurement
Transverse plane
Substitution to avoid:
   Trunk rotation
   Lifting of thigh from table
Goniometer:
   Axis through longitudinal axis of femur
   Shaft parallel to table
   Shaft parallel to lower leg

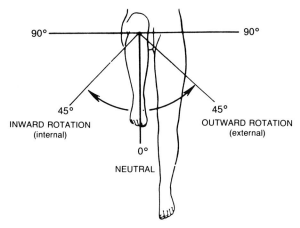

Figure 3–34

Hip, rotation. Rotation in flexion. Zero starting position: patient supine, hip and knee flexed 90° each, thigh perpendicular to transverse line across anterior-superior spines of pelvis. (From Measuring and recording of joint motion.[12] By permission of the publisher.)

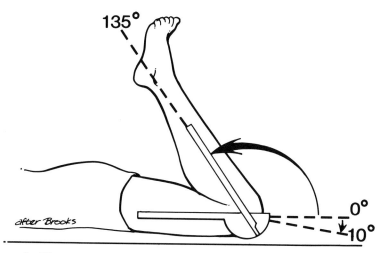

Figure 3–35

Knee flexion. (From Erickson et al.[13] By permission of the publisher.)

Position	*Measurement*
Prone (or supine with hip flexed if rectus femoris limits motion)	Sagittal plane
	Goniometer:
	Axis through knee joint
	Shaft along mid-thigh
	Shaft along fibula

Figure also demonstrates 10° of hyperextension.

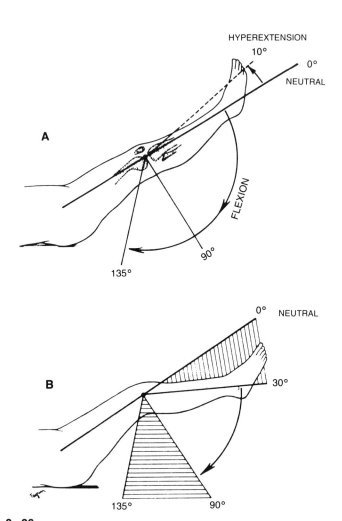

Figure 3–36

Knee. Zero starting position: extended straight knee with patient supine or prone. *A,* Flexion and hyperextension. *B,* Limited motion. Unshaded area is range of limited motion. (From Measuring and recording of joint motion.[12] By permission of the publisher.)

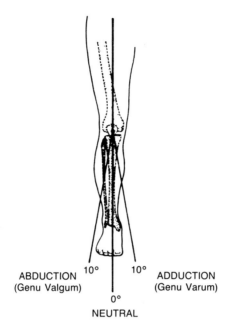

ABDUCTION   10°   10°   ADDUCTION
(Genu Valgum)   (Genu Varum)
0°
NEUTRAL

Figure 3-37
Knee, abduction and adduction—best measured in degrees and compared with opposite or normal knee. (From Measuring and recording of joint motion.[12] By permission of the publisher.)

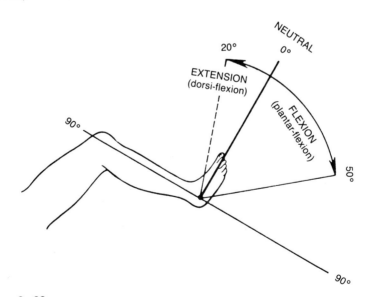

Figure 3-38
Ankle. Zero starting position: leg at right angles to thigh, foot at right angle to leg. Extension and flexion—best measured in degrees from right-angle neutral position and compared with opposite ankle. (From Measuring and recording of joint motion.[12] By permission of the publisher.)

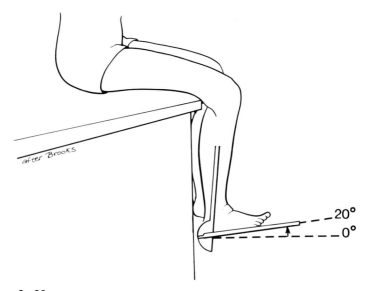

Figure 3–39

Ankle dorsiflexion. (From Erickson et al.[13] By permission of the publisher.)

Position
Sitting
Knee flexed to 90°
Foot at 90° angle to leg

Measurement
Sagittal plane
Goniometer:
    Axis on sole of foot
    Shaft along fibula
    Shaft along fifth metatarsal

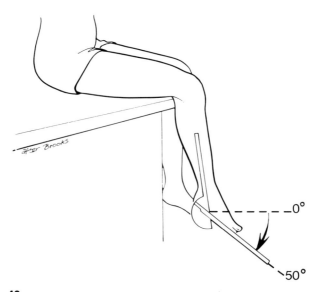

Figure 3–40

Ankle plantar flexion. (From Erickson et al.[13] By permission of the publisher.)

Position
Same as described for Figure 3–39

Measurement
Same as described for Figure 3–39

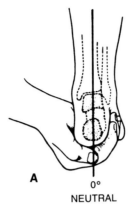

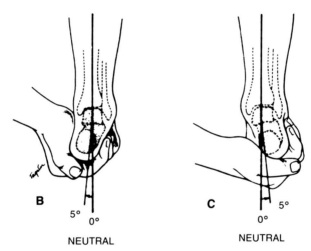

Figure 3–41
Hind part of foot (passive motion). *A*, Zero starting position: heel aligned with midline of tibia. *B*, Inversion. *C*, Eversion. (From Measuring and recording of joint motion.[12] By permission of the publisher.)

REFERENCES

1. Polley HF, Hunder GG. Rheumatologic interviewing and physical examination of the joints. Philadelphia: WB Saunders, 1978.
2. Hoppenfeld S. Physical examination of the spine and extremities. New York: Appleton-Century-Crofts, 1976.
3. Kapandji IA. The physiology of the joints: annotated diagrams of the mechanics of the human joints (translated by L.H. Honoré). 2nd ed. Vols 1–3. Edinburgh: E & S Livingstone, 1970.

4. Merritt JL, McLean TJ, Erickson RP, Offord KP. Measurement of trunk flexibility in normal subjects: reproducibility of three clinical methods. Mayo Clin Proc 1986; 61:192–197.
5. Kottke FJ, Stillwell GK, Lehmann JF, eds. Krusen's handbook of physical medicine and rehabilitation. 3rd ed. Philadelphia: WB Saunders, 1982.
6. Cyriax JH. Textbook of orthopaedic medicine. 7th ed. Vols 1 and 2. London: Baillière Tindall, 1978.
7. Ehrlich GE, ed. Rehabilitation management of rheumatic conditions. Baltimore: Williams & Wilkins, 1980.
8. Saunders HD. Evaluation, treatment and prevention of musculoskeletal disorders. Minneapolis: Viking Press, 1985.
9. Cailliet R. Soft tissue pain and disability. Philadelphia: FA Davis, 1977.
10. Medical knowledge self-assessment program in physical medicine and rehabilitation syllabus. Philadelphia: American Academy of Physical Medicine and Rehabilitation, 1977.
11. Cave EF, Roberts SM. A method for measuring and recording joint function. J Bone Joint Surg 1936; 18:455–465.
12. Measuring and recording of joint motion. Chicago: American Academy of Orthopaedic Surgeons, 1963.
13. Erickson RP, McPhee MC. Clinical evaluation. In: DeLisa JA, ed. Rehabilitation medicine: principles and practice. 2nd ed. Philadelphia: JB Lippincott, 1993: 51–95.

4 | Muscle Strength and Manual Muscle Testing

Lee D. Shibley

Mehrsheed Sinaki

The origins of muscle strength testing date back to Hippocrates[1] and early medicine. Archimedes' principles of density as a function of water volume displacement[1] identified differences between muscle densities of different people. During the Renaissance, Leonardo da Vinci first illustrated the human musculoskeletal system[1] and studied muscle and joint function.

Lister's germ theory advanced medicine beyond its pioneers,[1] and muscle testing became a tool to identify certain disease states and examine skeletal function. Currently, expensive computer-aided diagnostic techniques can confirm or deny a medical diagnosis based on simple manual muscle testing.

One of the pillars of physical examination, the manual muscle test is a subjective test of muscle function that can be standardized to provide data for objective physical examination. Mental status, central and peripheral nervous system function, and tendon, ligament, and joint function can also be assessed simultaneously.

TYPES OF MUSCLE CONTRACTION

Contraction of skeletal muscle can be classified according to the variables that are emphasized.[2] Muscle strength is defined as resistance against a predetermined force, with physiologic muscle contraction providing the resistance. Isometric contraction lacks net joint movement, whereas allowing joint movement identifies isotonic contraction. Joint and limb movement that is at constant velocity defines isokinetic contraction. Isometric muscle contraction is used in manual testing because the fewest variables are present and because of the ease of such testing, and thus it is the most reliable manual test.

GUIDELINES FOR MANUAL MUSCLE TESTING

For validity and reliability of muscle testing, several factors must be consistent. The tester's hand should be placed at the site just proximal to the next distal joint, relative to the muscle insertion. Joint position, usually at the middle or end range, should allow for maximal isometric contraction. Limbs being tested must have identical relationships to the resistance of gravity. Control of these factors allows for interpatient and intrapatient comparison of strength,[3] especially with equivalent limb length relative to gravity (Fig. 4–1, A). Adequate contraction time (2 to 5 seconds) and re-

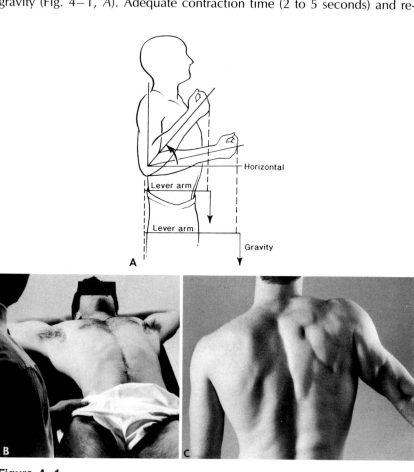

Figure 4–1

A, Joint-angle cosine contributes to effective strength. As the elbow joint-angle cosine decreases, so does the effective lever arm against which gravity provides resistance. Lever arm position and thus resistance against gravity should be considered when testing muscle strength. *B,* Cranial orientation of right iliac crest. Note the associated contraction of the right oblique abdominal muscles. *C,* Significant contraction of upper trapezius, substituting for abduction.

peated contractions are used to obtain consistent results. A thorough knowledge of muscle, nerve, and joint anatomy is essential for accurate manual muscle testing and interpretation.

Synergistic muscle contraction may confuse the practitioner into false interpretation of the results of a manual muscle test.[4] This substitution of proximal or distal muscles during manual testing must always be identified and eliminated from the testing procedure when possible.

For example, when the strength of the hip abductor is being tested, the quadratus lumborum should not be allowed to "hike" the pelvis cranially (Fig. 4–1 *B*); likewise, the upper trapezius must not be allowed to elevate the scapula when anterior, middle, and posterior deltoid strength is being tested (Fig. 4–1 *C*). Either of these substitute muscle contractions could partially or completely mask gluteus medius or deltoid weakness, respectively. By placing the hip in neutral flexion-extension-rotation with gluteus medius testing, the above-mentioned substitution can be avoided. Glenohumeral joint contracture or rotator cuff tear may present as a weak deltoid with the above-described trapezius substitution.

Data from muscle testing can be used to assess the status of the neurologic and musculoskeletal systems with the help of a knowledge of basic human anatomy. Knowledge of spinal segmental innervation and peripheral innervation can be used to differentiate muscle weakness caused by central or peripheral nervous system lesions. Knowledge of muscle origin and insertion and expected joint function can identify muscle, tendon, ligament, and joint abnormality.

NEUROLOGIC AND MUSCULOSKELETAL ASSESSMENT

Muscle weakness is often an indication of a neurologic disorder.[4] Trauma or disease to a peripheral nerve may impair the muscles fed by that nerve. Identification of both common spinal segmental and peripheral innervation allows identification of the nerve lesion (Tables 4–1 and 4–2). For example, an osteogenic sarcoma of the upper extremity near the lateral epicondyle would likely impair the extensor carpi radialis longus and brevis, extensor digitorum, and extensor indicus but spare the triceps brachii. A spinal nerve lesion at the level of the second and third lumbar segments would likely involve weakness of unilateral quadriceps femoris, adductor longus, and remaining adductor groups. A peripheral lesion involving the femoral nerve would present with quadriceps weakness but spare the adductors of the hip. Testing the strength of muscles from a common peripheral and central innervation allows the lesion to be differentiated as central or peripheral. The location of a peripheral nerve lesion can be identified according to the strength of the proximal and distal muscles fed by that nerve.

Because two muscles may effect similar action at one joint, isolating a single muscle with manual testing is often desirable. At the leg, both the gastrocnemius and the soleus muscles provide plantar flexion at the ankle.

TABLE 4–1

Common Segmental and Peripheral Innervations, Selected Nerves, and Muscles of the Arm[5, 6]

Segment	Peripheral Nerve	Muscle
C5, 6	Musculocutaneous	Biceps brachii
C5, 6		Brachialis
C5–7		Coracobrachialis
C5–8	Radial	Triceps brachii
C5, 6		Supinator
C6, 7		Abductor pollicis longus
C6, 7		Extensor pollicis brevis
C6, 7		Extensor carpi radialis longus, brevis
C7, 8		Extensor pollicis longus
C6–8		Extensor digitorum
C6–8		Extensor digiti minimi
C6–8		Extensor carpi ulnaris
C6, 7	Median	Pronator teres
C6, 7		Flexor carpi radialis
C7, 8		Palmaris longus
C7–T1		Pronator quadratus
C7–T1		Flexor digitorum superficialis
C7–T1		Flexor pollicis longus
C8–T1		Flexor digitorum profundus (radial portion)
C8–T1	Ulnar	Flexor digitorum profundus (ulnar portion)
C8–T1		Flexor carpi ulnaris

During assessment of the function of the posterior tibial nerve or trauma to the soleus muscle, gastrocnemius strength could mask soleus weakness. To avoid misinterpretation of the results of a manual test, gastrocnemius function must be diminished without soleus compromise. Because the gastrocnemius muscle spans both the knee and the talocrural joints but the soleus muscle spans only the talocrural joint, the function of these muscles can be differentiated.[2] Investigators have shown that skeletal muscle tension is

TABLE 4–2

Common Segmental and Peripheral Innervations, Selected Anteromedial Muscles, and Nerves of the Thigh[5, 6]

Segment	Peripheral Nerve	Muscle
L2, 3	Femoral	Sartorius
L2–4		Quadriceps
L2, 3		Pectineus
L3, 4	Obturator	Adductor magnus
L3, 4		Obturator externus
L3, 4		Adductor brevis
L3, 4		Gracilis
L2, 3		Adductor longus
L2, 3		Pectineus (occasionally)

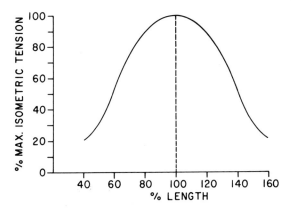

Figure 4–2
Length-tension relationship of skeletal muscle. When muscle is stimulated to contract at resting length (100%), it develops maximal isometric tension. If muscle length is increased or decreased, the amount of tension produced by nerve stimulation decreases. (From Eyzaguirre C. Physiology of the nervous system: an introductory text. Chicago: Year Book Medical Publishers, 1969. By permission of the publisher.)

a function of its length[7] (Fig. 4–2). As muscle length decreases, its ability to generate tension also decreases markedly.[2] The gastrocnemius can be placed in a shortened position by flexing the knee; this movement thereby allows soleus function to dominate ankle plantar flexion (Fig. 4–3). This length-tension relationship also exists at the hip joint, involving rectus fem-

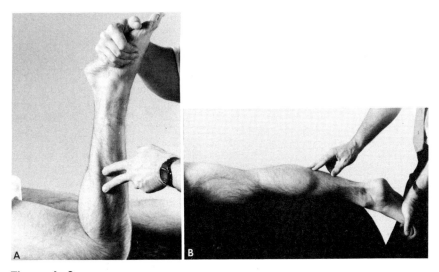

Figure 4–3
A and *B*, Soleus muscle is isolated from gastrocnemius by flexing the knee; this movement thus places the gastrocnemius in shortened position and uses the length-tension muscle relationship while patient is prone.

TABLE 4–3

Controlled Variables in Manual Muscle Testing

1. Manual contact just proximal to next distal joint, from point of muscle insertion
2. Isometric muscle contraction, avoiding undesirable substitution
3. Contraction time of 2 to 5 seconds
4. Joint position that allows maximal isometric contraction, usually at middle or end of available joint motion
5. Position of limb relative to gravity is consistent, right to left or over time
6. Serial testing, for consistency of results

oris-quadriceps strength as a function of hip-trunk angle (and thus rectus femoris length). Data have shown that the greatest knee extension torque is produced at a hip-trunk angle of 110° to 120° from horizontal.[8]

This length-tension relationship can differentiate two-joint muscles from one-joint muscles in the diagnosis of muscle or tendon injuries.[2, 9] Diagnostic and therapeutic injection, bracing considerations, and surgical referral rely on specific identification of contractile tissue and joint abnormality for appropriate rehabilitation.

CONTRACTILE VERSUS NONCONTRACTILE LESIONS

Contractile and noncontractile tissue can be differentiated[9] before or during a manual muscle test. Passive limb movement without muscle stretch will be pain-free in the presence of a tendon or a muscle lesion; the same maneuver will likely provoke pain with a noncontractile lesion such as ligament or joint capsule involvement.[9] Care must be taken in assessing passive joint motion to ensure complete muscle relaxation; pain with muscle contraction is indicative of a contractile lesion and could be misinterpreted as ligament or joint pain during passive testing. Occasionally, one of these structures is anesthetized by direct injection to assess joint mobility and muscle function fully. Pain provocation on active muscle contraction, passive muscle stretch, and direct palpation on the muscle or its tendon is indicative of a contractile lesion. Pain during a manual muscle test can induce the muscle to give way under manual pressure, and it therefore invalidates the test as a measure of strength.[3]

STRENGTH ASSESSMENT

Manual testing uses the strength of the examiner to assess the strength of the patient (Table 4–3). The use of manual contact, the choice of contact position on the patient's limb, and the position of the limb and of the joint are factors that affect the ability of the muscle to contract against resistance.[3] These variables need to be consistent for comparison of strength among patients and between different times of examination of the same patient. All of these variables should be kept constant; however, limb position relative to gravity is the variable that can be changed in order to grade the ability of the muscle to function at its joint (Fig. 4–4 A and Table 4–4).[3]

TABLE 4-4

Grading Systems for Manual Muscle Testing[10, 11]

Medical Research Council	National Foundation for Infant Paralysis	Lovett	Kendall	Aids to Investigation of Peripheral Nerve Injury
Strenuous muscle contraction, full joint motion, no giving way against gravity	0	Normal	100%	5
Obvious muscle contraction, full joint motion against gravity, mild giving way with resistance	1	Good	80%	4
Significant muscle contraction, full joint motion against gravity, but giving way against resistance	2	Fair	50%	3
Evidence of visible muscle contraction with joint motion less than full, with gravity eliminated and no resistance	3	Poor	20%	2
Evidence of slight muscle contraction or tendon tension, without joint motion	4	Trace	5%	1
No evidence of muscle contraction or tendon tension	5	Total paralysis	0%	0

TABLE 4-5

Upper Extremity Screening (Figure 4-4)[5, 6]

Muscle	Spinal Segments	Peripheral Nerve
Upper trapezius	Cranial nerve XI, C2-4	Spinal accessory, cervical roots
Deltoid	C-5	Axillary
Biceps brachii	C5, 6	Musculocutaneous
Brachioradialis	C5, 6	Radial
Triceps	C6, 7	Radial
Extensor pollicis longus	C7, 8	Radial
Extensor carpi ulnaris	C7, 8	Ulnar
Flexor pollicis longus	C6-8	Median
Opponens pollicis	C6-8	Median
Opponens digiti minimi	C-8, T-1	Ulnar

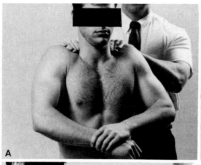
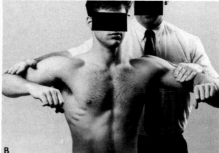
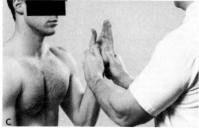

Figure 4–4

A, Upper trapezius muscle test position with antigravity scapular spine orientation and manual resistance placed just proximal to glenohumeral joints of shoulders. The patient's hands are unable to push from the examining table and influence the test results. *B,* Note the antigravity test position. Note the examiner's hand resistance just proximal to the next distal joint. The deltoid is visibly contracting without trapezius substitution. *C,* Testing of opponens pollicis and opponens digiti minimi. This test identifies function of the distal portions of the median and ulnar (motor) nerves.

Several muscle grading systems exist, depending on the examiner's field of specialization (Table 4–4). The system used by physical therapists[3] for evaluating muscle strength can assess both the static strength of the muscle and its ability to move a joint without resistance. Limb position relative to gravity is taken into account with the Kendall grading system,[3] pro-

TABLE 4–6

Lower Extremity Screening (Figure 4–5)[5, 6]

Muscle	Spinal Segments	Peripheral Nerve
Iliopsoas	L2, 3	Lumbar plexus
Adductor longus	L2, 3	Obturator
Quadriceps femoris	L3, 4	Femoral
Gluteus medius	L4, 5, S–1	Superior gluteal
Gluteus maximus	L–5, S1, 2	Inferior gluteal
Semitendinosus	L–5, S–1	Sciatic
Tibialis anterior	L4, 5, S–1	Superficial peroneal
Peroneus longus	L4, 5, S–1	Peroneal
Gastrocnemius	S1, 2	Posterior tibial

viding useful data of muscle strength and function, especially in the assessment of neurologic impairment and recovery.

SCREENING TESTS

After a thorough patient history is taken, a screening examination of the upper and lower extremities can be performed. This general screening examination can direct the clinician to more specific muscle testing to assess the musculoskeletal and nervous systems fully.

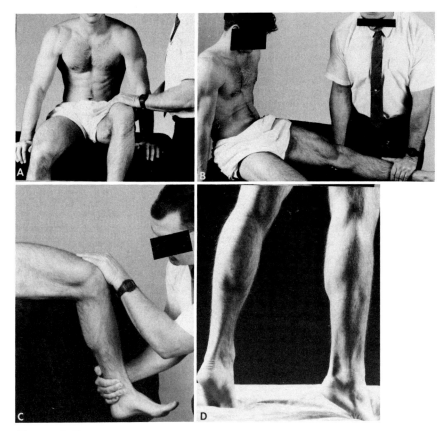

Figure 4–5
A, Iliopsoas test. Note the 90° trunk-femur angle to weaken the quadriceps and allow clear iliopsoas predominance. *B*, Quadriceps femoris test. Incorrectly testing the iliopsoas in this quadriceps test position allows the rectus femoris to ameliorate iliopsoas function. These test positions use the length-tension relationship. Compare this test position to that in *A*. *C*, Semitendinosus test. The patient may be positioned prone or standing for grading of strength. *D*, Gastrocnemius test. Toe-walking will test the gastrocnemius by raising the body's weight against gravity during plantar flexion. Heel-walking tests the tibialis anterior in a similar manner. Modifying gait can assess muscle function at the ankle.

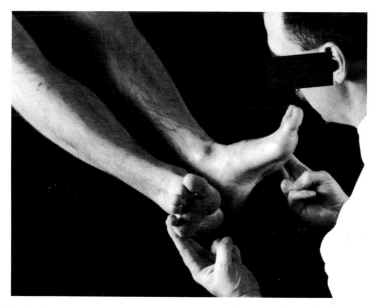

Figure 4–6
Ankle evertor (peroneus longus and brevis) testing. Notice the hand position; heels are touching.

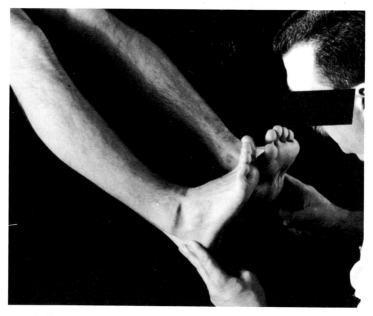

Figure 4–7
Ankle invertor (tibialis posterior) testing. Notice the hand position; toes are touching.

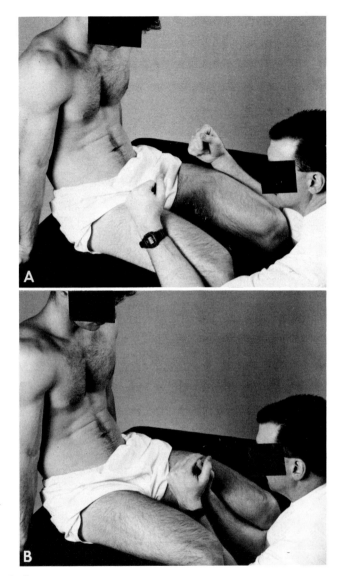

Figure 4–8
Hip abductor *(A)* and adductor *(B)* testing. Notice the examiner's mechanical advantage by using his shoulder muscles to test the powerful hip muscles while patient is seated.

Selected muscles of the upper extremities (Table 4–5) and lower extremities (Table 4–6) can be tested to provide this screening process. Proper selection of the extremity skeletal muscles to be tested allows efficient screening of the central and peripheral nervous systems as well as the musculoskeletal system. The effects of gravity can largely be ignored until specific testing is done. The results of the screening examination will direct

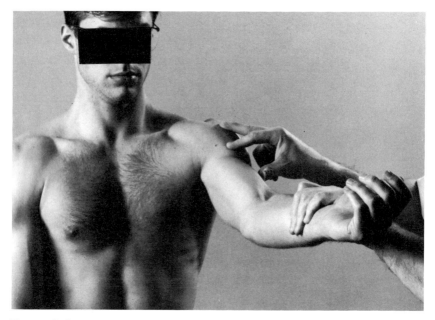

Figure 4–9
Speed test. This test will elicit painful weakness at the site of the biceps (long head) origin and aids in diagnosis of bicipital tendinitis.

the clinician to more specific evaluation of muscle strength, including control of limb position against gravity and grading[3] of muscle strength. Careful control of the previously mentioned variables will allow valid and accurate collection of data as the patient's muscle strength is examined further, as directed by screening.

Antigravity lever arm position (Fig. 4–4 A), manual resistance just proximal to the next distal joint (Fig. 4–4 B), testing of muscles fed by distal motor nerves to evaluate proximal peripheral nerve function (Fig. 4–4 C), use of muscle length-tension relationships (Fig. 4–5 A and B), and testing lower extremity muscles as functional groups rather than isolated muscles (Fig. 4–5 through 4–8) all aid the examiner during muscle and nerve function screening. Specific muscle-tendon tests can also be performed using the aforementioned principles and applied knowledge of human anatomy. For example, the long head of the biceps brachii can be placed on significant tension to stress its proximal tendon near the supraglenoid tubercle (Fig. 4–9). A more specific method of evaluating the hip abductors is antigravity evaluation; for this, the patient is positioned on his or her side and raises the leg from horizontal while the examiner's hand applies resistance at the distal femur.[3] These test may provoke pain when bicipital tendinitis is present.

REFERENCES

1. The World Book Encyclopedia. World Book, Inc. Vols 1, 12. Chicago: Scott Fetzer Company, 1985.

2. Norkin CC, Levangie PK. Joint structure and function: a comprehensive analysis. Philadelphia: FA Davis, 1983.
3. Kendall FP, McCreary FK. Muscles: testing and function. 3rd ed. Baltimore: Williams & Wilkins, 1983.
4. Kottke FJ, Stillwell GK, Lehmann JF. Krusen's handbook of physical medicine and rehabilitation. 3rd ed. Philadelphia: WB Saunders, 1982.
5. Hollinshead WH, Jenkins DB. Functional anatomy of the limbs and back. 5th ed. Philadelphia: WB Saunders, 1981.
6. Hollinshead WH, Rosse C. Textbook of anatomy. 4th ed. Philadelphia: Harper & Row, 1985.
7. Gowitzke BA, Milner M. Understanding the scientific bases of human movement. 2nd ed. Baltimore: Williams & Wilkins, 1980.
8. Cyriax J. Textbook of orthopaedic medicine. Vol 1. Diagnosis of soft tissue lesions. 8th ed. London: Ballière Tindall, 1982.
9. Richard G, Currier DP. Back stabilization during knee strengthening exercise. Phys Ther 1977; 57:1013–1015.
10. Janda V. Muscle function testing. Boston: Butterworths, 1983.
11. Pact V, Sirotkin-Roses M, Beatus J. The muscle testing handbook. Boston: Little, Brown and Company, 1984.

5

Muscle Innervation, Attachments, and Function

Mehrsheed Sinaki
Stephen W. Carmichael

Knowledge of the anatomy and innervation of muscles is necessary for the detection of muscle weakness. Muscle rehabilitation after nerve injury or traumatic injury to the central nervous system requires skill in kinesiology and a comprehension of the function of muscles. Although many books supply this information, this chapter provides the needed information in an accessible format without an extensive review of several anatomy textbooks. The innervation and anatomic origin and insertion of more than 100 muscles are described. The functions of these muscles are also summarized to provide an understanding of the kinesiology of joints.[1-3] Function is given in two formats. First is the classic "open-chain" function, in which the muscle acts on a freely moving limb. Second is the "closed-chain" function, in which the end of the limb is fixed; for our purposes, the hand is fixed in a position such as that when a patient supports himself or herself on crutches, and the foot is fixed on a surface as in standing (dynamic aspects such as walking and running are not considered). The closed-chain functions are offered as suggestions and are not based on original research; in many cases, muscles appeared to function as stabilizers and do not have actions directed proximally.

The open- and closed-chain concept relates to the "kinematic chain" introduced by Reuleaux[4] to refer to a mechanical system of links. In engineering, a kinematic chain is a closed system of links joined in such a manner that if any one link is moved on a fixed link, all of the other links will move in a predictable pattern. The skeletal links of the human body are generally not composed of closed links, rather they are open links because the distal ends of the limbs are free; at least this is how the system is classically considered in describing "actions" of muscles. However, in many circumstances the distal ends of the limbs are fixed and a system of closed links is created. In Table 5–1, we present an outline of both open and closed systems.

TABLE 5–1
Skeletal Muscles: Innervation, Origin, Insertion, and Kinesiology

Muscle	Innervation*	Origin	Insertion	Function Open Chain	Function Closed Chain
		Upper Limb			
Pectoralis major	Clavicular portion: lateral pectoral nerve, C5–7 Sternal portion: medial pectoral nerve, C8, T1	Medial half of clavicle, sternum, upper six costal cartilage	Lateral lip of intertubercular groove	Flexion and adduction of arm, abduction by clavicular fibers above 90°, depression, medial rotation	Stabilize arm, move trunk backward, assist in elbow extension
Pectoralis minor	Medial pectoral nerve, C8, T1	Ribs 2–5	Divides around subclavius muscle to coracoid process	Depression of shoulder downward and rotation of scapula	Stabilize shoulder, assist in lifting trunk
Sternocleidomastoid	Cranial nerve XI	Sternum, clavicle	Mastoid process	Raising of clavicle	Stabilize clavicle
Subclavius	Tiny branch from upper trunk, C5–6	First rib	Inferior surface of clavicle	Aid in retaining sternal end of clavicle in place	Stabilize clavicle (more importantly, serve as a soft tissue cushion between the most commonly fractured bone and major neurovascular structures)

(Continued.)

TABLE 5–1 (cont.)

Muscle	Innervation*	Origin	Insertion	Function Open Chain	Function Closed Chain
Trapezius	XI, C3–4 (mostly proprioception)	Ligamentum nuchae, cervical and thoracic spinous processes	Spine of scapula, acromion, lateral third of clavicle	Upper: elevation of shoulder rotation of scapula upward Lower: depression of scapula Mid: pulling shoulder back	Stabilize shoulder girdle
Levator scapulae	C3–4	Cervical transverse processes, C1–4	Superior angle of scapula	Elevation of scapula	Stabilize scapula, assist in moving cervical vertebrae
Rhomboideus minor	Dorsal scapular nerve, anterior ramus of C5	Lower ligamentum nuchae, C7 and T1	Medial border of scapula	Fixing of medial border, retraction of scapula, downward rotation of glenoid cavity	Stabilize scapula, assist in moving vertebral column
Rhomboideus major	Dorsal scapular nerve, anterior ramus of C5	Upper thoracic vertebrae	Medial border of scapula	Fixing of medial border, retraction of scapula, downward rotation of glenoid cavity	Stabilize scapula, assist in moving vertebral column

Muscle	Innervation	Attachment (origin)	Attachment (insertion)	Action	Function
Latissimus dorsi	Thoracodorsal nerve, C6, <u>7</u>, <u>8</u>	Lower thoracic and lumbar spinous processes, crest of ilium	Medial lip of intertubercular groove	Extension, internal rotation, and adduction of arm	Elevation and support of trunk, assist moving trunk forward
Serratus anterior	Long thoracic nerve, C5–7; anterior rami	Upper eight ribs, anterolateral chest	Medial border of scapula	Protraction of scapula, upward rotation of lateral angle	Elevation of ribs (inspiration)
Deltoid	Axillary nerve, C5–6	Clavicle, spine of scapula, acromion	Deltoid tuberosity of humerus	Abduction, adduction (anterior and posterior fibers), flexion, extension, external and internal rotation	Stabilize shoulder, may assist in extension (anterior fibers) or flexion (posterior fibers) of elbow
Supraspinatus	Suprascapular nerve, C4, <u>5</u>, **6**	Supraspinous fossa	Greater tubercle	Abduction of arm	Stabilize shoulder
Infraspinatus	Suprascapular nerve, C4, <u>5</u>, 6	Infraspinous fossa	Greater tubercle	External rotation of arm	Stabilize shoulder, assist forward movement of trunk
Teres minor	Axillary nerve, C5–6	Upper part of lateral border of scapula	Greater tubercle	External rotation of arm	Stabilize shoulder, assist forward movement of trunk
Teres major	Lower subscapular nerve, C5–6	Lateral border of scapula	Medial lip of intertubercular groove	Extension, internal rotation, adduction of arm	Stabilize shoulder, assist moving trunk forward

*Underlined numbers indicate the nerves that provide the main innervation.

(Continued.)

TABLE 5–1 (cont.)

Muscle	Innervation*	Origin	Insertion	Function — Open Chain	Function — Closed Chain
Subscapularis	Upper and lower subscapular nerves, C5–6	Subscapular fossa	Lesser tubercle	Internal rotation	Stabilize shoulder, assist moving trunk backward
Biceps brachii	Musculocutaneous nerve, C5–6	Short head: coracoid process. Long head: Supraglenoid tubercle	Tuberosity of radius (radial tuberosity)	Flexion of elbow and supination, flexion of shoulder	Stabilize arm, flex elbow, extend shoulder
Coracobrachialis	Musculocutaneous nerve, C5–6	Coracoid process	Humerus	Flexion and adduction of shoulder	Stabilize shoulder, extend shoulder
Brachialis	Musculocutaneous nerve, C5–6	Anterior humerus	Coronoid process and tuberosity of ulna	Flexion of forearm	Flex elbow
Triceps	Radial nerve, C5–8	Long head: scapula, infraglenoid tubercle. Lateral head: humerus. Medial head: humerus	Olecranon of ulna	Extends forearm. Long head: extension and adduction of shoulder	Extend elbow, flex shoulder, assist in elevating trunk
Anconeus	Radial nerve, C6–7	Lateral epicondyle	Ulna	Extension of forearm	Stabilize elbow
Palmaris longus	Median nerve, C7–8, T1	Medial epicondyle	Palmar aponeurosis	Flexion of wrist and pronation	Stabilize wrist

Muscle	Innervation	Origin	Insertion	Function	Stabilization
Flexor carpi radialis	Median nerve, C6–7	Medial epicondyle	Base of second metacarpal	Flexion of wrist, pronation, radial abduction	Stabilize wrist, extend elbow
Flexor carpi ulnaris	Ulnar nerve, C8, T1	Medial epicondyle and ulna	Pisiform bone	Flexion of wrist, ulnar abduction	Stabilize wrist, extend elbow
Flexor digitorum superficialis	Median nerve, C7–8, T1	Humeroulnar head: medial epicondyle, coronoid process of ulna; Radial head: upper half of radius below radial tuberosity	Base of middle phalanx of medial 4 digits	Flexion of proximal interphalangeal joint	Stabilize wrist, hand
Flexor digitorum profundus	Median nerve, ulnar nerve, C7–8	Proximal two-thirds of ulna	Base of distal phalanges	Flexion of distal interphalangeal joint of 2nd and 3rd digits; Flexion of distal interphalangeal joint of 4th and 5th digits	Stabilize wrist, hand
Flexor pollicis longus	Median, anterior interosseous branch, C7–8, T1	Anterior surface of radius and interosseous membrane	Distal phalanx of thumb	Flexion of distal phalanx	Stabilize wrist, thumb
Pronator quadratus	Median nerve, C7–8, T1	Ulna	Radius	Pronation	Stabilize forearm, flex elbow
Pronator teres	Median nerve, C6–7	Humerus, coronoid process of ulna	Lateral side of radius	Flexion of elbow and pronation	Stabilize elbow, flex elbow

*Underlined numbers indicate the nerves that provide the main innervation.

(Continued.)

TABLE 5-1 (cont.)

Muscle	Innervation*	Origin	Insertion	Function Open Chain	Function Closed Chain
Brachioradialis	Radial nerve, C5–6	Lateral border of humerus above epicondyle	Distal radius	Flexion of elbow (pronation or supination)	Flex elbow
Extensor carpi radialis longus	Radial nerve, C6–7	Above lateral epicondyle	Base of second metacarpal	Extension and abduction of wrist	Stabilize wrist
Extensor carpi radialis brevis	Radial nerve, C6–7	Lateral epicondyle	Base of third metacarpal	Extension of wrist; abduction and supination of forearm	Stabilize wrist
Extensor digitorum	Radial nerve, C6–7	Lateral epicondyle	Middle and distal phalanges 2,3,4,5	Extension of fingers, principally at metacarpal, phalangeal, and interphalangeal joints	Stabilize wrist, hand
Extensor digiti minimi	Radial nerve, C6–7	Lateral epicondyle	Middle and distal phalanges of fifth finger	Extension and abduction of fifth finger	Stabilize wrist, hand
Extensor carpi ulnaris	Radial nerve, C6–7	Lateral epicondyle and ulna	Base of fifth metacarpal	Extension and ulnar abduction of wrist	Stabilize wrist. flex elbow

Muscle	Innervation	Attachments	Function	Stabilize
Supinator	Radial nerve, C6–7	Humeral: lateral epicondyle Ulnar: radial collateral and annular ligaments	Anterior surface of radius	Supination	Stabilize elbow
Abductor pollicis longus	Radial nerve, C6–7	Radial and interosseous membrane and ulna	Base of first metacarpal	Extension and external rotation of first metacarpal	Stabilize wrist
Extensor pollicis brevis	Radial nerve, C6–7	Radius and interosseous membrane	Proximal phalanx of thumb	Extension of metacarpophalangeal joint, abduction of metacarpal, assist in radial abduction of wrist	Stabilize wrist, thumb
Extensor pollicis longus	Radial nerve, C6–7	Ulna and interosseous membrane	Distal phalanx of thumb	Extension of interphalangeal joint of thumb and first metacarpophalangeal joint, extension of wrist	Stabilize wrist, thumb
Extensor indicis	Radial nerve, C6–7	Ulna	Distal second metacarpal, joins extensor digitorum	Extension of all joints of index finger	Stabilize wrist, hand

*Underlined numbers indicate the nerves that provide the main innervation.

(Continued.)

TABLE 5–1 (cont.)

Muscle	Innervation*	Origin	Insertion	Function	
				Open Chain	Closed Chain
Lumbricals (4)	Median nerve, 1, 2 (C8, T1); ulnar nerve, 3, 4 (C8, T1)	Tendons of flexor digitorum profundus	Extensor aponeurosis	Flexion of metacarpophalangeal joints, extension of proximal and distal interphalangeal joints	Stabilize hand
Abductor pollicis brevis	Median nerve, C8, T1	Trapezium and flexor retinaculum	Base of proximal phalanx (some on extensor pollicis longus tendon)	True abduction of thumb	Stabilize thumb
Opponens pollicis	Median nerve, C8, T1	Trapezium and flexor retinaculum	Dorsal side of first metacarpal	Opposition	Stabilize thumb
Flexor pollicis brevis	Superficial: median nerve, C8, T1; Deep: ulnar nerve, C8, T1	Superficial: flexor retinaculum; Deep: second and third metacarpals	Radial side of base of proximal phalanx	Flexion of metacarpophalangeal joint of thumb; adduction and opposition of thumb	Stabilize thumb
Adductor pollicis	Ulnar nerve, C8, T1	Transverse head: third metacarpal; Oblique head: capitate and trapezoid	Ulnar side of base of proximal phalanx of thumb	Adduction and flexion of thumb	Stabilize thumb

Muscle	Innervation	Attachment	Attachment	Function	Function
Abductor digiti minimi	Ulnar nerve, C8, T1	Pisiform	Ulnar side of base of proximal phalanx of fifth digit	Abduction of fifth digit	Stabilize fifth finger
Flexor digiti minimi brevis	Ulnar nerve, C8, T1	Flexor retinaculum and hamate	Proximal phalanx of fifth digit (more on palmar surface)	Flexion at metacarpophalangeal joint of fifth digit	Stabilize fifth finger
Palmar interossei (3)	Ulnar nerve, C8, T1	Second, fourth, and fifth metacarpals	Extensor tendons	Adduction of second, fourth, and fifth digits to middle finger; flexion of metacarpophalangeal joints; extension of interphalangeal joints	Stabilize hand
Dorsal interossei (4)	Ulnar nerve, C8, T1	First: first and second metacarpals; Second: second and third metacarpals; Third: fourth and fifth metacarpals; Fourth: fourth and fifth metacarpals	First: base of proximal phalanx of index (radial side); Second and third: base of proximal phalanx of middle, radial, and ulnar; Fourth: proximal phalanx of ring finger (ulnar side)	Abduction of second, third, and fourth fingers; flexion of metacarpophalangeal joints; extension of interphalangeal joints	Stabilize hand

(Continued.)

TABLE 5–1 (cont.)

Muscle	Innervation*	Origin	Insertion	Function Open Chain	Function Closed Chain
Opponens digiti minimi	Ulnar nerve, C8, T1	Flexor retinaculum, hamate bone	Ulnar side of fifth metacarpal	Cupping of hand	Stabilize hand
			Lower Limb		
Gluteus maximus	Inferior gluteal nerve, L5–S2	Sacrum, dorsal sacroiliac ligament, ilium, sacrotuberous ligament	Iliotibial tract, gluteal tuberosity	Extension, external rotation, adduction (when extended)	Stabilize hip, knee; tilt pelvis back (raise the pubis)
Gluteus medius	Superior gluteal nerve, L4–S1	Lateral surface of ilium	Greater trochanter	Abduction and external rotation of femur Anterior fibers: flexion, internal rotation	Prevents pelvis from dropping on unsupported side
Gluteus minimus	Superior gluteal nerve, L4–S1	Ilium	Greater trochanter	Posterior fibers: extension and external rotation Abduction and internal rotation at hip	Prevents pelvis from dropping on unsupported side
Tensor fascia lata	Superior gluteal nerve, L4–S1	Iliac crest	Iliotibial tract	Abduction, internal rotation, flexion of thigh	Stabilizes hip, knee
Piriformis	Ventral rami, S1, S2	Anterior surface of sacrum	Inner surface of upper part of greater trochanter	Lateral rotation and abduction (if hip flexed)	Stabilizes hip, retraction of contralateral hip

Muscle	Innervation	Origin	Insertion	Action	Stabilization
Obturator internus	Nerve to obturator internus and superior gemellus, L5–S2	Inner surface of pelvis and obturator foramen	Trochanteric fossa	Lateral rotation and abduction (if hip flexed)	Stabilizes hip, retraction of contralateral hip
Gemellus superior	Nerve to obturator internus and superior gemellus, L5–S2	Ischial spine	Obturator internus tendon then inserts into trochanteric fossa	Lateral rotation and abduction (if hip flexed)	Stabilizes hip, retraction of contralateral hip
Gemellus inferior	Nerve to quadratus femoris and inferior gemellus, L4–S1	Ischial tuberosity	Obturator internus tendon then inserts into trochanteric fossa	Lateral rotation and abduction (if hip flexed)	Stabilizes hip, retraction of contralateral hip
Quadratus femoris	Nerve to quadratus femoris and inferior gemellus, L4–S1	Ischial tuberosity	To femur just below greater trochanter	External rotation and adduction of thigh	Stabilizes hip, retraction of contralateral hip
Obturator externus	Obturator nerve, L3–4	Outer surface of pelvic obturator foramen	Medial side of trochanteric fossa	External rotation and adduction of thigh	Stabilizes hip, retraction of contralateral hip
Semitendinosus	Tibial nerve (sciatic), L4–S2	Ischial tuberosity	Medial side of tibial tuberosity (pes anserinus)	Extension of hip, flexion of knee	Stabilizes hip, knee, tilt pelvis back

(Continued.)

TABLE 5–1 (cont.)

Muscle	Innervation*	Origin	Insertion	Open Chain	Closed Chain
				\<Function\>	
Semimembranosus	Tibial nerve (sciatic), L4–S2	Ischial tuberosity	Medial tibial condyle	Extension of hip, flexion of knee	Stabilizes hip, knee, tilt pelvis back
Biceps femoris	Long head: tibial nerve, L4–S2 Short head: common peroneal (fibular) nerve, L4–S2	Long head: ischial tuberosity Short head: linea aspera	Head of fibula	Long head: hip extension, knee flexion Short head: knee flexion only	Stabilizes hip, knee, tilt pelvis back
Sartorius	Femoral nerve, L2–3	Anterior superior iliac spine	Medial side of tibial tuberosity (pes anserinus)	Hip flexion, external hip rotation, knee flexion	Stabilizes hip, knee, tilt pelvis back
Rectus femoris	Femoral nerve, L3–4	Anterior inferior iliac spine	Patellar tendon	Hip flexion, knee extension	Stabilize hip, tilt pelvis forward (lower the pubis), extend knee (raise body)
Vastus medialis	Femoral nerve, L3–4	Medial lip of linea aspera, anterior femur	Patellar tendon	Knee extension	Extend knee (raise body)
Vastus lateralis	Femoral nerve, L3–4	Lateral lip of linea aspera	Patellar tendon	Knee extension	Extend knee (raise body)
Vastus intermedius	Femoral nerve, L3–4	Anterior, medial, and lateral femur	Patellar tendon	Knee extension	Extend knee (raise body)

Muscle	Innervation	Attachment	Attachment	Function	Function
Articularis genus	Femoral nerve, L3–4	Front of femur	Upper part of synovial membrane of knee joint	Drawing synovial membrane up	Draw synovial membrane up
Psoas major	Lumbar plexus and femoral nerve, L2–4	Transverse processes and bodies of lumbar vertebrae	Lesser trochanter	Hip flexion, external rotation of femur, hip adduction	Stabilize hip, tilt pelvis forward (lower the pubis)
Iliacus	Femoral nerve, L2–4	Inner surface of ilium	Lesser trochanter	Hip flexion, external rotation of femur, hip adduction	Stabilize hip, tilt pelvis forward (lower the pubis)
Psoas minor	Femoral nerve, L2–4	T12–L1 vertebrae	Superior ramus of pubis	Upward rotation of pelvis	Stabilize pelvis, tilt pelvis back (raise the pubis)
Pectineus	Femoral nerve, L3–4 (sometimes from obturator nerve)	Superior ramus of pubis	Femur below lesser trochanter	Hip flexion and adduction	Stabilize hip, tilt pelvis forward (lower the pubis)
Adductor longus	Obturator nerve, L2–3	Pubic tubercle	Medial lip of linea aspera	Flexion and adduction at thigh, external rotation	Stabilize hip, tilt pelvis forward (lower the pubis)
Adductor brevis	Obturator nerve, L2–3	Pubis and inferior ramus	Between lesser trochanter and linea aspera	Flexion and adduction at hip, external rotation	Stabilize hip, tilt pelvis forward (lower the pubis)
Adductor magnus	Anterior part, obturator nerve; ischiocondylar portion, sciatic nerve, L3–S1	Inferior ramus of pubis and ischium, ischial tuberosity	Linea aspera, adductor tubercle	Adduction and flexion at hip, extension at hip along with hamstrings	Stabilize hip, tilt pelvis

(Continued.)

TABLE 5–1 (cont.)

Muscle	Innervation*	Origin	Insertion	Function — Open Chain	Function — Closed Chain
Gracilis	Obturator nerve, L2–3	Inferior ramus of pubis and ischium	Medial side of tibial tuberosity (pes anserinus)	Adduction at hip, flexion at knee	Stabilize hip, knee, tilt pelvis forward (lower the pubis)
Gastrocnemius flex	Tibial nerve, S1–2	Medial and lateral epicondyles of femur	Calcaneus	Plantar flexion, knee flexion	Tilt leg back, flex knee
Soleus	Tibial nerve, L5–S2	Soleal line of tibia, upper third of posterior surface of fibula	Calcaneus	Plantar flexion	Tilt leg back
Plantaris flex	Tibial nerve, L4–S1	Lateral epicondyle of femur	Calcaneus	Plantar flexion	Tilt leg back, flex knee (weak)
Popliteus	Tibial nerve, L4–S1	Lateral epicondyle of femur	Posterior surface of tibia	Internal rotation of leg on femur, knee flexion	Rotatory stabilizer, external rotation of femur on tibia ("unlocking" the knee)
Flexor hallucis longus	Tibial nerve, S1–2	Posterior aspect of fibula	Distal phalanx of big toe	Flexion of big toe	Lift anterior foot
Flexor digitorum longus	Tibial nerve, S1–2	Posterior aspect of tibia	Distal phalanx of lateral four toes	Flexion of lateral four toes	Lift anterior foot
Tibialis posterior	Tibial nerve, L5–S1	Tibia (posterior surface) and fibula (medial surface)	All tarsals (except talus) and base of second, third, and fourth metatarsals	Adduction, inversion, plantar flexion	Tilt leg medially and back

Muscle	Innervation	Origin	Insertion	Function	Function
Tibialis anterior	Deep fibular nerve, L4–S1 (common "peroneal" nerve and its branches are known as "fibular")	Lateral surface of tibia	Medial cuneiform and first metatarsal	Inversion and dorsiflexion of foot	Tilt leg medially and forward
Lumbricals (4)	First, medial plantar nerve, L5, S1; others by lateral plantar nerve, S1–2	Flexor tendons	Medial proximal phalanges	Flexion of metatarsophalangeal joints	Stabilize anterior foot
Plantar interossei	Lateral plantar nerve, S1–2	Third, fourth, and fifth metatarsals	Medial side of proximal phalanges	Adduction	Stabilize anterior foot
Dorsal interossei	Lateral plantar nerve, S1–2	*Metatarsal Interossei* 1, 2: First 2, 3: Second 3, 4: Third 4, 5: Fourth	First: medial side of 2 Second: lateral side of 2 Third: lateral side of 3 Fourth: lateral side of 4	Abduction	Stabilize anterior foot
Flexor digitorum brevis	Medial plantar nerve, S1–2	Calcaneus and both intermuscular septa	Four tendons, medial phalanx of lateral four toes	Flexion of four lateral toes	Lift anterior foot

(Continued.)

TABLE 5–1 (cont.)

Muscle	Innervation*	Origin	Insertion	Function	
				Open Chain	Closed Chain
Abductor digiti minimi	Lateral plantar nerve, S1–2	Calcaneus	Lateral side of proximal phalanx of fifth toe	Abduction of fifth toe	Stabilize fifth ray
Flexor hallucis brevis	Medial plantar nerve, S1–2	Cuneiform bones	Both sides of first proximal phalanx	Flexion of big toe	Lift anterior foot
Adductor hallucis	Lateral plantar nerve, S1–2	Oblique: second and third metatarsals Transverse: third, fourth, and fifth metatarsophalangeal joints	Base of proximal phalanx of big toe with lateral head of flexor hallucis brevis	Adduction of big toe	Stabilize first ray
Flexor digiti minimi brevis	Lateral plantar nerve, S1–2	Cuboid and base of fifth metatarsal	Plantar surface of proximal phalanx	Flexion of little toe	Stabilize fifth ray
Quadratus plantae	Lateral plantar nerve, S1–2	Calcaneus	Lateral side of long flexor tendons	Assist flexion of four lateral toes	Stabilize foot
Extensor hallucis brevis	Deep fibular nerve, L5–S1	Larger medial part of extensor digitorum brevis	Base of proximal phalanx of big toe	Extension of big toe	Extend big toe
Extensor digitorum longus	Deep fibular nerve, L5–S1	Lateral condyle of tibia, anterior surface of fibula	Medial and distal phalanges of lateral four toes	Extension of four lateral toes, dorsiflexion of foot	Tilt leg forward
Extensor hallucis longus	Deep fibular nerve, L5–S1	Anterior surface fibula	Distal phalanx of big toe	Extension of big toe, weak dorsiflexion	Tilt leg forward

Muscle	Innervation	Origin	Insertion	Function	
Peroneus tertius	Deep fibular nerve, L5–S2	Lateral slip of extensor digitorum longus	Lateral side of fifth metatarsal	Eversion and dorsiflexion of foot	Tilt leg laterally and forward
Peroneus longus	Superficial fibular nerve, L5–S1	Lateral surface of fibula	Base of first metatarsal and adjacent medial cuneiform	Eversion of foot	Tilt leg laterally
Peroneus brevis	Superficial fibular nerve, L5–S1	Lateral surface of fibula	Dorsal part of base of fifth metatarsal	Eversion of foot	Tilt leg laterally
Abductor hallucis	Medial plantar nerve, S1–2	Calcaneus and medial intermuscular septum	Medial side and flexor surface of proximal first phalanx	Flexion of metatarsophalangeal joint, abduction of big toe	Lift and stabilize first ray
Extensor digitorum brevis	Deep fibular nerve, S1–2	Upper surface of calcaneus	Three tendons to second, third, and fourth toes, along with long extensor tendon	Extension of toes, except little toe	Extend middle three toes

The terminology in this chapter is that most commonly used. We have also incorporated anglicized versions of the Latin muscle names in *Nomina Anatomica.*[5-7]

REFERENCES

1. Jenkins DB. Hollinshead's functional anatomy of the limbs and back. 6th ed. Philadelphia: WB Saunders, 1991.
2. Gowitzke BA, Milner M. Scientific bases of human movement. 3rd ed. Baltimore: Williams & Wilkins, 1988.
3. Hollinshead WH. Anatomy for surgeons. Vol 3. The back and limbs. 3rd ed. Philadelphia: Harper & Row, 1982.
4. Reuleaux F. Theoretische Kinematik: Grundig einer theorie de maschinenwesens. Braunschweig: IF Vieweg und Sohn, 1875. (Also, translated by ABW Kennedy. The kinematic theory of machinery: outline of a theory of machines. London: Macmillan Publishing Company, 1876.)
5. Nomina anatomica. 6th ed. Authorised by the Twelfth International Congress of Anatomists in London, 1985, together with Nomina histologica third edition, Nomina embryologica, third edition. Revised and prepared by subcommittees of the International Anatomical Nomenclature Committee. Edinburgh: Churchill Livingstone, 1989.
6. Gardner ED. Gardner-Gray-O'Rahilly anatomy: a regional study of human structure. 5th ed. Philadelphia: WB Saunders, 1986.
7. Pansky B. Review of gross anatomy. 5th ed. New York: Macmillan Publishing Company, 1984.

PART III

Rehabilitation in Neurologic Disorders

6

Rehabilitation After Stroke

Mehrsheed Sinaki
Peter T. Dorsher

Cerebrovascular accidents (strokes) are syndromes of persistent neurologic damage to the cerebrum or brainstem due to vascular pathologic processes. Stroke is a common cause of death and disability; its incidence is about 141 per 100,000 per year.[1]

In stroke patients with rehabilitation potential, it is important that they reach their maximal level of independence because a return to community living is then usually possible. Hemiplegia is one of the disorders for which patients with stroke are most frequently referred for rehabilitation.

CAUSE OF STROKE

The basic processes that account for most strokes are thrombosis, thromboembolism, embolism, and hemorrhage. Hemorrhage may be intracerebral or subarachnoid. Cerebral thrombosis causes about 75% of strokes.[1] Survival is poorest for patients with stroke caused by intracerebral hemorrhage (Table 6–1). [2] The intensity of the rehabilitation program should be adjusted according to the cause of stroke. If the cause is a hypertensive intracerebral hemorrhage, the first goal should be to control the hypertension. Meanwhile, a mild, slowly progressive rehabilitation program can be initiated (that is, passive range of motion and positioning) until the patient's condition becomes stable. In cases of completed post-thrombotic and embolic stroke, range of motion and progressive ambulation should be started as soon as they are tolerated by the patient.

TABLE 6–1
Survival to 30 Days After Stroke in
Residents of Rochester, Minnesota,
1975–1979

Type of Stroke	Survival (%)
Cerebral infarction	84
Subarachnoid hemorrhage	63
Intracerebral hemorrhage	42

Data from Garraway et al.[2]

REHABILITATION

The primary concerns of rehabilitation are evaluation of the patient's potential for improvement with intensive rehabilitation (Table 6–2). These goals should be realistic. They should also be flexible because the patient's neurologic status and degree of deficits usually change with time. The best results are obtained when the patient and family participate as team members in setting the rehabilitation goals.

The emotional reactions of the hemiplegic patient to loss of control of the body may be overwhelming; the degree of depression, anxiety, fear, frustration, anger, or sometimes senility may prevent the patient from being able to participate in the rehabilitation process. It is important to be aware of the patient's premorbid personality, occupation, and skills and of family and social relationships.

Early Phase (Table 6–3)

The patient may have an altered level of consciousness or be unable to participate actively in care during the early phase of treatment.

TABLE 6–2
Factors to Consider in Evaluation of a Patient's Potential for Rehabilitation After Stroke

Exercise tolerance
  Weakness, stiffness, cardiopulmonary insufficiency, reaction to drugs
Cognition, behavior
  Level of consciousness, emotional status, behavior, communication, memory,
    motivation
Motor deficit
  Weakness, spasticity, contracture
Sensory deficit
  Vision, hearing, proprioception, discrimination, cortical integration
Postural control
  Sitting, standing, walking

TABLE 6-3

Common Complications After Stroke

Early
    Pressure sores
    Urinary retention or incontinence
    Bowel incontinence or constipation
    Urinary tract infection
    Depression
    Deep venous thrombosis
    Pulmonary atelectasis or pneumonia
    Language disorders
Late
    Spasticity and contractures
    Shoulder-hand syndrome
    Central pain
    Seizure disorders

Nursing Care

Pressure sores can be prevented by using a water mattress and changing the patient's position every 2 hours during the day and every 4 hours during the night. Persons involved in the patient's care should be instructed in the principles of positioning in bed. The desired positioning principles are as follows: (1) a small pillow is placed by the greater trochanter of the plegic hip when the patient is supine; (2) a pillow is placed in the axilla of the plegic side, abducting the arm up 60° to 90° when the patient is supine, and the hand is elevated higher than the elbow; and (3) the plegic leg is elevated, and the foot is higher than the knee because of the effect of gravity. When the patient is supine a footdrop splint is used when indicated (Fig. 6-1). Supportive positions should be used to prevent overstretch of the neurovascular plexus and glenohumeral joint of the flail shoulder during sitting or transfer activities. When palmar grasp reflex is present, the resting-hand splint (Fig. 6-2) should be modified to avoid increasing the flexor digitorum tone through palmar stimulation (Fig. 6-3).

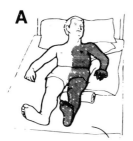 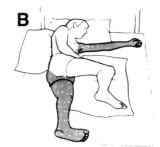

Figure 6-1
Proper positioning principles for patients with hemiplegia. Shaded area is affected side. *A,* When supine. *B,* When lying on affected side. Arm needs to be abducted and extended to avoid rotator cuff injury.

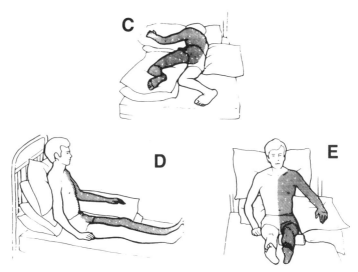

Figure 6–1 (cont.)

C, When lying on unaffected side. D and E, When sitting in bed. (From Seymour R, ed. Home exercises for the patient with hemiplegia. Lexington, Kentucky: Allied Health Publications, University of Kentucky, 1983. By permission of the publisher.)

Range-of-Motion Exercises

Passive range-of-motion exercises are used to prevent contractures and stiffness. When the upper extremity has marked weakness with severe involvement of the shoulder girdle muscles, the glenohumeral joint needs to be supported during range-of-motion exercises. This support prevents glenohumeral subluxation and injury to the rotator cuff by the subluxed head of the humerus.

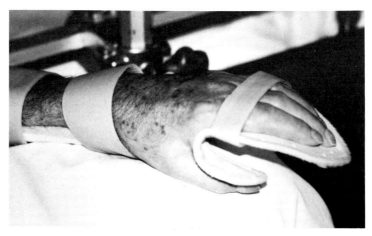

Figure 6–2

Resting-hand splint with palmar contact.

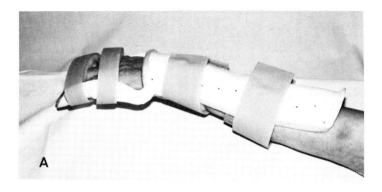

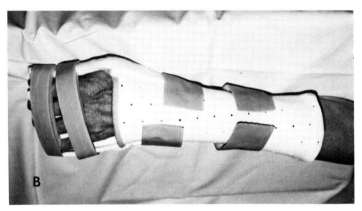

Figure 6-3
A and *B*, Resting-hand splint with elimination of palmar contact to avoid palmar grasp reflex during stretching and resting.

Urinary Tract and Bowel

Infections of the urinary tract should be prevented. Treatment is required if they occur. If the patient is incontinent of urine and if the bladder sphincter is flaccid, an external condom catheter is used in men and an indwelling catheter is used in women. External catheters are changed every day, and indwelling catheters are changed every 2 weeks. If urinary retention is a problem, intermittent catheterization is performed four times a day. Urine specimens for culture need to be obtained weekly while the patient is hospitalized (Table 6-4). The amount of residual urine after voiding needs to be determined when spontaneous voiding returns to ensure that high amounts of residual urine (more than 90 mL) or "overflow" voiding is not occurring. A fluid intake of 1,600 to 1,800 mL a day improves constipation and regulates urinary output. The care of neurogenic bladder or uninhibited bladder is described in detail in Chapter 15. Bowel movement should be encouraged every other day or even daily if this has been the premorbid pattern. Overall, every effort should be made to prevent fecal impaction. In cases of constipation, a high-fiber diet and a stool

TABLE 6–4
Management of Neurogenic Bladder in Stroke Patients

Findings	Treatment, by Sex	
	Male	Female
Flaccid bladder and sphincter, urinary incontinence	Ambulating: condom catheter In bed: urinal Avoid indwelling catheter if possible	Indwelling catheter (change every 2 weeks)
Spastic sphincter or urinary retention	Intermittent catheterization every 3 hours; later extend interval to every 4 hours or four times daily Methantheline (Banthine), 15 mg two times daily*	Intermittent catheterization every 3 hours; later extend interval to every 4 hours or four times daily Fluid intake: 1,600 mL/day Methantheline (Banthine), 15 mg two times daily*
All cases	Urine culture weekly	Urine culture weekly

*Use the lowest effective dose because this drug can increase constipation.

softener are recommended. If these measures are unsuccessful, use of glycerin or bisacodyl (Dulcolax) suppositories can be considered. Long-term bladder and bowel problems are uncommon except in bilateral strokes.

Emotional Lability
Emotional problems should be recognized and dealt with to avoid a delay in the rehabilitation process.

Deep Venous Thrombosis
Elastic stockings should be worn to prevent deep venous thrombosis of the lower extremities, especially during ambulatory activities. Early detection of phlebitis and application of proper treatment are important. Trauma to the lower extremities should be avoided during transfer activities. The risk of deep venous thrombosis is obviously low in patients who are receiving anticoagulant treatment for cerebrovascular disease or cardiac disease (in cases of cardiogenic emboli). In other patients, subcutaneously administered heparin (5,000 U every 12 hours) may have a beneficial preventive effect. Pneumatic sequential compression devices for the legs also decrease the risk of venous thrombosis (see Fig. 9–7).

Respiratory Care
A dependent position, lack of deep breathing, and accumulation of secretions in the alveoli contribute to the development of pulmonary atelec-

tasis or pneumonia. Incentive deep-breathing exercisers are used when a patient's cooperation permits. Respiratory therapy and postural drainage are indicated in most cases.

Speech and Language

Problems with communication can vary from disturbances of articulation (dysarthria) to disorders of comprehension or programming of language (dysphasia). Early evaluation of communication problems and initiation of proper measures and speech therapy are of utmost importance.

Late Phase (Table 6–3)

In this phase, patients participate more actively in physical therapy and occupational therapy training sessions.

Training in Activities on the Mat

Mat activities include turning, rolling, sitting, and kneeling. Motor re-education should be based on the following points.

(1) The affected side should be activated, and therefore stimulated, with correct postures and with passive and active movements.

(2) The patient should be positioned in postures that inhibit spasticity (for example, a lateral prone position with the involved side up and the head turned to the affected side is useful to inhibit the spasticity of the extensor muscles in the leg and flexor muscles in the arm).

(3) Passive and active exercises of paralyzed limbs should be started early after stroke and continued into the late phase. These are significant sources of exteroceptive and proprioceptive stimuli.

(4) Passive and active movements should be started in the trunk and subsequently be performed in the shoulder and hip. The movements should gradually be extended from these proximal joints to joints that are more distal.

(5) Restoring righting reactions, equilibrium reactions, weight on the affected side, and postural adaptation against gravity should accompany the performance of passive and active exercises. Neuromuscular facilitation techniques are used to elicit a refined movement, and eventually that movement can be performed volitionally.[3, 4] Once this is accomplished, the movement is repeated and polished until it becomes permanent.[5]

Brachial Plexus and Rotator Cuff Injury in the Flail Upper Extremity

The flaccid hemiplegic shoulder needs to be protected from undue strain to avoid rotator cuff injury, which could initiate the development of "hemiplegic shoulder-hand syndrome" and frozen shoulder. The following principles are recommended for the treatment of shoulder-hand syndrome: (1) proper positioning of the upper extremity (Figs. 6–1 and 6–4), (2) antiedema measures (see Chapter 27), (3) passive or active-assisted range-of-

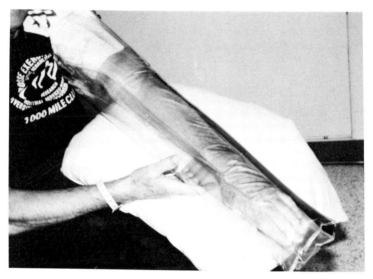

Figure 6–4
Air splint for decreasing edema of upper extremity while stretching it.

motion exercises, (4) pain reduction with analgesics or a trial of transcutaneous electrical nerve stimulation, and (5) proper support of the hemiplegic shoulder with a lapboard for the wheelchair (see Fig. 6–11) and a shoulder sling or similar support for ambulation. In some cases, application of a mild, localized heat, such as ultrasound, to the painful shoulder will decrease pain. Heat to the whole upper extremity should be avoided to prevent an increment of edema.

Thalamic Pain

Occasionally, some hemiplegic patients who also have suffered injury to the thalamic nuclei complain of disturbing unilateral sensory symptoms. These symptoms are persistent and aggravated by stress and fatigue. They are described as burning, drawing, swelling, tingling, and hurting sensations. When the involved extremities are touched, a disagreeable, unpleasant sensation is produced, and the patient exhibits a "touch-me-not" attitude. The sensory stimuli become blocked or distorted at the damaged thalamus and are perceived as painful and distressing sensations at the sensory cortex. This distressing pain can significantly interfere with rehabilitation efforts. In many patients, this pain syndrome gradually improves. In some patients, pain may be reduced by anticonvulsant medications, such as carbamazepine (Tegretol) or phenytoin (Dilantin). Amitriptyline (Elavil) alone or in combination with fluphenazine (Prolixin) is also often helpful, as may be some of the benzodiazepine derivatives. The prolonged use of phenothiazines (such as fluphenazine) should be avoided because it may lead to parkinsonism and, even more disturbingly, to tardive dyskinesias, especially in elderly patients.

Seizure Disorder

A seizure disorder is not a rare complication of cerebral infarction. The residual atrophic region may emanate epileptiform activity leading to partial or generalized seizures. When this occurs, treatment with anticonvulsants should be instituted.

Use of the Upper Extremity for Self-Care and Activities of Daily Living

Patients should be instructed to initiate use of the upper extremity even if the function is not coordinated (Fig. 6–5). Even small accomplishments bring them closer to achieving independence.

Ambulatory Activities

Gait training starts with attaining sitting balance and progresses to standing balance and then walking. Learning to transfer in and out of a bed and chair facilitates self-care and is initiated as soon as it is tolerated by the patient (Fig. 6–6). There are different schools of thought regarding use of ankle-foot orthoses for gait training and also different methods for gait training. Gait training may be applied with the therapist holding and positioning the hemiplegic arm and without use of any devices for ambulation. Gait training may also be secured and applied more safely with use of an ankle-foot orthosis and parallel bars. Later, a broad-based cane or other assistive devices can be introduced.

Anosognosia, Unilateral Neglect, and Homonymous Hemianopia

Specific methods of treatment are used to overcome the deficits of body image, space perception, and unilateral neglect resulting from parietal lobe damage. Intensive training by an occupational therapist is needed. One source of stimulus is placement of a radio or a television be-

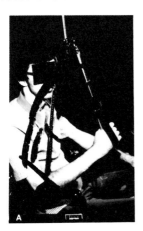 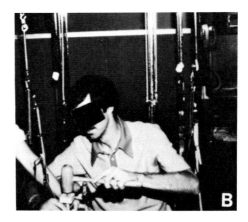

Figure 6–5
A and *B*, Patient using deltoid aid (Rancho Los Amigos overhead suspension sling) on hemiplegic side to aid performance of bimanual activities.

side the neglected side. Perception can also improve with weight bearing after proper splinting of the affected area. Stimulation of the proprioceptors of the joints is an effective feedback mechanism. In most cases, the perception of a limb may return if the physical treatment program is geared to its function.[6]

Orthoses in Adults With Hemiplegia

The prognosis for functional use of the upper limb after a severe stroke with hemiplegia is generally poor; however, the prognosis for ambulation is relatively good. Approximately two-thirds of adult patients with hemiplegia after a cerebrovascular accident will have less function of the upper ex-

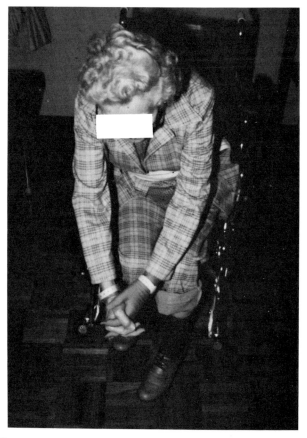

Figure 6–6
Patient, in order to stand, is instructed to extend the hemiplegic left upper extremity with help of unaffected hand. This maneuver facilitates extension of affected knee for weight bearing.

tremities; however, 70% will be able to ambulate with orthotic assistance or external support for the lower extremity. Different types of ankle-foot orthoses are used for ambulatory activities in hemiplegic patients (see Fig. 9–9; Fig. 6–7). Ambulation starts with training in sitting balance and advances to standing balance and gait training. Hemiplegic patients may or may not need assistive devices for ambulation. Many hemiplegic patients ambulate with use of a cane and an ankle-foot orthosis on the hemiplegic side (short leg splint or brace). In some cases, a shoulder hemisling is used to support the shoulder and arm of a patient with a flail upper extremity; it should be used in selected cases.

If the plegic hand is developing severe spasticity and flexion contractures, splinting needs to be considered. The flail wrist may require only a cock-up splint. The resting-hand and wrist splints are made of molded Orthoplast and may be applied over the dorsal-volar aspect of the extremity, according to the patient's condition. Resting-hand splints with contact on the dorsum of the hand decrease the palmar grasp reflex in spastic upper

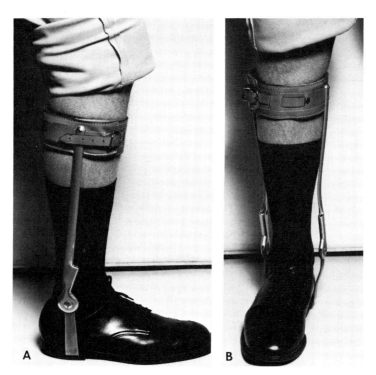

Figure 6–7
Lateral *(A)* and anterior *(B)* views of double-upright ankle-foot orthosis used for moderate to severe weakness of dorsiflexors of ankles. (From Sinaki M. Rehabilitation. In: Mulder DW, ed. The diagnosis and treatment of amyotrophic lateral sclerosis. Boston: Houghton Mifflin Professional Publishers, 1980:169–193. By permission of John Wiley & Sons.)

extremities (Fig. 6–3). Other types of splints are the Bobath digital spreader, hand cone, and Isotoner glove (for certain indications).

The following are some of the most popular arm slings and supports used: (1) neurodevelopmental treatment (NDT) sling, (2) Roylan sling, (3) Bobath sling (Fig. 6–8), (4) hemihook harness (Fig. 6–9), (5) Mayo sling, (6) deltoid aid (Rancho Los Amigos overhead suspension sling) (Fig. 6–5), (7) gutter splint (Fig. 6–10), and (8) foam wedge combined with a lapboard (Fig. 6–11).

The following are some of the common wheelchair features and adaptive equipment used for patients with hemiplegia:[7] (1) desk-type armrests and lapboards with wedge-shaped hand supports to decrease edema in the hand (Fig. 6–11), (2) elevating leg rests, (3) detachable footrests and leg rests, (4) seat cushion or pad, (5) brake handle extension, (6) lapboard, (7) lap belt, (8) low chair or hemichair, and (9) deltoid aid (Rancho Los Amigos overhead suspension sling) (Fig. 6–5).

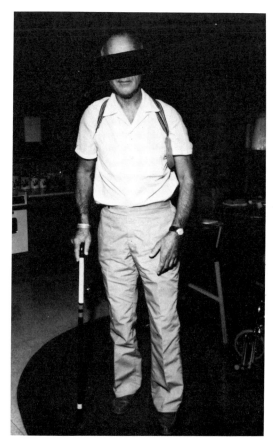

Figure 6–8
Bobath sling, used to decrease pain in left shoulder with moderate weakness of shoulder girdle musculature.

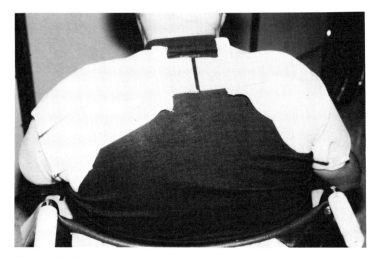

Figure 6–9
Hemihook harness.

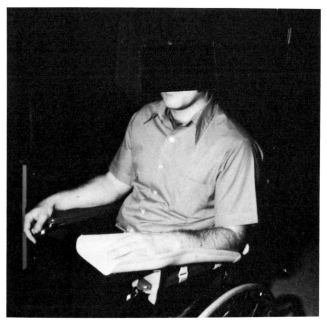

Figure 6–10
Gutter splint, applied to arm of chair.

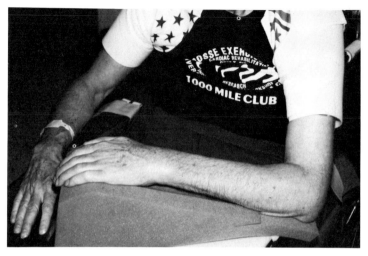

Figure 6–11
Wedge-shaped resting cushion, used to decrease edema in hands of patients with hemiplegia.

Psychometric Tests

Shortly after a stroke, as part of the evaluation of the potential for rehabilitation, the patient's cognitive abilities are evaluated. Detailed psychometric tests are deferred until a patient's medical condition and level of cooperation permit. These tests are useful in most cases to help individualize appropriate methods of teaching for each patient.

Dismissal Planning

Secondary prevention of stroke is essential because the recurrence rate is up to 10% per year. Although aging is the single most important risk factor for stroke, proper management of hypertension and diabetes helps minimize the risk of recurrence. Because coexistent coronary artery disease is common, weight reduction, treatment of elevated serum lipid values, and cessation of smoking are issues to address before dismissal.[8] Patients should be given antiplatelet or anticoagulant medications as appropriate. Before dismissal, a follow-up date should be established and the patient should be referred for vocational rehabilitation if appropriate. Follow-up management may include a neurologic evaluation, a cardiovascular workup, and reevaluation of neurogenic bladder and bowel. A follow-up examination and consultation with the patient and family allow the physicians to remain informed about the implementation and continuation of proper care after dismissal.

REFERENCES

1. Matsumoto N, Whisnant JP, Kurland LT, Okazaki H. Natural history of stroke in Rochester, Minnesota, 1955 through 1969: an extension of a previous study, 1945 through 1954. Stroke 1973; 4:20–29.
2. Garraway WM, Whisnant JP, Drury I. The changing pattern of survival following stroke. Stroke 1983; 14:699–703.
3. Bobath B. Adult hemiplegia: evaluation and treatment. 2nd ed. London: William Heinemann Books, 1978.
4. Johnstone M. Restoration of motor function in the stroke patient: a physiotherapist's approach. New York: Churchill Livingstone, 1978.
5. Stonnington HH. Rehabilitation in cerebrovascular diseases. Primary Care, March 1980; 7:87–106.
6. Redford JB, Harris JD. Rehabilitation of the elderly stroke patient. Am Fam Physician 1980; 22:153–160.
7. Kottke FJ, Stillwell GK, Lehmann JF, eds. Krusen's handbook of physical medicine and rehabilitation. Philadelphia: WB Saunders, 1982.
8. Goldberg G, Berger GG. Secondary prevention in stroke: a primary rehabilitation concern. Arch Phys Med Rehabil 1988; 69:32–40.

7

Traumatic Brain Injury

Robert W. DePompolo

Referred to as the silent epidemic by groups such as the National Head Injury Foundation, traumatic brain injury has been little recognized by the general population despite ever-growing numbers of persons suffering from this problem (Fig. 7–1). It is the major cause of death in persons involved in motor vehicle accidents, and it is estimated to cost billions of dollars per year for medical care and loss of productivity in the United States. The incidence rate of head trauma in the United States is approximately 300 per 100,000 population.[1] In addition, because of continued improvement in the acute care of patients with traumatic brain injury, the number of patients surviving severe head injuries has increased. Therefore, the management of patients with traumatic brain injury has become an important issue not only to medical personnel but also to society as a whole.

PREVENTION

The first point to be made regarding traumatic brain injury is the issue of preventing new injuries from occurring. Educating the persons at highest risk (those 15 to 30 years of age) as well as the general population to use safety restraints when riding in cars, to wear helmets when riding motorized and nonmotorized bikes, and to avoid driving after drinking alcohol may save needless tragedies. Physicians should play an active role in this process and use their position to influence the behaviors of their communities.

PREDICTING OUTCOME

Information regarding outcome based on the injury is useful for planning the appropriate medical intervention as well as for counseling the pa-

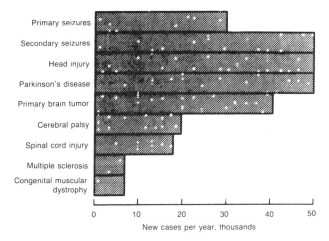

Figure 7–1

Estimated yearly incidence of persons left with disability after head injury compared with incidence of other important neurologic diseases, excluding cerebrovascular disease (which accounts for 450,000 cases yearly). (From NHIF Goals. The silent epidemic. Framingham, Massachusetts: National Head Injury Foundation, June 1984. By permission of the Foundation.)

tient and the patient's family. The need for an accurate prognosis is important. Factors that have been shown to be somewhat predictive of outcome include the patient's age, the duration of coma, the duration of posttraumatic amnesia, the clinical picture, and certain laboratory data.

The role that age plays in outcome is controversial. It has been traditionally believed that given the same extent of brain injury, the patient who is younger than 18 years has a better outcome than the patient who is older than 18 years. However, in some studies, extremely young patients (infants) seem to have a worse outcome than the adult group of patients with brain injury.

Both the duration of coma and the duration of posttraumatic amnesia are related to outcome. Jennett and Teasdale[2] found that coma of longer than 2 weeks generally resulted in some physical dependency, coma of longer than 1 month resulted in death or in a persistent vegetative state in 50% of patients, and coma of longer than 2 months resulted in death or a persistent vegetative state in 70% of patients. When they studied the duration of posttraumatic amnesia, they found that if it was less than 14 days 83% of the patients had a good recovery, and if it was more than 28 days only 27% had a good recovery and 30% were severely disabled.

The extent of brain injury obviously is a significant factor in outcome. However, it might be difficult to evaluate the extent of damage early after head injury. Computed tomographic scans may not reveal a more diffuse type of injury to the brain. Brainstem-evoked potentials are of some help in predicting outcome.

Certain clinical factors, defined by Jennett and Teasdale[2] in their

Glasgow coma scale, are predictive of outcome. The Glasgow coma scale is based on clinical observations of eye movement, motor function, and verbal output. Each category is scored according to the level of performance; the lowest possible score is 3 and the highest is 15 (Table 7–1). Outcome studies based on scores obtained early in the acute phase of traumatic brain injury show that this scale has some predictive value. In addition to predicting ultimate outcome, the Glasgow coma scale also helps standardize the assessments made by the different medical and paramedical staff caring for a patient.

In general, although predicting outcome in patients with traumatic brain injury is important for treatment, establishing firm criteria has been difficult. Certain factors are useful for suggesting outcome; however, assessment of the ultimate outcome is difficult, especially early in the course of the disorder.

MANAGEMENT

Improved acute medical management of patients with traumatic brain injury has resulted in less morbidity and mortality. A few texts[2–4] have outlined the critical areas of concern. Medical complications that can occur include posttraumatic seizures, hydrocephalus, diabetes insipidus, inappropriate antidiuretic hormone secretion, heterotopic bone formation, and thrombophlebitis.

The specific problems of chronic management of patients with traumatic brain injury vary, depending on the severity of injury. The basic initial rehabilitation problem areas include nutrition, bladder and bowel dysfunction, joint range of motion, skin care, respiratory status, and cognitive stimulation.

The nutritional concerns depend on the patient's level of alertness and ability to swallow. A comatose patient or one with brainstem involvement may be unable to handle oral intake. The initial treatment is usually intravenous maintenance. This probably is adequate for the first few days after injury. If the patient's status remains unchanged, other forms of nutrition need to be considered. The general course is either a nasogastric feeding tube or total parenteral nutrition. Both of these feeding techniques are satisfactory for a few weeks. They allow time for possible recovery and eventual oral feeding. Currently, nasogastric tube feedings are preferred if there are no contraindications. If the patient remains in a coma or persistent vegetative state or continues to be unable to swallow safely, the usual recourse is a feeding gastrostomy or feeding gastrojejunostomy tube. Current techniques allow the gastrostomy tube to be placed with a percutaneous insertion method and local anesthesia.

If the patient shows improvement in the level of alertness and has no major brainstem involvement, oral feedings are possible. If the patient has problems with the oral phase of swallowing, a soft mechanical diet may be preferable to liquids because patients can control soft foods and form a bolus better than they can with liquids.

TABLE 7–1

Glasgow Coma Scale

Clinical Observation	Examiner's Test	Patient's Response	Assigned Score
Eye opening	Spontaneous	Opens eyes on own	4
	Speech	Opens eyes when asked to in a loud voice	3
	Pain	Opens eyes when pinched	2
	Pain	Does not open eyes	1
Best motor response	Commands	Follows simple commands	6
	Pain	Pulls examiner's hand away when pinched	5
	Pain	Pulls a part of body away when pinched	4
	Pain	Flexes body inappropriately to pain (decorticate posturing)	3
	Pain	Body becomes rigid in an extended position when pinched (decerebrate posturing)	2
	Pain	Has no motor response to pinch	1
Verbal response (talking)	Speech	Carries on a conversation correctly and tells examiner where and who he or she is and the month and year	5
	Speech	Seems confused or disoriented	4
	Speech	Talks so examiner can understand, but makes no sense	3
	Speech	Makes sound that examiner cannot understand	2
	Speech	Makes no noise	1

From Rimel and Jane.[3] By permission of the publisher.

Bladder and bowel function may be a management problem, again depending on the severity of head injury. Initially, a comatose patient will most likely have an indwelling urethral catheter for bladder drainage. As medical problems stabilize and neurologic status improves, the approach to the bladder will need reconsideration. Depending on the location of the central nervous system damage, spontaneous voiding may or may not occur. The bladder dysfunction that commonly occurs with cortical damage is an uninhibited bladder. However, other types of bladder dysfunction are not unusual, depending on the location of the central nervous system lesion. An uninhibited bladder may not be a management problem if a condom catheter can be worn. Continued episodes of urinary incontinence generally are not tolerated for long periods before the skin in the perineal area breaks down. Bowel control may also be a problem. The extent of the bowel program depends on the patient's level of consciousness, the severity of damage, and the type of nutritional support.

Maintaining joint range of motion may present a special problem if increased muscle tone exists. A physical therapist may be of significant help in maintaining joint motion through appropriate positioning techniques for the upper and lower extremities and joint range-of-motion exercises. Splinting or inhibitory casting of an extremity may be necessary, depending on the amount of abnormal muscle tone and whether strong synergistic patterns are developing.

Skin care in an immobile patient is also a concern. Such a patient should be repositioned at least every 2 hours by the nursing staff. Skin care also involves preventing irritation from excess moisture resulting from incontinence and sweating. Skin creases that are not kept dry may also be areas of skin breakdown. An air mattress, foam cushion, or water mattress on the bed may prevent bed sores. A sheepskin mattress pad may prevent shear stresses on the skin when the patient is moved around in bed.

Respiratory status may be of concern if the injury involves the brainstem. Cheyne-Stokes respiration, tachypnea, and ataxic respiration can occur with brainstem lesions. Acute respiratory failure requiring ventilation may occur in severe injuries. The respiratory status can also be compromised by aspiration due to poor oral control, and atelectasis may develop secondary to poor ventilation. Patients may require assistance from the nursing staff for coughing. Chest physiotherapy may help prevent pneumonias.

The best approach to the amount and type of stimulation in a patient with resolving coma is somewhat controversial. Providing some degree of visual, tactile, taste, auditory, and olfactory stimulation in a controlled setting is reasonable if only to document the patient's response consistently. In addition, such stimulation may induce a quicker recovery. As coma resolves, cognitive rehabilitation should begin.

It is not unusual for a patient with a closed head injury to move through a state of recovery marked by agitation. When agitation does develop, other possible causes should be ruled out, such as metabolic imbalance, pulmonary embolism, and septicemia. Agitation secondary to head injury can be a difficult management problem. Medications, restraints, and environmental controls are some of the ways to deal with this problem. Appropriate control of the environment is a preferable first step to determine whether it is sufficient to manage the agitation. It is the most difficult but perhaps the most satisfying means of controlling agitation. The patient should be in a structured, consistent, safe environment. If medications are used, the side effects must be clearly understood by the physician. Multiple drugs have been tried, including dopamine agonist, stimulants, antidepressants, anticonvulsants, phenothiazine, and haloperidol. Because of concern that these drugs may have a negative impact on cognitive recovery, they are used only when necessary. If restraints are used, they should be appropriate and properly fitted.

REHABILITATION TEAM

Physical Therapy

Often, a patient has a plegic or paretic extremity secondary to the traumatic brain injury. In addition to the role of maintaining range of motion outlined above, the physical therapist is involved in muscle reeducation, strengthening exercises, and exercises directed toward retraining of coordination. Mobility retraining, including gait, transfers, and mobility in bed, may be another area of involvement. Because the deficits vary with the severity of traumatic brain injury, treatment programs must be individualized.

Occupational Therapy

The occupational therapist addresses the areas of activities of daily living such as dressing, hygiene, and feeding and also helps evaluate swallowing difficulties and suggests therapeutic intervention. Cognitive and perceptual functioning can be evaluated and treatment directed toward improvement of a patient's adaptation to these deficits. The occupational therapist may address the issues of disorientation and confusion by helping the team provide the appropriate structure and consistency to the patient's environment. When upper-extremity motor function is impaired secondary to central nervous system damage, the occupational therapist can facilitate maximal use of the arms or hands through functional activities.

Speech Pathology

Patients may demonstrate a speech disorder such as aphasia, dysarthria, or apraxia, depending on the area of central nervous system injury, and require speech therapy. Also, difficulty with prosody can occur. Because communication is a cognitive function, the speech therapist may work in conjunction with the occupational therapist and psychologist to optimize intellectual functioning in many related areas. In some rehabilitation settings, the speech pathologist assesses and treats dysphagia.

Psychology

The psychologist, in conjunction with the occupational therapist and speech pathologist, is the third member of the treatment team who can help direct the rest of the team's efforts in the area of cognitive and perceptual dysfunction. During the recovery stages, the psychologist can provide estimates of cognitive function and, as the deficits stabilize, can administer specific batteries of psychometric tests to define the areas of limitation better. In addition to the standard Wechsler Adult Intelligence Scale, the psychologist can offer other tests to isolate certain areas of cognitive dysfunction. In a patient with a behavioral or emotional problem, the psychologist may counsel the patient or help the rehabilitation team coordinate its efforts more effectively.

Social Service

The social worker may help with arranging financing and obtaining needed equipment. A comprehensive outline of the family structure and the patient's previous work situation and educational experiences can be provided by the social worker. This information can be helpful to the rehabilitation team for setting expectations and goals. The social worker may also provide support and education to family members and interface among the physician, the therapist, and the family to ensure that questions are being answered appropriately. Other areas of social work involvement include dismissal planning, regardless of the disposition. If the patient is dismissed home, the social worker helps to mobilize the appropriate community resources to provide maximal care for the patient and support for the family. If the disposition is elsewhere, the social worker can help the family locate the best possible alternative housing situation, whether it be a nursing home, sheltered housing, or other chronic care facility. The social worker may also coordinate services with the department of vocational rehabilitation, if appropriate.

Recreation Therapy

Recreation can be used as a tool to facilitate team goals in the areas of motor retraining, cognitive rehabilitation, endurance training, and emotional or behavioral programming. In addition, the recreation therapist helps with issues relating to reentry into the community, including redeveloping avocational interests and social skills. Through trips outside the institution, the patient can be exposed to the community in a protected, gradational fashion.

Rehabilitation Nursing

The nursing staff is an important factor in providing consistency and structure to the patient's daily activities by reinforcing what the patient learns in occupational therapy, in terms of activities of daily living, and in physical therapy, in terms of transfers and mobility. The nursing staff has a significant impact on educating the patient and family, reinforcing orientation, and addressing any behavioral or emotional problems. Finally, the training that might be needed for bowel or bladder function rests heavily on the nursing staff.

Physician

The physician is instrumental not only for managing the medical problems that arise but also for coordinating the efforts of the different team members to establish appropriate goals. The physician has a unique role in counseling the patient and the patient's family to ensure that all questions are answered and that all issues are addressed.

Other

Other possible team members include a dietitian, chaplain, pharmacist, and tutor (for school-age children). No individual team member has exclusive dominion over any particular area of care; the substantial amount of overlap is extremely helpful for reinforcing what is being trained. Therefore, each member should work as part of the team, and the team should set joint goals and approach intervention in a coordinated manner.

REENTRY INTO THE COMMUNITY

Rehabilitation does not stop when a person with brain injury leaves the acute inpatient rehabilitation setting. In some ways, it is just beginning. The transition back into the community may take many routes, require multiple resources, and consume months to years of time.

During the past few years, the diverse needs of persons with brain injury as they reenter society have been more clearly defined, and creative, new resources have been developed, including long-term residential programs, outpatient (community-based) day programs, and group homes.

Vocational issues were initially addressed through sheltered workshops and vocational counseling. These resources also have expanded to include enclave work, job coaching, and other types of on-the-job training and support.

For successful reentry into the community, coordination and cooperation of multiple community-based resources are needed. Persons with brain injury may require all or none of these services as they recover.

CONCLUSION

The rehabilitation of patients with traumatic brain injury demands the teamwork of several different qualified rehabilitation specialists. This may be a devastating injury to both the patient and the patient's family, and the ultimate level of recovery depends to some extent on how aggressively and appropriately rehabilitation services are used. Beyond acute rehabilitation, this patient population has a complex set of needs for community resources, including outpatient rehabilitation, protective housing, vocational retraining, and family and patient support groups.

REFERENCES

1. Annegers JF, Grabow JD, Kurland LT, Laws ER Jr. The incidence, causes, and secular trends of head trauma in Olmsted County, Minnesota, 1935–1974. Neurology 1980; 30:912–919.
2. Jennett B, Teasdale G. Management of head injuries. Philadelphia: FA Davis, 1981.
3. Rimel RW, Jane JA. Characteristics of the head-injured patient. In: Rosenthal M, Griffith ER, Bond MR, Miller JD, eds. Rehabilitation of the head-injured adult. Philadelphia: FA Davis, 1983:9–21.
4. Cooper PR, ed. Head injury. 2nd ed. Baltimore: Williams & Wilkins, 1987.

8

Multiple Sclerosis

John H. Noseworthy
Mehrsheed Sinaki

Multiple sclerosis (MS) is the most common relapsing or progressive inflammatory demyelinating disease affecting the white matter of the central nervous system. Approximately 250,000 persons in the United States are known to have the disease. Perhaps an additional 75,000 to 125,000 cases are unrecognized. The clinical course of MS is both extremely variable and largely unpredictable, particularly in the early phases of the disease.[1] Until the cause is found, progress toward finding an effective treatment will be dependent on the results of randomized, blinded, and placebo-controlled clinical trials.

CLINICAL FEATURES AND DIAGNOSIS

The symptoms of MS typically have their onset between the ages of 15 and 50 years, although the first symptoms develop earlier or later in life in approximately 10% of cases. The female:male ratio is approximately 2:1. The mean age at onset is approximately 30 years; in women, the onset of symptoms occurs approximately 2 years earlier (on average). Symptoms of acute attacks of MS usually evolve over hours or days and then plateau, most commonly for a period of 3 to 6 weeks; gradual improvement or resolution occurs over 6 to 12 weeks, although there is considerable variability in the behavior of an acute exacerbation. The symptoms correspond directly to the sites of conduction slowing and block within white matter tracts. The most common clinical patterns are those reflecting dysfunction of the optic nerves (optic neuritis—central visual blurring, color desaturation, eye pain with movement, afferent pupillary defect, reduced visual acuity, central scotoma, and often the subsequent development of optic atrophy), brainstem (internuclear ophthalmoplegia—diplopia and oscillopsia, facial numbness, facial myokymia, central vertigo, hearing loss, and pseudobulbar and bulbar palsy), and spinal cord (Lhermitte's symptom [cervical spinal cord], "sensory cord" [the development of a slowly progressive numbness or tingling first affecting one limb and, thereafter, a second limb and often the trunk], the "useless hand syndrome" [impaired proprioception and incoordination without weakness], monoplegia, paraplegia, or diplegia, and disturbance of bowel, bladder, and sexual function). Fatigue (new or worsening) frequently accompanies an acute attack, as does heat sensitivity and worsening of symptoms late in the afternoon and early evening when central body temperature is at its highest. In slowly progressive MS (for example, chronic progressive myelopathy), symptoms gradually worsen over periods of months. Typical symptoms include slowly developing weakness (footdrop, impaired intrinsic hand function), loss of proprioception and vibratory sense usually without a marked spinothalamic deficit (for example, no sensory level), and progressive bowel and bladder dysfunction.

The diagnosis of MS remains primarily a clinical one.[2, 3] Accepted diagnostic criteria emphasize the documentation of evidence of white matter dysfunction separated in both time and space (for example, two separate sites such as the optic nerve and spinal cord) with clinical documentation of at least one anatomic site of impairment. Evoked potentials and, more recently, magnetic resonance imaging (MRI) (Fig. 8–1) may provide evidence of the second lesion in space but not in time (laboratory-supported probable MS). The finding of oligoclonal banding or increased synthesis of IgG in the cerebrospinal fluid provides supportive laboratory evidence for the diagnosis.

A single episode of central nervous system dysfunction suggestive of inflammatory-demyelinating disease is insufficient to make a diagnosis of MS even when the clinical features closely resemble those seen in "typical" MS attacks. Lhermitte's symptom, optic neuritis, and brainstem or spinal cord (incomplete or complete transverse myelitis) involvement alone should prompt a search for other diagnostic possibilities. Considerations should include hereditary diseases (Leber's optic atrophy, familial cavernous hemangioma, spinocerebellar atrophies, hereditary spastic paraparesis, adrenomyeloneuropathy, metachromatic leukodystrophy, and Eldridge's leukodystrophy), congenital malformations at the craniocervical junction (such as Chiari malformation), inflammatory and autoimmune diseases (sarcoidosis, Sjögren's syndrome, Behçet's disease, systemic lupus erythematosus, systemic and isolated central nervous system vasculitis), infectious diseases (neurosyphilis, human immunodeficiency virus, tropical spastic paraparesis [human T-cell lymphoma/leukemia virus-1], Lyme disease, viral transverse myelitis, epidural abscess, acute disseminated encephalomyelitis), vascular disease (cerebral and spinal arteriovenous malformations, ischemic optic neuritis), metabolic disease (subacute combined degeneration of the spinal cord, pyridoxine toxicity), degenerative disc disease (spondylotic myelopathy), neoplastic and paraneoplastic syndromes, idiopathic diseases (multiple systems atrophy, Wartenberg's migratory sensory neuritis), and psychiatric disease (somatization disorder, conversion reaction).

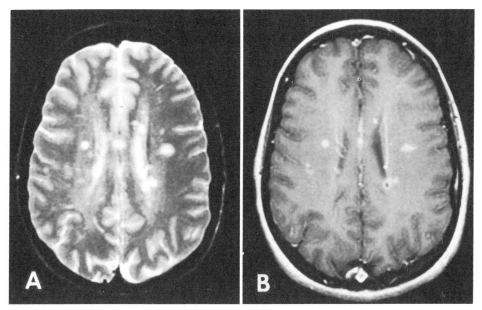

Figure 8–1

A, T2-weighted cranial magnetic resonance imaging scan, demonstrating multiple focal areas of abnormal signal in the cerebral hemispheric white matter bilaterally in a patient with active, relapsing-progressive multiple sclerosis. *B,* Magnetic resonance imaging scan obtained after gadolinium administration, demonstrating contrast enhancement in many of the lesions shown in *A.* This finding indicates active inflammation-demyelination (blood-brain barrier disruption).

ETIOLOGY AND MECHANISMS OF THE DISEASE

The cause of MS remains unknown. The marked geographic variability in the prevalence of the disease (areas of high, medium, and low frequency roughly paralleling the distance from the equator) has been taken as evidence for an environmental agent such as a virus.[4] Alternatively, this north-south gradient could reflect differences in gene pools (for example, patients of Scandinavian origin [high-risk zone] tend to migrate to areas sharing a similar climate; the reverse is true for patients migrating from tropical areas). Viral isolation-transmission studies have isolated more than 10 putative "MS viruses" in the past 4 decades. Subsequent studies have failed to confirm these exciting preliminary reports. Further supportive evidence for a virus as either the cause or the triggering agent in this disease includes the observations that at least 25% of acute attacks are triggered by a viral infection, the demonstration of shared peptide sequences between viruses and central nervous system antigens, the occurrence of acute monophasic inflammatory-demyelinating disease after a virus infection (acute disseminated encephalomyelitis), and a large number of animal models that share similarities with human MS. Recently, studies in twins have suggested that genetic factors play a role in disease susceptibility in that the risk for development of MS in a monozygotic twin of a patient with MS is at least 15- to 20-fold higher than that of a dizygotic twin or an HLA-identical sibling. It is likely that there is no single MS susceptibility gene, but, as is also probably the case for other putative autoimmune diseases (such as type I diabetes mellitus, rheumatoid arthritis), susceptibility to MS may be polygenic. Candidate genes include the HLA-DR, GM-allotype, and T-cell receptor genes.

The primary event in the pathogenesis of the disease, as mentioned, is unknown. One possible sequence of events is as follows. Presumably, a viral agent or some other exogenous "trigger" factor causes primary, cross-reactive immunization with either myelin basic protein or another central nervous system antigen.[5] Central nervous system antigen-specific T cells are generated, and in response to this immune activation, interferon- α, β, and γ are produced. Virus infection and interferon-γ production induce Ia expression on central nervous system endothelium, astrocytes, and microglia, permitting these resident central nervous system cells to act as potential sources for antigen presentation to circulating activated cells of the immune system. T cells presumably recognize the putative MS antigen in the context of these class II (Ia) antigens. T-cell activation results, and subsequently there is amplification of the nonspecific immune response. This results in disruption of the blood-brain barrier, cytotoxic edema, lymphocytic (B- and T-cell) and macrophage penetration into the central nervous system with disturbed saltatory conduction, conduction slowing, temporal dispersion, and conduction block resulting in neurologic symptoms and signs. In the course of this immune response, there is further central nervous system injury from complement, lipid peroxidation, and cellular- and humoral-mediated immune damage. Presumably, in the chronic phase of the disease there are repeated episodes of disruption of the blood-brain barrier with ongoing inflammation, demyelination, and gliosis. Again, the triggering factors for this ongoing, low-grade, inflammatory-demyelinating, and subsequently gliotic process remain incompletely defined.

There is almost no evidence for a disturbance in the systemic immune response of patients with MS. There is conflicting evidence for altered T-cell immunity. Variations in the percentage of helper and suppressor-cytotoxic T-cell ratios have been reported during different phases of the disease by different investigators. In 90% of patients with clinically definite MS, there is evidence for the production of antibodies of limited, but as yet unidentified, antigen specificity (oligoclonal banding) and increased IgG synthesis within the central nervous system (cerebrospinal fluid studies) suggesting chronic B-cell activation. Additional indirect evidence that MS may be immunologically mediated is derived from the finding that one of the best experimental animal models of the disease, relapsing experimental allergic encephalomyelitis (EAE), is a T-cell-mediated disease.

PATHOLOGY

The gross and microscopic extent of pathologic changes far exceed the clinical expression of MS. In advanced cases there is cortical atrophy, and on gross inspection one sees discrete visible and palpable regions of scarring (plaque) extending to the surface of the parenchyma. Serial sections often show the predilection for these macroscopic areas of demyelination and gliosis to be located in the periventricular regions of the deep cerebral hemispheric white matter and the optic nerves.

The microscopic pathologic features of the active, chronic MS lesions are poorly demarcated borders, concentrations of inflammatory cells in perivascular, parenchymal, and meningeal locations, astrocytic hypercellularity, and proliferations of foamy macrophages and proliferating oligodendrocytes. Macrophages are seen immediately adjacent to naked axons (demyelination). There is interstitial edema, and special stains reveal the presence of neutral fat, esterified cholesterol, and expression of class II antigens on the surface of the endothelial cells, astrocytes, and microglia and interferon-γ on the surface of astrocytes. At the plaque border, class I-expressing CD8-positive (suppressor-cytotoxic) and CD4-positive (helper-inducer) T cells are seen. At the center of the plaque, fewer T cells are seen, but class I- and II-positive endothelial cells and class II-negative astrocytes can be identified by special stains. Chronic, inactive MS plaques have sharply demarcated borders and are generally acellular. Oligodendrocytes are absent at the center of the demyelinated plaque but are present at the border and may show morphologic changes suggesting attempts at remyelination. There is mild-to-moderate axon loss and an abundance of fibrillary, hypertrophic astrocytes (gliosis).

NATURAL HISTORY OF THE DISEASE

Overall, two-thirds of cases follow a relapsing-remitting course initially. This percentage is higher in young patients; more than 80% of patients begin with a relapsing-remitting course when their first symptom occurs before the age of 30 years. Approximately 60% of patients begin with a progressive form of the disease when their first symptom occurs after the age of 40 years. With time, many patients enter a progressive phase of the disease with either slow, progressive worsening (chronic-progressive) or apparent slow progression punctuated by infrequent, acute attacks of the illness (relapsing-progressive disease). Within 5 years of onset, evidence of progressive disease develops in approximately 12% of patients whose illness was initially relapsing-remitting; by 10 years, this percentage increases to approximately 40%. Almost 50% of patients who have had the illness for 15 years show evidence of chronic progression.[6]

The course of the disease remains unpredictable for each individual, although a large number of attacks during the first 2 years of the disease, a short first interattack interval, and a relatively brief time to develop evidence of a fixed, moderate degree of disability (Expanded Disability Status Scale [EDSS], 3.0) are somewhat predictive of more aggressive relapsing-remitting disease. The mean duration from disease onset to the need for unilateral assistance for walking (EDSS, 6.0) is approximately 15 years in large series. Currently, there is no clinical or laboratory factor that will reliably predict eventual clinical outcome (natural history) or response to intervention with an experimental treatment. Studies are currently under way in several centers to determine whether serial magnetic resonance imaging can be used to prognosticate at an early stage.

THERAPY

The search for an effective treatment has been severely hampered by ignorance of the cause of the disease.[7] If the triggering antigen(s) could be identified, immunologic tolerance could presumably be induced and further tissue damage prevented. If one or several viruses were definitively identified, vaccination programs could reduce the development of new cases and nonspecific and specific antiviral strategies could be developed to attenuate the illness in those already affected. With the identification of one or several specific antigens, a number of treatment approaches could be developed to interfere with the presentation of this peptide by major histocompatibility (MHC) antigen-expressing, antigen-presenting cells (macrophages, astrocytes, microglia, endothelial cells?) to the T-cell receptor of activated lymphocytes. Each of these components of the trimolecular complex (T-cell receptor, antigen, MHC molecule on the surface of the antigen-presenting cell) could be modified in an attempt to down-regulate the immune response. Blocking peptides that bind to the MHC receptor or T-cell receptor but fail to activate the T cell could be generated. Anti-sense DNA and RNA could be used to block the synthesis of these triggering peptides. If it is shown that there is a limited and homogeneous T-cell response in MS, anti-idiotypes could be generated to regulate the concentration of important T-cell receptor idiotypes, and immune-mediated ablation of specific T cells could be attempted. Monoclonal antibodies directed against important MHC binding peptides could be administered intermittently.

Recent, exciting work in experimental allergic encephalomyelitis suggests that it is possible to prevent and attenuate this animal model of MS by both synthetic T-cell receptor peptide immunization and the administration of peptide analogs of the encephalogenic myelin basic protein epitopes that bind MHC but do not activate T cells. An effective treatment strategy would probably reduce or prevent the migration of activated lymphocytes through the disrupted blood-brain barrier, prevent the proliferation of immunologically activated T cells and macrophages within the central nervous system, reduce the local amplification of the immune response, and down-regulate the expression of class II surface antigens by endothelial cells, astrocytes, and microglia. The production of the many, nonspecific soluble mediators of inflammation would be diminished, as would the intrathecal production of antibody. Remyelination would need to be encouraged and gliosis prevented.

Most of the clinical trials recently completed or currently under way are designed to evaluate the efficacy of antigen nonspecific immunosuppression. Corticotropin (ACTH) and corticosteroids both help to stabilize the blood-brain barrier and reduce MHC expression. Immunosuppressive agents ablate activated T cells, and antiedema and anti-inflammatory agents reduce the concentration of the diffusible products of the immune response and correct conduction block.

Exacerbations

Patients with MS should be instructed to seek medical attention if either new neurologic symptoms develop or they experience a return or worsening of previously experienced ones. It is important that an intercurrent illness (such as a urinary tract infection) be promptly and thoroughly treated (pseudoexacerbation). Patients should be instructed to rest as much as possible during an attack. Neurologic opinion is divided about the use of ACTH and corticosteroids for the short-term management of acute exacerbations. Recent evidence suggests that these treatments are similar in efficacy. Synthetic ACTH, 25 to 60 units, can be infused over an 8-hour period and then tapered over a 2- to 3-week period. Alternatively, a 3- to 5-day course of intravenously administered methylprednisolone (500 to 1,000 mg/day) can be administered on either an inpatient or an outpatient basis, and many neurologists recommend following this therapy with a tapering course of orally administered prednisone (60 to 80 mg/day for 7 to 14 days, tapered by 10 mg every 3 to 5 days thereafter). Others omit methylprednisolone and simply administer prednisone orally. Experience suggests that these steps hasten the time to recovery. Whether the degree of recovery is influenced by these forms of intervention is less clear.

Many multicenter clinical trials are either planned or under way to assess whether copolymer-1, recombinant interferon-β, or sulfasalazine reduces the frequency of attacks, the subsequent development of permanent neurologic damage, or the development of progressive disease in patients with relapsing-remitting MS.

Progressive Disease

As mentioned above, MS can be progressive from onset, particularly if the first symptoms develop later in life. In patients with initially relapsing-remitting MS, the time of onset of the progressive phase of the disease is often less clear-cut. Currently, there is no proven therapeutic intervention that will prevent, slow, or halt the development of further progression in these cases, although several trials (completed and in progress) have been designed to address this important area. Whenever possible, patients with progressive disease should be encouraged to consider enrollment in such trials because there is some evidence to suggest that participation is beneficial even to patients randomized to receive a placebo. During the past decade, most such trials have addressed whether nonspecific suppression of the immune response can slow the progression of MS. Treatments that have received the greatest attention include cyclophosphamide, azathioprine, plasma exchange, cyclosporin A, interferon, copolymer-1, total lymphoid irradiation, and dietary measures. Again, opinion differs, but most would agree that none of these treatments predictably prevent further neurologic deterioration.

One important lesson from these trials is that the rate and degree of neurologic deterioration are not uniform or predictable between patients. Periods of apparent rapid worsening are often followed by spontaneous (placebo-induced?) apparent stabilization. Recent evidence suggests that clinical estimates of disease activity frequently underestimate the degree and extent of disease activity as measured by serial magnetic resonance imaging studies. Continued disease activity as measured by serial magnetic resonance imaging is common during periods of apparent stabilization in patients with both relapsing and progressive disease. Clinical trials testing various nonspecific approaches to immunosuppression are still under study (cyclophosphamide, total lymphoid irradiation, azathioprine, mitoxantrone, psoralen with long-wave ultraviolet radiation, and others). Several new approaches to treatment are being developed, including peptide immunotherapy, T-cell vaccination, and the use of human chimeric monoclonal antibodies against T-cell surface antigens. Other classes of drugs that should be considered for trials include the five aminosteroids and the macrolide FK506.

SYMPTOMATIC TREATMENT AND REHABILITATION

Vision

Impairment of vision may occasionally be partially helped with corrective lenses. An eye patch is recommended for patients with diplopia; the patch is alternated from eye to eye every 2 days. Patients who are blind should be referred to services for the blind and should learn Braille reading.

Paroxysmal Symptoms

Virtually all of the common symptoms experienced by patients with MS can occur paroxysmally, including paresthesias, numbness, pain (such as trigeminal neuralgia), weakness, incoordination, visual blurring, aphasia, dysarthria, and diplopia. A few paroxysmal phenomena are so unique to MS that their presence should suggest the diagnosis. Paroxysmal tonic seizures (painful, tetanic posturing of the face or, more commonly, one or more extremities lasting up to 2 to 3 minutes), often preceded by momentary pain or tingling in the affected limb, can recur several times in the course of the day and may be precipitated by movement or hyperventilation. Spells of paroxysmal ataxia and dysarthria generally last less than 1 to 2 minutes but may recur dozens of times in the course of a day and can similarly be precipitated by hyperventilation, talking, or movement. Each of these paroxysmal events can be troublesome for periods of weeks or months, but generally they cease spontaneously. Both are readily treated with a low dose of either carbamazepine, phenytoin, or baclofen.

Fatigue

Most patients with MS are troubled by fatigue at some point in their illness. This symptom can be overwhelming and disabling, even in patients who are otherwise well with limited, or indeed, no evidence of permanent neurologic disability. This symptom is difficult to characterize, but most patients describe their fatigue as being different from that experienced before the onset of their illness. Despite regular periods of rest and other attempts at energy conservation, fatigue can limit the patient's activities significantly. Some patients notice a modest improvement in their symptoms with amantadine (100 mg once or twice daily). If no benefit is noticed after 3 to 4 weeks of taking this medication, its use can be stopped because it will not be helpful. Side effects include livedo reticularis, insomnia, nightmares, gastrointestinal upset, and headache. Most patients tolerate this medication well. Pemoline may also provide moderate relief of symptoms of fatigue. Anecdotal reports that clonazepam, fluoxetine, and deprenyl selegiline are useful in this condition have not been confirmed by controlled trials. Other causes of fatigue (depression, sleep disorder, hypothyroidism, anemia) should be judiciously excluded.

Pain

Acute pain syndromes (trigeminal neuralgia, Lhermitte's symptom, segmental limb pain) are both less common and generally more easily treated than the chronic pain syndromes that occur in MS. Recurring episodes of trigeminal neuralgia (unilateral or bilateral) often respond to medical measures such as carbamazepine, phenytoin, and baclofen, either alone or in combination. Patients with MS generally tolerate high doses of these drugs less well than do patients with other neurologic disorders. In drug-resistant cases, surgical measures, including percutaneous radiofrequency heating lesions, or glycerol injection may be needed. Microvascular decompression of the trigeminal nerve is not warranted because the site of origin of the pain of MS is within the central nervous system (pons). Lhermitte's symptom (electrical shocklike sensations radiating up or down the spine or into one or more limbs with neck flexion or extension) rarely requires treatment, although in troublesome cases a low dose of either carbamazepine or phenytoin will often be helpful. This symptom can persist for many months. Acute segmental pain may signal an acute, inflammatory-demyelinating lesion at a root entry zone and, as such, may respond to ACTH or corticosteroids.

Chronic pain develops in up to 50% of patients with long-standing disease. Burning, dysesthetic extremity pain occurs in up to half of such cases. This symptom may be worse at night and can be both disabling and extremely resistant to current approaches to treatment. Tricyclic antidepressants, carbamazepine, baclofen, transcutaneous electrical nerve stimulation, and clonazepam can be tried either alone or in combination. Resistant cases may benefit from a multidisciplinary approach utilizing behavior modification, psychologic strategies, relaxation and stretching exercises, and "stretch-and-spray" techniques together with the medications outlined above. Other more treatable causes of chronic pain, including mechanical low back pain, facet disease, cervical and lumbar radiculopathies, and myofascial-tension myalgia pain syndromes, are common, particularly in patients with a moderate degree of disability.

Spasticity

Patients with moderate and advanced corticospinal tract impairment notice, in addition to weakness, reduced fine motor control, slowness of movement, and, at times, troublesome extensor spasms and clonus. Extensor spasms are often present at night and can be precipitated with movement. They are generally painless. Spasticity can be augmented through nociceptive input into the central nervous system. Therefore, a sudden increase in spasticity may indicate development of urinary tract infection, decubitus ulcers, constipation, deep venous thrombosis, or other irritative conditions. Lower extremity flexor spasms typically occur only in patients with a moderate-to-marked degree of paraparesis or paraplegia. They can be extremely troublesome and painful, and when severe they can interfere with peroneal care in bedridden patients. Lower extremity clonus can generally be easily controlled by simply instructing patients and their caregivers to avoid postures that excessively stretch the patellar and Achilles tendons.

Patients with a mild increase in extensor tone may respond to low doses of baclofen (5 to 10 mg, two to four times daily), although higher doses are needed in more severe cases (such as 20 mg, four times daily). A low dose of benzodiazepine at bedtime is often helpful for nocturnal spasms. Benzodiazepine dependence is rare in such cases. Stretching exercises used twice daily and relaxation exercises may reduce extensor tone and can be particularly helpful at bedtime. In addition to the prevention of joint contracture, stretching may modulate spasticity by decreasing primary spindle afferent activity.[8] Antispasticity medications rarely result in improved fine motor control or speed of movement and may temporarily worsen strength in a dose-dependent fashion. It is particularly important to consider this effect in patients dependent on an increase in extensor tone for ambulation. A short course of corticosteroids may be helpful for reducing recently acquired spasticity. The continuous infusion of intrathecal baclofen or narcotics may be useful in severely disabled patients and should be considered before proceeding with irreversible treatment such as intrathecal phenol injection, adductor and hamstring tendon release, posterior rhizotomy, and longitudinal myelotomy. These destructive approaches to spasticity control can be justified only in paraplegic patients who have lost control of bowel and bladder function. Physical modalities such as application of cold, electrical stimulation, and inhibitive positioning through proper splinting are recommended[9] (Table 8–1).

Tremor and Ataxia

Severe appendicular and axial (titubation) tremor rarely responds well to medical management. Clonazepam, propranolol, isoniazid, primidone, and weighted bracelets may be tried, but the results are rarely gratifying. Anecdotal reports of success with stereotactic thalamotomy in patients with disabling unilateral arm tremor require confirmation. Ataxia, when appendicular, may be reduced through application of small weights (1 to 2 lb) to the distal areas of the extremities. In truncal ataxia, weight can be applied to improve balance, and in this case it may be applied to the anterior or posterior aspect of the chest (Fig. 8–2). Use of a long cane to increase the base of support also improves the patient's stability of gait.

Cognitive and Emotional Disturbances

Traditionally, neurologists have paid little attention to the changes in higher cortical function which occur in MS. In early reports, euphoria and

TABLE 8–1
Some of the Rehabilitation Measures for Patients With Multiple Sclerosis

Symptom or Sign	Management
Spasticity	Range-of-motion exercises, corrective positioning
	Stretching
	Drugs (baclofen, dantrolene, diazepam)
	Motor blocks, phenol blocks, neurectomy, tenotomy
	Prevention of nociceptive stimuli
Pain	Transcutaneous electrical nerve stimulation
	Stroking massage
Fatigue	Rest during the day
	Avoidance of exertional activities
	Reduction of spasticity
Weakness	Assistive device
	Moderate reduction of spasticity
	Energy-saving measures
Bowel and bladder dysfunction	Care of neurogenic bladder, as described in Table 8–2
	Bowel care
	High-fiber diet
	Fluid intake of 1,800 to 2,000 mL/day
	Prevention of fecal impaction
	Glycerin or bisacodyl (Dulcolax) suppositories (every other day)
	If diarrhea present: 1 tablespoon of Kaopectate after each loose bowel movement and decrease in fluid intake to 1,600 mL/day

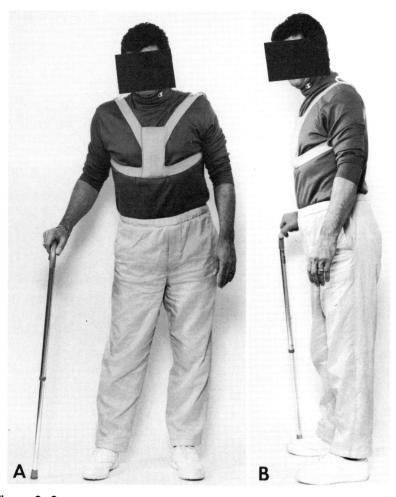

Figure 8–2

A and *B*, Patient with truncal ataxia who has a tendency to fall backward. After application of Posture Training Support with weight in the pouch (1.75 lb), the patient was independent in gait and able to walk without assistance.

depression were emphasized. Many neurologists are still reticent to recommend neuropsychologic studies in their patients, recognizing that such deficits, once identified, are likely to be largely irreversible, may contribute to the frustration and despair experienced by the patient, and may contribute to marital and job insecurity. On a more positive note, if problems with memory and conceptual reasoning have developed as a result of MS (problems with language and praxis are much less common), family members and employers can try to anticipate the kinds of situations that would be frustrating to the patients and should be vigilant for errors in judgment and performance that could occur as a consequence of these deficits. Cognitive and perceptual impairments may require psychometric and functional testing for evaluation of the intensity of the deficit and the patient's safety in the home environment. Reactive depression and anxiety states are much more common than euphoria. Suicide is alarmingly common in patients with a mild-to-moderate degree of neurologic dysfunction from MS. In advanced cases, pseudobulbar affect with pathologic laughter and crying (emotional incontinence) occurs and may respond favorably to a low dose of a tricyclic antidepressant.

Bowel and Bladder Dysfunction

The prevalence of bowel and bladder symptoms increases with the duration and degree of disability in this disease. Management of the neurogenic bowel and bladder is similar regardless of the cause. Important, treatable causes of bowel and bladder dysfunction must always be considered and treated appropriately (particular attention is applied to exclude early bowel carcinoma in patients older than 40 years and repeated vigilance is kept for urinary tract sepsis throughout the patient's life).

Patients should develop a regular pattern of bowel emptying. This can be facilitated by instructing the patient to attend to the awareness of rectal distention with prompt evacuation (for example, after exercise, after caffeine ingestion, postprandially). Increasing the intake of fiber and, when needed, dietary supplementation with senna or psyllium hydrophilic mucilloid and infrequent use of glycerine suppositories (once or twice weekly) are often sufficient. The use of bowel stimulants (bisacodyl suppositories and enemas) should be minimized.

Bladder dysfunction can be more difficult to manage. The symptoms of bladder dysfunction correlate poorly with disturbances in physiology. Problems with both bladder storage and emptying commonly coexist. Urodynamic studies reveal that the most common pattern of bladder dysfunction is bladder-sphincter dyssynergia. Management of the neurogenic bladder in patients with MS is summarized in Table 8–2.

Patients with small-capacity bladders with detrusor muscle hyperreflexia are often helped by anticholinergic medications (oxybutynin chloride, propantheline bromide, and tricyclic antidepressants), but their use should be restricted to times when the patient will have limited access to toilet facilities (such as during social events or traveling). Anticholinergics at bedtime can reduce the severity and frequency of nocturia and nocturnal incontinence. Patients with bladder hypotonia and overflow incontinence may benefit from a cholinergic medication (carbachol, bethanecol chloride), but problems with proper relaxation of the external urethral sphincter (seen in patients with spasticity and bladder-sphincter dyssynergia) limit their use.

Intermittent self-catheterization (together with anticholinergics) is successful in patients who have preserved proprioception and dexterity. Occasionally, complex combinations of medications (anticholinergics, α-

TABLE 8-2

Management of Neurogenic Bladder in Multiple Sclerosis

	Management
Result of urodynamic studies	
	Men
Flaccid bladder sphincter, urinary sphincter, urinary incontinence	Ambulatory: condom catheter In bed: urinal to avoid indwelling catheter; if necessary, increase fluid intake to > 2,000 mL/24 hr; change catheter every 4 wk
	Women
	Indwelling catheter, change every 4 wk; trial of bethanecol (Urecholine; 15 mg four times/day) Note: In some cases, both men and women with severe flaccid bladder disturbances may benefit from intermittent self-catheterization
Spastic bladder sphincter	Intermittent catheterization every 6 hr after attempts at voiding. If residual volume exceeds 90 mL, intermittent catheterization is continued. If catheterized volume exceeds 500 mL, catheterization is done every 4 hr until there is compliance with fluid intake schedule. Patients with very resistant spastic bladders (frequent voiding, frequent incontinence) who can be taught intermittent self-catheterization may benefit from the combination of self-catheterization and moderate- to high-dose anticholinergics
Bladder detrusor and sphincter dyssynergia	Oxybutynin chloride (Ditropan; 5 to 10 mg two or three times a day as needed) and intermittent catheterization
Fluid intake	1,800 mL/24 hr: 400 mL with each meal, 200 mL in mid-morning, 200 mL in mid-afternoon, nothing after 8:00 p.m.
Voiding schedule	Attempted voiding every 3 hr during the day, intermittent catheterization
Suppressive treatment	Trimethoprim-sulfamethoxazole, orally p.m. (Septra, one double-strength, p.m.)
Urine culture	Weekly in hospital, monthly when indwelling catheter is changed

adrenergic blockers, or antispasticity drugs) may be needed for patients with bladder-sphincter dyssynergia. Urethral meatotomy and bladder neck resection may result in persistent urinary incontinence requiring the use of a condom catheter with a leg bag in men or an indwelling Foley or suprapubic catheter in women. Recent innovative urologic approaches to this problem include urinary diversion procedures (ileal conduit) and the creation of an artificial subcutaneous pouch (Koch or Indiana pouch) that can be catheterized by the patient through a surgically created stoma in the lower anterior abdominal wall.

SUMMARY

During the earliest stages of MS, patients and their families should be provided with sufficient information about their disease to permit them to make appropriate plans for their future. They should be reassured that MS follows a relatively benign course for many patients for many years and that there is reason for hope through scientific research. Much can be done to control troublesome symptoms in patients with transient and permanent sequelae of MS, often through the cooperative efforts of a multidisciplinary team of interested physicians, paramedical personnel, and family members.

REFERENCES

1. Matthews WB, Compston A, Allen IV, Martyn CN. McAlpine's multiple sclerosis. 2nd ed. Edinburgh: Churchill Livingstone, 1991.
2. Poser CM, Paty DW, Scheinberg L, et al, eds. The diagnosis of multiple sclerosis. New York: Thieme-Stratton, 1984.
3. Swanson JW. Multiple sclerosis: update in diagnosis and review of prognostic factors. Mayo Clin Proc 1989; 64:577–586.
4. Wynn DR, Rodriguez M, O'Fallon WM, Kurland LT. Update on the epidemiology of multiple sclerosis. Mayo Clin Proc 1989; 64:808–817.
5. Rodriguez M. Multiple sclerosis: basic concepts and hypothesis. Mayo Clin Proc 1989; 64:570–576.
6. Weinshenker BG, Bass B, Rice GPA, et al. The natural history of multiple sclerosis: a geographically based study. I. Clinical course and disability. Brain 1989; 112:133–146.
7. Noseworthy JH. Therapeutics of multiple sclerosis. Clin Neuropharmacol 1991; 14:49–61.
8. Merritt JL. Management of spasticity in spinal cord injury. Mayo Clin Proc 1981; 56:614–622.
9. Erickson RP, Lie MR, Wineinger MA. Rehabilitation in multiple sclerosis. Mayo Clin Proc 1989; 64:818–828.

9

Motor Neuron Disease

Mehrsheed Sinaki
Donald W. Mulder

The term "motor neuron disease" describes diseases whose principal common feature is a progressive dysfunction of the primary motor neurons (anterior horn cells). The diseases are insidious in onset, and progression is often slow. No intervention has been shown to modify the course of degeneration of the anterior horn cells. Supportive and symptomatic therapy has allowed many affected patients to lead productive and fulfilling lives. The disorders (Table 9–1) have been classified according to the age of the patient at onset, clinical course, and outcome. Confusion about the usage of the various terms was recently reviewed by Williams and Windebank.[1]

Most of the syndromes are rare, and a full description can be found in standard neurologic textbooks. Werdnig-Hoffmann disease, or infantile progressive muscular atrophy, is a rare disease of the motor neurons that begins before age 2 years and usually leads to death in early childhood. Onset of disease in childhood and early adolescence is designated as Kugelberg-Welander disease, or juvenile proximal muscular atrophy. In adolescence, the disease tends to be most prominent in proximal muscles and to have a very long clinical course. This form of the disease is often mistaken for one of the limb-girdle dystrophies. The adolescent and infantile forms sometimes overlap and then cannot be differentiated. In the rare syndrome of juvenile progressive bulbar palsy (bulbar palsy of Fazio-Londe), symptoms are limited to the musculature of the throat. Muscular atrophy may be limited to the anterior horn cells in a few adjacent segments (Sobue), often in the lower cervical area. This gives rise to weakness in adjacent muscles of the upper extremity, which does not spread to other musculature.

The most common of the diseases of the motor neurons is amyotrophic lateral sclerosis (ALS). In ALS, the pathologic condition is not limited to the anterior horn cells. The laterally placed motor pathways (pyramidal tracts)

TABLE 9–1

Primary Motor Neuron Diseases

Infantile progressive muscular atrophy
  (Werdnig-Hoffman disease)
Juvenile proximal muscular atrophy
  (Kugelberg-Welander disease)
Juvenile progressive bulbar palsy
  (Fazio-Londe atrophy)
Segmental spinal muscular atrophy (Sobue)
Amyotrophic lateral sclerosis
  Sporadic form
  Familial form
  Guamanian form
Primary lateral sclerosis

are also involved. Primary lateral sclerosis is a syndrome manifested by signs of corticospinal tract involvement without evidence of lower motor neuron involvement.

EPIDEMIOLOGY AND INCIDENCE

ALS is an adult-onset, chronic, progressive disease that increases in frequency with age. The average age at onset is about 60 years, and the average age at death is about 64 years. The incidence of the disease is reported to be 1.8 per 100,000 population. It accounts for about 1 in every 1,000 adult deaths.[2] The patient is most commonly male (male:female ratio, 1.6:1).

The cause of the disease remains unknown, although 5% or more of patients have other family members who have the disorder. The disorder is inherited as an autosomal dominant trait in 5% to 10% of patients.[3] The unusual incidence of ALS on the island of Guam has been reported to be related to local environmental factors. Williams and Windebank[1] recently reviewed the proposed causes.

SYMPTOMS AND SIGNS

The initial manifestations are often asymmetric progressive muscular atrophy and weakness associated with hyperreflexia and sometimes with Babinski signs. The patient initially may have signs of only anterior horn cell involvement, and the pyramidal tract signs become evident later in the course of the disease. Pyramidal tract signs may never be apparent because of the overwhelming flaccid paralysis. Difficulty with talking and swallowing is the presenting complaint in about 30% of patients with ALS. Dysarthria may be flaccid, spastic, or mixed flaccid and spastic. Regardless of where the signs and symptoms are first noted, the weakness with atrophy and fasciculations spreads and eventually involves all of the striated muscles other than the muscles subserving ocular movement and cardiac function. Surprisingly, affected patients do not have signs of dysfunction of their nervous system other than the motor system. The disease is progressive, and the patient dies of dysphagia, respiratory failure, or inanition. The average life expectancy from the onset of symptoms is less than 3 years. Rarely, patients with ALS have lived for more than 20 years from the time of onset. In a few patients, the presenting symptom is only that of involvement in the upper motor system. Such patients, in our experience, have another disease (such as multiple sclerosis or primary lateral sclerosis). In most cases, ALS is rapidly progressive. It is an incurable disorder. Many physicians and also patients and their families equate the diagnosis with a loss of hope for the future, an attitude that results in a nihilistic approach to therapy.

Postpolio weakness has many similarities to ALS. Thus, many of the rehabilitation measures used for ALS can also be applied to patients with postpolio weakness.

PATHOLOGIC FINDINGS

Pathologically, the primary features of ALS are degeneration and loss of the anterior horn cells in the spinal cord. These are associated with a massive loss of Betz cells and other pyramidal cells from the precentral cortex. The corticospinal tracts are then depleted of large myelinated fibers (Fig. 9–1).[4] In addition, many abnormalities of the fine structure of the nervous system have been identified in patients with ALS, and although some of them are commonly found, none are diagnostic of the disease.[1]

The diagnosis is dependent on the history and examination of the patient. There is no definitive laboratory test (Table 9–2). It is imperative to differentiate other causes of motor system dysfunction for which there is definitive therapy (Table 9–3).[3] Patients who are suspected of having ALS should have a complete neurologic and medical evaluation, including, in every instance, an electromyographic examination with nerve conduction studies (Table 9–4).

LABORATORY DATA

Electromyographic examination characteristically shows normal nerve conduction studies or only slightly slow conduction velocities. Needle electrode examination usually shows "neurogenic" changes, including irritability, fibrillation potentials, fasciculation potentials, and large polyphasic, rapidly firing motor unit potentials. The degree of the changes noted depends on the stage of progression of the disease. Ordinarily, denervation

TABLE 9–2
Clinical Features of Amyotrophic Lateral
Sclerosis

Lower motor neuron signs and symptoms
  Muscle atrophy, cramps, fasciculations,
    and weakness
  Flaccid dysarthria, dysphagia, and
    dyspnea
Upper motor neuron signs and symptoms
  Clonus, increased reflexes, spasticity of
    muscles, and weakness
  Abnormal reflexes such as Babinski signs
    and positive sucking responses
  Pseudobulbar palsy with spastic
    dysarthria and dysphonia
Signs and symptoms not regularly a part of
  the disease
  Sensory loss
  Bladder dysfunction
  Impairment of eye movements
  Extrapyramidal disease
  Mental impairment

should be noted in at least three extremities before a definite electromyographic diagnosis of motor neuron disease is made. The serum creatine kinase value is elevated in about half of patients, but its elevation does not correlate with the stage, the severity, or the rate of progression of the disease.[5] ALS is usually diagnosed by careful clinical and electromyographic

TABLE 9–3
Actual Clinical Syndromes of 46 Patients
Initially Diagnosed as Having Amyotrophic
Lateral Sclerosis

Syndrome	No. of Patients
Upper cervical cord lesion	16
Focal atrophy of upper extremities	9
Inflammatory neuropathy	5
Fasciculations with minimal atrophy	4
Myopathy	3
Multiple sclerosis	2
Miscellaneous*	7

*One each with Shy-Drager syndrome, parkinsonism, arsenical myelopathy, stenosis of the neural canal of the lumbar spine, multiple lacunar infarcts of the brain, brain tumor, and brachial plexus neuropathy. From Mulder.[3] By permission of Amyotrophic Lateral Sclerosis Association.

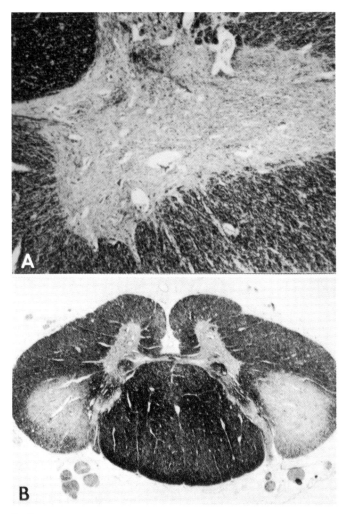

Figure 9–1
Loss of anterior horn cell *(A)* and demyelination of pyramidal tracts *(B)* of motor neurons. (From Okazaki.[4] By permission of the publisher.)

examinations. Thus, a muscle biopsy is needed only infrequently to diagnose ALS.

COURSE OF REHABILITATION AFTER DIAGNOSIS

The success of rehabilitation depends on the active participation of the patient and his or her family as full partners in the therapeutic program. This approach requires that the physician deal directly and honestly with

TABLE 9-4

Tests Needed in Patients Suspected of
Having Amyotrophic Lateral Sclerosis

Determination of:
  Complete blood cell count
  Erythrocyte sedimentation rate
  Automated biochemistry screen values
  Muscle enzyme (alanine
    aminotransferase, creatine kinase)
    values
  Cryoglobulins
Serum protein electrophoresis
Urinalysis
Electrocardiography
Chest radiography
Cerebrospinal fluid examination
Electromyography and nerve conduction
  studies
Cerebral computed tomography
Myelography

From Williams and Windebank.[1] By permission of
Mayo Foundation.

the patient about the illness and its clinical course. It is always difficult and often agonizing for the physician to discuss this fatal illness. We have found, as others have described, that the patient is able to deal effectively with the disease and to help decide how intensive a therapeutic effort is indicated only when this direct approach is used. This discussion must take place when it is most appropriate for the patient.[6]

We have found it useful to classify patients according to the rapidity of progression of the illness, the site of onset of the disease, and the stage of disability. Approximately half of patients with ALS live for more than 3 years from the onset of their illness, and 10% of these live for 10 years or more.[7] Obviously, these patients must be treated differently from the 50% of patients who die within 3 years of onset. Patients with a long clinical course have a remarkable capacity to compensate for motor unit loss, and this may enable them to continue with daily activities for years.[8]

In our experience, a well-designed physical therapy program can keep muscles from disuse atrophy and overuse fatigue. In some cases, the exercise derived from completion of daily activities and required ambulation is adequate. Prolonged and strenuous programs of physical therapy in such instances are inadvisable.

With progression of the disease and variation in the distribution of weakness, the rehabilitation techniques should be modified after careful neurologic and physiatric evaluations.

Prescribed exercises range from simple range-of-motion and stretching techniques to mild, nonstrenuous strengthening exercises (Figs. 9-2 through 9-5). Visits with the occupational therapist and use of adaptive

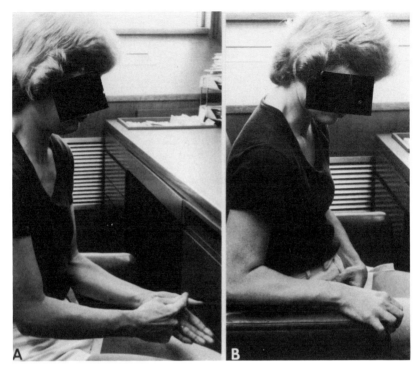

Figure 9–2

Isometric strengthening exercises. *A*, Manual resistance is applied to strengthen thumb abductor muscle. *B*, Resistance is applied against arm of chair to strengthen right flexor digitorum profundus (finger flexor) muscle. (From Sinaki.[12] By permission of Elsevier Science Publishers B.V. [Biomedical Division].)

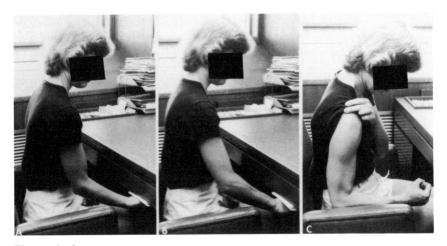

Figure 9–3

Isometric strengthening exercises. *A*, Resistance is applied against a heavy object (a desk in this instance) to strengthen wrist flexor muscle. Note that palm is up. *B*, Same exercise to strengthen wrist extensor muscle. Note that palm is down. *C*, Resistance is applied against arm of chair to lateral aspect of elbow to strengthen right shoulder abductor muscles (deltoid and supraspinatus). (From Sinaki.[12] By permission of Elsevier Science Publishers B.V. [Biomedical Division].)

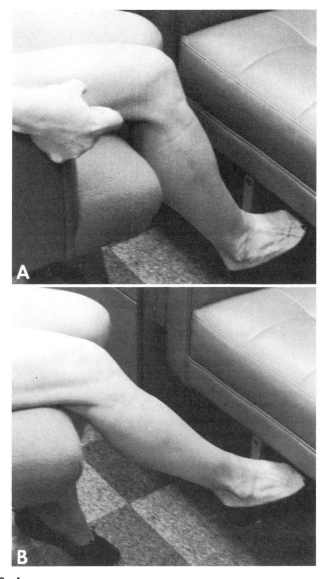

Figure 9–4

Isometric strengthening exercises. *A,* Subject attempts to lift heavy object to strengthen ankle dorsiflexor muscle. *B,* Subject attempts to lift heavy object with knee straight to strengthen quadriceps muscle. Each contraction lasts for a count of three, and subject may try 5 to 10 contractions. (From Sinaki.[12] By permission of Elsevier Science Publishers B.V. [Biomedical Division].)

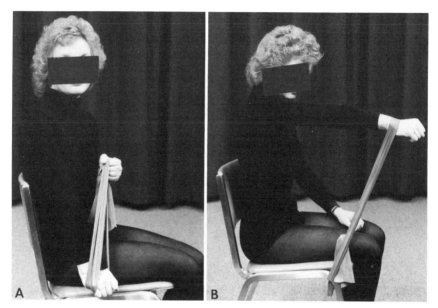

Figure 9–5
A and B, Mild strengthening exercises, performed with an elastic band (such as Theraband). (From Sinaki.[12] By permission of Elsevier Science Publishers B.V. [Biomedical Division].)

equipment are of utmost importance for increasing independence at the early stages of disease (Fig. 9–6). During the later stages, every effort should be made to improve the patient's quality of life and facilitate care by the family.

Overprescribing physical therapeutic measures can be avoided by considering rehabilitation measures according to the stage of disability of the patient. As with any progressive neuromuscular disease, one should prevent further complicating the course by the effect of immobility. Such complications consist of weakness secondary to lack of use, osteopenia, constipation, thrombophlebitis, contractures, pressure sores, and pulmonary infections. Physical exercise not only improves circulation and prevents stiffness but also promotes relaxation and a sense of well-being in the patients.

SYMPTOMATIC TREATMENT

The variability in the distribution of weakness in patients with ALS requires that rehabilitation techniques be individualized.[9, 10] The progression of the illness requires continuous modification of treatment for each patient. Patients with a long clinical course have a remarkable capacity to compensate for motor unit loss,[7] which may enable them to continue daily activities for years. Patients with a slow clinical course continue to have

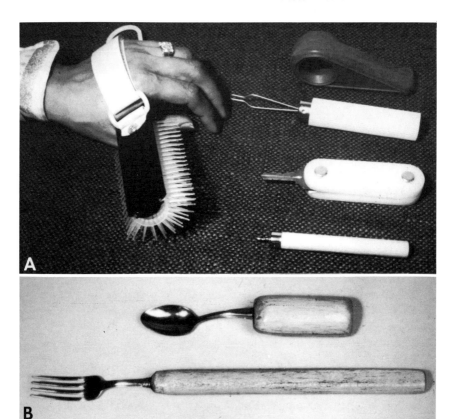

Figure 9–6
A and *B,* Various assistance devices used by patients with weakness in upper extremities to help maintain independence in self-care. (From Sinaki.[12] By permission of Elsevier Science Publishers B.V. [Biomedical Division].)

slow progression throughout their illness, whereas those whose illness has been rapidly progressive can be expected to continue to deteriorate rapidly.

Bulbar Paralysis

Brainstem involvement or so-called bulbar symptoms may occur during any stage of ALS. About 20% of patients with ALS present with prominent bulbar abnormalities. The prognosis should be based on the rapidity of the clinical course and not on the site of onset of symptoms. Breathing difficulty is the most serious complication of ALS. It is often accompanied by bulbar symptoms but is not necessarily a part of these symptoms. Because of the involvement of the bulbar musculature about the throat, the patient has difficulty with speaking and swallowing, and respiration is

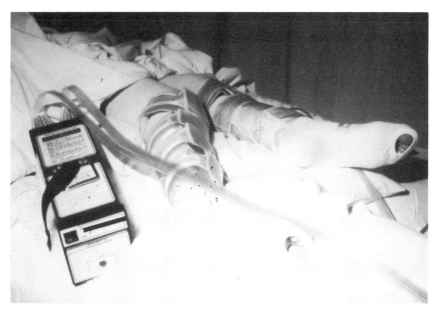

Figure 9–7
Use of thromboguards to assist circulation in lower extremities. (From Sinaki.[12] By permission of Elsevier Science Publishers B.V. [Biomedical Division].)

eventually compromised. Not only the diaphragm but also all of the muscles of breathing, including the auxiliary muscles, become involved. The problem may be compounded by obstruction of the airway because of bulbar symptoms. If the illness is slowly progressive, the patient may be able to function with a simple chest respirator. The use of more sophisticated respiratory aids, such as tracheostomy and permanent respirators in patients who are already totally paralyzed, must be discussed in detail with the patient and family to determine whether these measures are appropriate.

The patient's difficulty with eating can be assisted with very careful feeding techniques, such as using a long-stemmed spoon so that food can be placed in the posterior part of the pharynx, and eating substances that can be easily swallowed. For example, many patients are able to obtain adequate nourishment from formula diets that are available commercially as liquids, solids, or soft foods. If these formulas are unsatisfactory, tube feeding has proved to be an excellent solution for patients who are unable to eat. Gastrostomy, particularly with the Janeway technique, can be a satisfactory approach for patients who are psychologically able to accept it.

One of the most serious complaints is a patient's inability to handle saliva. The patient with a serious swallowing deficit experiences considerable psychologic and physical distress. Many patients use suction devices. Others have attempted to use medications to dry up secretions; unfortunately, this approach has led to more tenacious secretions and, thus, to ever more difficulty (Table 9–5). Selective operation may diminish the flow of the salivary secretions. Cricopharyngeal myotomy has been suggested, but we have not had sufficient experience with this procedure to allow proper evaluation of its place in therapy. In one study, 64% of a group of patients benefited from this procedure.[11]

Dysarthria and Problems With Communication

Dysarthria and, finally, anarthria are serious complaints. For the patient with a degenerative neuromotor speech disorder, the speech pathologist should intervene at critical points during the course of the disease to maximize the patient's communication efforts. As the illness progresses, the use of supplementary electronic amplifications of the voice may be helpful, and sometimes speech therapy is of value. Many patients find that the most satisfactory method of communication is by writing,

TABLE 9–5

Treatment of Common Symptoms of Motor Neuron Disease*

Symptom	Treatment
Constipation	Hydration
	High-fiber diet
	Stool softener (e.g., docusate sodium [Colace])
	Suppositories (e.g., bisacodyl [Dulcolax], glycerol)
Cramps	Quinine (200 mg at bedtime)†
	Phenytoin (Dilantin)†
Spasticity	Baclofen (Lioresal)
Sialorrhea	Amitriptyline (10 mg four times daily)†
	Hyoscyamine sulfate (0.125 mg four times daily)†
	Trihexyphenidyl hydrochloride†
Dysphagia	Slow eating
	Food that is easy to swallow
	Frequent meals
	Caloric supplementation (e.g., Ensure, Isocal)
	Pureed food
	Percutaneous gastrostomy
Dysarthria	Speech therapy
	Writing (e.g., Magic Slate)
	Alphabet cards
	Typewriters (Canon Communicator)
	Computerized communication devices

*For patients with motor neuron disease, we use medications cautiously because of untoward side effects.
†Titrate to effective dose.
From Sinaki M, Litchy WJ, Mulder DW. Motor neuron disease. Curr Ther Intern Med 1987; 2:1325–1329. By permission of B.C. Decker.

perhaps with the use of Magic Slate or similar communication boards. For patients whose illness is only slowly progressive, it is appropriate to consider the use of elaborate electronic devices with which the patient can communicate.[12]

STAGING FOR AXIOAPPENDICULAR INVOLVEMENT

Patients with primary involvement of the axial and appendicular muscles are of particular concern when rehabilitation techniques are considered. We have found that the illness can generally be divided into stages, each of which demands a somewhat different rehabilitation approach.

In general, most patients with ALS go through three phases (Table 9–6 and Fig. 9–8).[13] During phase 1, the independent phase, the patient is ambulatory with or without assistive devices. This phase starts when ALS is diagnosed and the patient has minor weakness. During this phase the patient's needs range from psychologic support for the patient and family to application of hand splints or leg braces. This phase is completed when the patient is fatigued easily to the point that a wheelchair is needed for some ambulatory activities. This phase consists of stages I, II, and III.

At phase 2, the partially independent phase, the patient is confined to a wheelchair. Early in this phase, the patient is mostly independent in activities of daily living. Later in this phase, the patient becomes mostly dependent in self-care activities. This phase consists of stages IV and V.

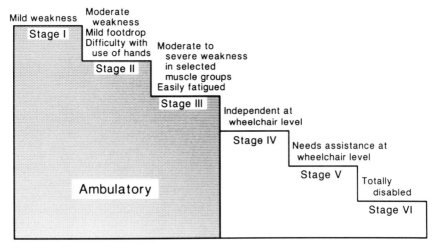

Figure 9–8
Characteristics of patients with amyotrophic lateral sclerosis, by stage of disease.

Phase 3, the dependent phase, is the final stage. The patient totally depends on the physical and emotional strength of his or her family. The patient needs proper facilities to accommodate care at home. At this phase, prevention of life-threatening complications of immobility is important.

TABLE 9–6

Exercise and Rehabilitation Programs for Patients With ALS, According to Stage of Disease

	Stage, Characteristics	Treatment
	Stage I Patient is ambulatory, independent in ADL Mild weakness, clumsiness	Encourage ROM exercises, normal activities Encourage nonstrenuous strengthening of unaffected muscles to compensate for weakened muscles Discourage strenuous exercise to strengthen already weakened muscles because it leads to increased fatigue and disability Psychological support is very important*
Phase 1, independent	*Stage II* Patient is ambulatory Moderate selective weakness Slightly decreased independence in ADL (e.g., difficulty climbing stairs, raising arms, or buttoning clothing)	Substitute fastening tape (Velcro) for buttons Encourage use of ankle-foot orthoses, wrist and thumb splints Encourage cautious, selective nonstrenuous strengthening for unaffected muscles and stretching exercises to avoid contractures; advise to avoid overuse and fatigue
	Stage III Patient is ambulatory Moderately decreased independence in ADL Easily fatigued with long-distance ambulation Severe selective weakness in ankles, wrists, hands, or neck extensors	Keep patient physically independent as long as possible Encourage deep-breathing exercises to strengthen auxiliary muscles of respiration Prescribe wheelchair—standard or battery operated with proper modifications Apply nuchal support (Figs. 9–15 and 9–16) to improve posture and gait

(Continued.)

TABLE 9–6 (cont.)

	Stage, Characteristics	Treatment
Phase 2, partially independent	*Stage IV* Patient is confined to wheelchair Able to perform ADL Severe lower extremity weakness (± spasticity)† Moderate upper extremity weakness Hanging-arm syndrome with shoulder pain and sometimes edema in the hand	Heat, massage, and application of shoulder splint Preventive anti-edema measures Passive ROM exercises to the weakly supported joints Encourage isometric strengthening of the few remaining uninvolved muscles
	Stage V Patient is in wheelchair Increasingly dependent in ADL Severe lower extremity weakness (Fig. 9–7), ‡ moderate to severe upper extremity weakness Possible skin breakdown	Encourage family to learn proper transfer and positioning principles Encourage modifications at home to aid patient's mobility and independence Water mattress or waterbed is helpful
Phase 3, dependent	*Stage VI* Patient is bedridden Completely dependent in ADL	For dysphagia, use soft diet, long spoons, or tube feeding For accumulated saliva, use suction, medications, surgery to decrease flow For dysarthria, use palatal lifts, electronic speech amplification For breathing difficulty, clear airway or use tracheostomy or respirator

*Sedatives or tranquilizers (such as diazepam) may cause depression.
†Spasticity may serve as a splinting effect for ambulation; if it is severe, try the smallest dose of baclofen that is effective.
‡Thrombophlebitis in flaccid lower extremities can be prevented by avoiding trauma; by applying passive ROM (twice a day), elastic stockings, dorsal and plantar flexion every 2 or 3 hours, and thromboguards (Fig. 9–7); or by using a trial of subcutaneous heparin (5,000 U every 12 hours) in selected cases.
Abbreviations: ADL, activities of daily living; ROM, range of motion.
From Sinaki M, Litchy WJ, Mulder DW. Motor neuron disease. Curr Ther Intern Med 1987; 2:1325–1329. By permission of B.C. Decker.

Phase 1 (Independent Phase)

Stage I

The patient is ambulatory and is able to care for himself or herself and accomplish the activities of daily living. There is mild weakness or clumsiness of the musculature. The patient usually does not need any therapy beyond psychologic support and encouragement. Instruction in the development of auxiliary muscles to support the already weakened muscles may be necessary. Customary daily physical activities and general range-of-motion exercises are usually advised. It is useful to advise the patient to avoid immobility and to attempt strengthening of the unaffected muscles as substitutes for those that have been impaired.

Stage II

Moderate weakness is present in selected muscle groups (for example, mild footdrop on one or both sides). The patient often has difficulty climbing stairs, elevating the arms, or using the hands (especially for fine motor activities such as buttoning garments). The use of a few assistive devices will improve the patient's fine hand function during activities of daily living (see Fig. 17–10). Measures such as ankle-foot orthoses to assist with dorsiflexion of the feet may be needed. These devices help the patient to walk better and also provide good mechanical support for the stability of the ankles (Fig. 9–9). A less expensive variety of ankle-foot orthosis can be purchased off the shelf and is available in small, medium, and large sizes (Fig. 9–10). Such a device is mainly used as a splint for persons who have weak but not totally paralyzed or severely affected dorsiflexors. Occupational therapists can be of significant help to these patients not only by making the appropriate hand splints but also by helping them learn to use and apply the various assistive devices for independence in self-care. Passive exercises of the joints are of value for preventing contractures. Weakness of the abductor pollicis brevis muscle may be aided by the addition of an extra splint that places the thumb in apposition to obtain more effective use of the hand for small movements (Figs. 9–11 and 9–12). With this method, the patient has a stronger grip, and the hand can be used more effectively.[9]

Stage III

The patient is ambulatory but has severe weakness in selected muscle groups. Such a patient often has severe footdrop and pronounced weakness and atrophy of the intrinsic muscles of the hand and is often unable to rise from a chair without help. This stage requires, in addition to the previously described techniques, measures and devices such as lightweight ankle-foot orthoses, wrist and hand splints (Figs. 9–13 and 9–14), and high-seated or electrically powered height-adjustable chairs to assist with getting in and out of a chair. Assistive respiratory exercises with a blow-bottle or incentive deep-breathing exercises (such as a Triflo device) may help to maintain the functional capacity for respiration. If the weakness is

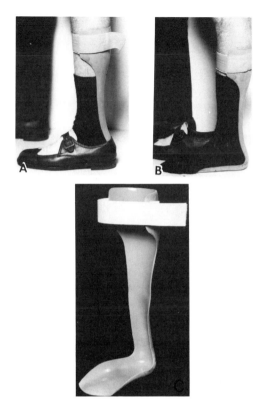

Figure 9-9

Examples of lightweight ankle-foot orthoses. *A* through *C,* Custom-made posterior leaf-spring brace. (*A* and *B,* From Sinaki.[10] By permission of John Wiley & Sons. *C,* From Sinaki and Mulder.[9] By permission of Mayo Foundation.)

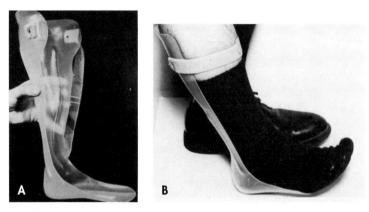

Figure 9-10

Ankle-foot orthoses. *A,* Alimed orthosis, commercially available in small, medium, and large sizes. *B,* Alimed splint can be used by patients who have footdrop but incomplete paralysis of foot dorsiflexor muscles. Patient can attempt some dorsiflexion. Alimed splints are not as strong a support as posterior leaf-spring braces. (From Sinaki and Mulder.[9] By permission of Mayo Foundation.)

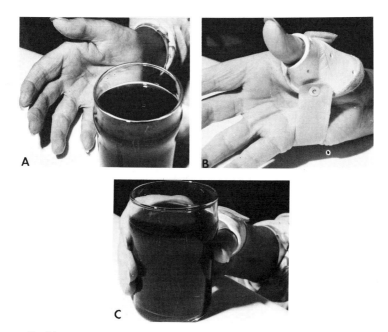

Figure 9–11

Patient with weakness and atrophy of thenar muscles. *A,* Without a splint, patient is unable to stabilize thumb to hold glass. *B,* After application of thumb-shell splint, which helps to stabilize thumb in apposition. *C,* With splint, patient has effective cylinder grasp and is able to hold glass. (From Sinaki and Mulder.[9] By permission of Mayo Foundation.)

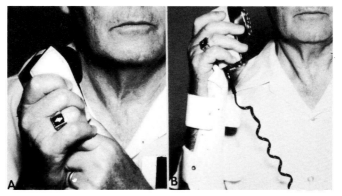

Figure 9–12

Patient with weakness of wrist extensor and intrinsic hand muscles. *A,* Patient is unable to hold electric razor with one hand. *B,* After application of wrist-extension splint with thumb-shell addition, patient can hold electric razor effectively with one hand. (From Sinaki and Mulder.[9] By permission of Mayo Foundation.)

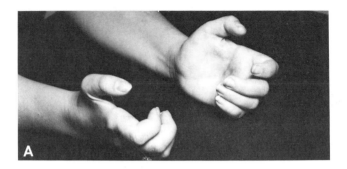

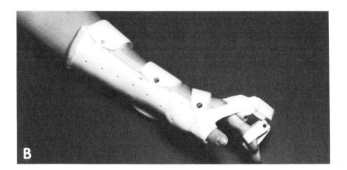

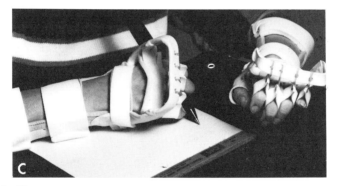

Figure 9–13

A, Patient with severe atrophy and weakness of thenar muscles and of finger and wrist extensors. *B*, Static wrist-extension splint with thumb-shell addition coupled with dynamic finger-extension device. *C*, Complex but practical splint enables patient to do certain (even fine) movements, such as writing. (From Sinaki.[10] By permission of John Wiley & Sons.)

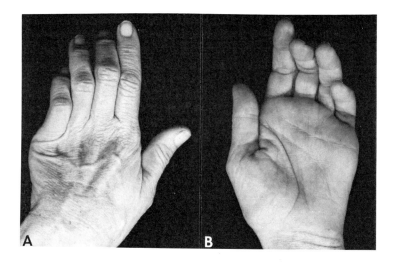

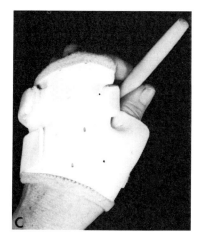

Figure 9–14
A and *B*, Claw-hand deformity in a patient with amyotrophic lateral sclerosis. *C*, Hand splint used for rehabilitation.

of such magnitude that walking for any distance is difficult, a wheelchair should be used for long trips, shopping, or for other activities outside the home.[14] Table 9–6 shows the characteristics of each stage and the indications for implementing a feasible exercise program in patients with motor neuron disease. Weakness of the selected muscle groups may necessitate application of special supports to the weakly supported joints in order to facilitate and prolong the patient's independence in ambulatory activities (Figs. 9–15 through 9–17).

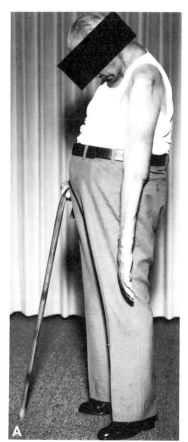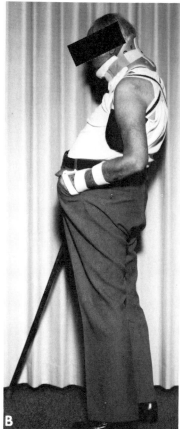

Figure 9–15

A, Patient with weakness of extensor nuchal muscles. *B*, Application of cervical collar (Philadelphia collar) to improve posture and independence in activities of daily living.

Phase 2 (Partially Independent Phase)

Stage IV

The patient is confined to a wheelchair because of progression of the illness. Severe weakness of the lower extremities is present, and the upper extremities have moderate involvement. At this stage, a patient can perform most activities of daily living from the wheelchair. Many patients prefer electrically powered chairs. However, a wheelchair should be ordered by the physician after consideration of all aspects of a patient's disability in order to obtain the most appropriate equipment for that patient. An electrically powered wheelchair that allows the patient to activate power keys to provide propulsion and to turn the chair in different directions may be required. Various such wheelchairs that can be conveniently transported are now available. Passive exercises are particularly important to prevent con-

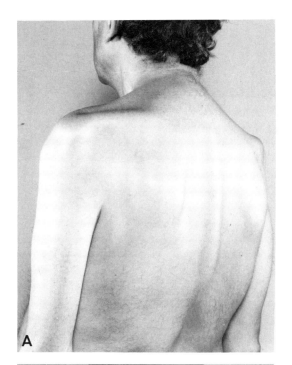

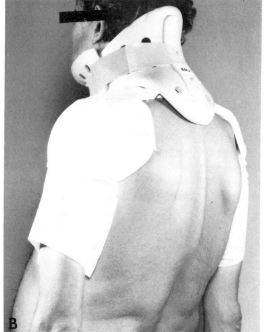

Figure 9–16

A, Patient with weakness of shoulder girdle and extensor nuchal musculature. *B,* Combined application of hemihook shoulder sling and cervical collar (Philadelphia collar) to compensate for weakness and to decrease discomfort.

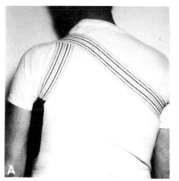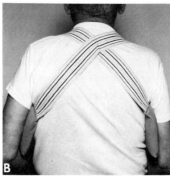

Figure 9–17
Shoulder slings. *A*, Bobath shoulder sling used to decrease sagging of shoulder and to reduce stretch on brachial and axillary neurovascular bundle. *B*, Modified Bobath sling used for bilateral shoulder-girdle weakness (so-called hanging-arm syndrome). (From Sinaki.[10] By permission of John Wiley & Sons.)

tractures and to retard the changes secondary to disuse. It is often necessary to instruct the family in the application of such exercises. The physiatrist must review the uninvolved musculature to determine whether there are muscles the patient could strengthen to assist in maintaining independence.[9]

Stage V

The patient is in a wheelchair and is dependent. Weakness of the lower extremities is pronounced, and weakness of some of the muscle groups of the upper extremities is moderate or pronounced. The patient requires devices for assistance in transferring in and out of the wheelchair, such as a lift (Hoyer). The family must be instructed in the technique of transferring a patient into and out of bed. The bathroom should be modified so that it can be used with a wheeled shower chair; a hand-held shower is helpful. A water mattress is helpful for preventing pressure sores, as is a synthetic sheepskin. Patients often complain about the pain associated with lying in bed and being unable to move for hours at a time; therefore, the principles of proper positioning should be taught to increase the patient's comfort and to reduce the possibility of contractures. For weakness of the shoulder girdle muscles, the use of arm splints or a resting arm splint while the patient is in a wheelchair will decrease the painful stretch on the brachial plexus and add to the patient's comfort.[9, 10]

Phase 3 (Dependent Phase)

Stage VI

The patient is bedridden and is unable to perform any of the useful activities of daily living or of self-care and needs maximal assistance. Proper mattresses and beds must be available, and the family must be assisted and instructed in the care of the patient. The most severe symptoms are often due to bulbar involvement. The techniques used are very similar to those essential for the care of any quadriplegic patient, except that the patient with ALS does not have bladder involvement.

PYRAMIDAL INVOLVEMENT

Another component of ALS, involvement of the pyramidal pathways, results in hyperreflexia and spasticity. These symptoms, surprisingly, constitute only a small portion of the patient's complaints, if the dysphonia that occurs with pronounced spasticity is excluded. Simple rehabilitation methods are usually sufficient. In ambulatory patients, the spasticity of the lower extremities may serve as a splinting effect and may help the patient to walk better.[9] Management of spasticity may consist of daily range of motion exercises and stretching, antispasticity medications, motor point blocks, and splinting. The lowest effective dose of antispasticity drugs, such as baclofen, is recommended.

Finally, emotional support of the patients and their families must be addressed at any stage of the disease. Reactive depression is not uncommon, but suicide is rare. Counseling and planning for the future must begin at the early stages. Chapters of the ALS Society and the Muscular Dystrophy Association are helpful not only for providing emotional support but also for extending specific help to both the patient and the physician.[6]

REFERENCES

1. Williams DB, Windebank AJ. Motor neuron disease (amyotrophic lateral sclerosis). Mayo Clin Proc 1991; 66:54–82.
2. Juergens SM, Kurland LT, Okazaki H, Mulder DW. ALS in Rochester, Minnesota, 1925–1977. Neurology 1980; 30:463–468.
3. Mulder DW. Commentary. In: The diagnosis and treatment of amyotrophic lateral sclerosis. Boston: Houghton Mifflin Professional Publishers, 1980:79–82.
4. Okazaki H. Fundamentals of neuropathology: morphologic basis of neurologic disorders. 2nd ed. New York: Igaku-Shoin, 1989.
5. Sinaki M, Mulder DW. Amyotrophic lateral sclerosis: relationship between serum creatine kinase level and patient survival. Arch Phys Med Rehabil 1986; 67:169–171.
6. Sinaki M, Litchy WJ, Mulder DW. Motor neuron disease. Curr Ther Neurol Dis 1987; 2:255–258.
7. Mulder DW, Howard FM Jr. Patient resistance and prognosis in amyotrophic lateral sclerosis. Mayo Clin Proc 1976; 51:537–541.
8. Brown WF. Functional compensation of human motor units in health and disease. J Neurol Sci 1973; 20:199–209.
9. Sinaki M, Mulder DW. Rehabilitation techniques for patients with amyotrophic lateral sclerosis. Mayo Clin Proc 1978; 53:173–178.
10. Sinaki M. Rehabilitation. In: Mulder DW. The diagnosis and treatment of

amyotrophic lateral sclerosis. Boston: Houghton Mifflin Professional Publishers, 1980:169–193.

11. U KS, Norris FH Jr, Denys EH, Lebo CP. Surgery in patients with amyotrophic lateral sclerosis: experience with cricopharyngeal myotomy in 100 cases (abstract). Excerpta Medica International Congress Series 1977; 427:45.

12. Brandenburg SA, Vanderheiden GC. Communication, control and computer access for disabled and elderly individuals: resource book. Communication Aids. Boston: College Hill Press, 1987.

13. Sinaki M. Exercise and rehabilitation measures in amyotrophic lateral sclerosis. Excerpta Medica International Congress Series 1988; 769:343–368.

14. Sinaki M. Physical therapy and rehabilitation techniques for patients with amyotrophic lateral sclerosis. In: Cosi V, Kato AC, Parlette W, Pinelli P, Poloni M, eds. Amyotrophic lateral sclerosis: therapeutic, psychological, and research aspects. New York: Plenum Press, 1987:239–252.

10

Neuropathic Disease

Jon B. Closson

This chapter reviews the management of neuropathic diseases. No attempt is made to classify these entities; standard neurology textbooks dealing with these topics generally contain a classification. Therapeutic principles and options for both sensory neuropathies and motor deficits are discussed. Also, specific approaches to a representative neuropathic disease, the Guillain-Barré syndrome, are reviewed. Those for amyotrophic lateral sclerosis are outlined in Chapter 9.

Some basic principles apply to all patients with one of these entities. First, use of the interdisciplinary team is helpful. Some of the diseases strike during the peak of economic and family responsibilities, and some are fatal within a short time. Therefore, all possible resources and support need to be marshaled to help the patient and family. Second, every effort should be made to maintain or regain function and to strive for as much independence as possible, both in mobility and in activities of daily living.

THERAPY FOR SENSORY INVOLVEMENT

Patients with peripheral neuropathies generally have both sensory and motor involvement, although not to an equal degree. The sensory involvement is likely not to be the same in all the senses. Most commonly, patients complain of some form of decreased sensation (numbness) or some type of pain.

The therapeutic approach may need to be multifaceted. The benefits of oral analgesics are usually less than optimal, and narcotics are rarely, if ever, indicated.

The use of heat or cold for pain relief requires great caution, especially when sensation is decreased. Radiant heat provides superficial heat and is probably the safest form because the skin can be observed during the therapy. Deeper heat, such as short wave diathermy or ultrasound, may be unsafe because the feedback about pain that is needed for its regulation is diminished. Tepid, swirling water may be helpful. The use of cold is of limited value for pain control.

Massage techniques, especially desensitization massage, may be helpful, particularly in the presence of positive symptoms in the distal extremities.

Transcutaneous electrical nerve stimulation is effective in some cases. There are no hard-and-fast rules regarding the use of either "high" or "low" stimulation; a trial of both may be warranted. Likewise, placement of the electrodes proximally or distally is a matter of trial.

One of the most important tasks when dealing with a patient with decreased sensation is that of education. This includes providing information not only about the disease, its course, and prognosis but also about how to protect the skin from damage due to environmental factors. For example, one complication of loss of pain and proprioception is a neurogenic foot ulcer. Patients with insensate feet are subject to localized ischemic necrosis and skin breakdown from weight bearing or poor-fitting footwear. Walking without frequently checking the skin of the weight-bearing or contact areas may result in ischemia ulcer formation, gangrene, abscess formation, and, in some cases, osteomyelitis. Treatment consists of prevention or removal of risk factors, early recognition of inflammation, and, if an ulcer develops, meticulous wound care. Attention to proper footwear is essential. The patient needs to be reminded that damage can occur from temperature changes (hot or cold) as well as from trauma.

THERAPY FOR MOTOR INVOLVEMENT

The effects of peripheral neuropathy on motor function can be the result of one problem or a combination of problems. Muscular weakness can be due to an abnormality in the motor pathway. Weakness also results from immobility; normal persons confined to bed rest lose about 3% of their initial strength per day.[1] Patients can also lose joint mobility due to either a lack of muscle power or the development of contractures of soft tissues about the joint; either one of these problems or a combination can result in decreased flexibility and mobility.

Therapy can be instituted at any point in the course of the disease. However, reversing the limitations imposed by joint contractures is difficult because it is prolonged and there may be less than full return of motion or function. Therefore, prophylactic measures (that is, range of motion) should be used, even when the involvement is mild.

The methods described in the section on sensory neuropathies can be used to treat motor involvement. However, in addition to providing pain relief (if present), some of these measures can be used to improve flexibility and mobility.

As long as sensation is intact, the deeper heat treatments (short wave diathermy and ultrasound) can be beneficial. Because of the effect of heat on collagen, short wave diathermy and ultrasound are especially helpful for treating joint contractures. Specifically, the application of ultrasound to an affected area accompanied and followed by prolonged stretch of the contracted tissues is the most effective noninvasive technique available.[2]

If spasticity is present, application of cold or heat may reduce muscle tone.

Exercises can be an important part of the treatment of patients with peripheral neuropathies and primary motor involvement. Maintaining flexibility is important. Each peripheral joint should be put through its full range of motion once daily. Depending on the degree of weakness, the range should be applied either by the therapist (passive) or with assistance from another person (active assisted).

In the presence of joint contractures, prolonged stretch by traction or proper positioning should be tried. Depending on the response, it may need to become a lifelong activity.

The question of strengthening in the presence of neuropathic disease is currently of considerable controversy. Submaximal strengthening (avoidance of fatigue during exercise) is believed to be generally safe. Maximal strengthening during the acute phase and early convalescence is to be avoided. Therefore, a specific, well-supervised program is important.

As strength improves, muscle reeducation should be instituted. This can be accomplished under the specific guidance of a physical therapist. Biofeedback techniques may be effective.

Orthoses may be needed during the course of the illness or after it. Many orthoses are available for both the upper and the lower extremities to help maintain proper alignment and to help compensate for weakness in muscle groups. These can be either static (no motion in the orthosis) or dynamic. In dynamic orthoses, power to move the appliance is provided, at least in part, by some external source (for example, rubber bands or springs).

Likewise, gait aids may be needed to provide stability or to compensate for a lack of muscle strength. Gait aids include canes, crutches, walkers, and wheelchairs.

SPECIFIC APPROACHES

There are many neuropathic diseases, and no attempt has been made to detail a program for each. However, a suggested program is outlined for the Guillain-Barré syndrome (see Chapter 11).

The Guillain-Barré syndrome is a sensory-motor polyneuropathy that can affect any striated muscle in the body. Because about two-thirds of patients recover completely and 25% have some residual deficit, intervention with principles of physical medicine and rehabilitation is important.

When paralysis is present, particular attention needs to be paid to positioning and posture. Resting splints can help maintain proper alignment. All peripheral joints should be put through their full range of motion daily to prevent contractures. Preventive measures to avoid pressure sores must be instituted. Special attention needs to be directed toward bowel and bladder function (see Chapter 15).

As recovery progresses, all the skills of the rehabilitation team are needed—physical therapist, occupational therapist, recreational therapist, medical social worker, psychologist, and physiatrist. Recovery depends, to some extent, on the severity of the initial involvement and can take up to 2 years. Attempts to strengthen too rapidly can result in relapses. Pain is sometimes a significant problem, and if the measures outlined above are ineffective, medications may be needed. Other authors have outlined rehabilitation principles for neuropathic diseases.[3, 4]

In conclusion, knowledge of the basic course and prognosis of neuropathic diseases is essential for deciding what needs to be done and when.

REFERENCES

1. Kottke FJ. The effects of limitation of activity upon the human body. JAMA 1966; 196:825–830.
2. Lehmann JF, de Lateur BJ. Diathermy and superficial heat and cold therapy. In: Kottke FJ, Stillwell GK, Lehmann JF, eds. Krusen's handbook of physical medicine and rehabilitation. 3rd ed. Philadelphia: WB Saunders, 1982:275–350.
3. Vignos PJ Jr. Physical models of rehabilitation in neuromuscular disease. Muscle Nerve 1983; 6:323–338.
4. Fowler WM Jr, Taylor M. Rehabilitation management of muscular dystrophy and related disorders. I. The role of exercise. Arch Phys Med Rehabil 1982; 63:319–321.

11

Guillain-Barré Syndrome

Bahram Mokri
Mehrsheed Sinaki

Guillain-Barré syndrome (acute inflammatory demyelinating polyradiculo-neuropathy) is an acutely or subacutely evolving inflammatory polyradiculoneuropathy that commonly involves cranial nerves.[1-3] It is presumed to be an autoimmune disorder with antecedent triggering events in one-half to two-thirds of cases. There is progressive and relatively symmetric flaccid paralysis with mild sensory symptoms and signs. Completion of the course is within 1 to 3 weeks, and recovery is satisfactory in more than 85% of cases. Death is now uncommon, but when it occurs it is often due to respiratory failure.

The syndrome was first described by Landry, a French physician, in 1859 and was later described in more detail in 1916 by two French neurologists, Guillain and Barré. In 1976, in connection with vaccination for swine flu in the United States, it gained more publicity.

EPIDEMIOLOGY AND INCIDENCE

The syndrome occurs at any age from infancy to old age and has a bimodal age distribution. The main peak is among young adults.[3] The second smaller peak occurs in persons who are in the middle 40s to middle 60s. There is only a slight male preponderance. It occurs sporadically at all seasons of the year. The mean annual incidence is about 1.7 per 100,000 population. It is the most common cause of acute weakness in patients younger than 40 years.

PATHOLOGY AND PATHOGENESIS

Initially, endoneurial mononuclear cell infiltration and focal segmental demyelination occur. Axons are typically spared, but axonal degeneration does occur in severe lesions. In later stages there is remyelination by Schwann cells, and axonal regrowth occurs in some cases with axonal degeneration and denervation.[4]

Guillain-Barré syndrome is presumed to be an autoimmune disorder of delayed hypersensitivity. It resembles experimental allergic neuritis. The exact mechanism of its development is unknown. The role of an inciting event is unclear. The antigen that causes this disease is unknown. One-half to two-thirds of patients have a preceding illness, usually an upper respiratory tract infection and, less commonly, gastroenteritis. The symptoms of neuropathy appear 1 to 4 weeks after resolution of the preceding illness. Certain well-recognized viral diseases (viral hepatitis, infectious mononucleosis) and mycoplasmal pneumonia have been recognized as preceding illnesses. In 5% to 10% of instances the patient has a history of operation 1 to 6 weeks before the onset of the neuropathy. This syndrome may occur in immunocompromised patients, those with lymphomas or systemic lupus erythematosus, or those who have undergone organ transplantation.[1]

SYMPTOMS AND SIGNS

Muscle Weakness

Weakness, which is usually symmetric, is the most common presenting symptom. It often begins from the lower extremities and then spreads to other areas. The intensity of weakness reaches its maximum often within a few days or, occasionally, a few weeks. Usually the weakness is greater distally, but occasionally it is greater in the proximal musculature. Respiratory muscle weakness may occur, and in one-fourth of cases it may become severe enough to necessitate the use of a respirator. The interval between the onset of the first symptoms to the appearance of respiratory failure may range from 2 days to 3 weeks. Bulbar manifestations are seen in 85% of cases. Facial nerves are the most commonly involved cranial nerves; occasionally, this involvement is accompanied by facial myokymia. The facial weakness may be unilateral; when bilateral, it is usually symmetric. Dysphagia and dysarthria are not uncommon. Extraocular muscle weakness is infrequent.

The involvement of sphincters and incontinence of bowel and bladder are very uncommon but do occur in some severe cases. Such involvement usually presents as transient incontinence or retention.

Sensory Symptoms

Occasionally, limb paresthesias may be the initial symptom and may precede weakness. Many patients with Guillain-Barré syndrome report distal sensory symptoms, even those whose muscle weakness is primarily proximal. A mild distal "stocking/glove" sensory loss can be detected in one-third of cases. Subjective sensory symptoms are usually more prominent than objective sensory signs. When objective sensory changes are detected, sensations of vibration and position are lost more often than those of touch, pain, or temperature. Occasionally, impairment of the sensations of vibration and position is marked and sensory ataxia is significant (the "ataxic form" of Guillain-Barré syndrome).

Reflexes

Muscle stretch reflexes and cutaneous reflexes may be diminished but are often absent. Preservation of reflexes in significantly weak muscles should cast doubt on the diagnosis of Guillain-Barré syndrome.

Papilledema

Papilledema occurs only occasionally. It is presumed to be due to increased intracranial pressure resulting from respiratory embarrassment, high cerebrospinal fluid protein content, or disturbed cerebrospinal fluid absorption.

Pain

Pain of slight to moderate intensity and in the form of muscle tenderness or sensitivity of nerves may occur in less than one-third of patients.

Autonomic Dysfunction

Sinus tachycardia occurs in more than 50% of severe cases. It may or may not respond to carotid stimulation. Orthostatic hypotension can be present, and in rare cases syncope may be the presenting complaint. Hypertension is also found in some cases. Episodes of parasympathetic hyperactivity, such as facial flushing, bradycardia, and a tightening sensation in the chest and abdomen, may occur. Loss of sweating is noted in some cases, as is Horner's syndrome. Also noted are vasomotor changes and disturbances of thermal regulation.

Fisher's Syndrome

This is a variant of Guillain-Barré syndrome manifested by ophthalmoplegia, ataxia, and areflexia. The course is benign, and spontaneous recovery usually takes place.[5] In occasional patients, respiratory distress requiring assisted ventilation has developed.

CEREBROSPINAL FLUID FINDINGS

Cerebrospinal fluid pressure is usually normal. In severe cases, increased pressure may sometimes be noted.

The protein concentration of cerebrospinal fluid is usually normal during the first few days. Then it often begins to rise steadily, sometimes to as high as 1,000 mg/dL. It may remain high for some months, even through the recovery phase.

The cerebrospinal fluid cell count is usually normal, but in about 20% of cases a pleocytosis of 10 to 50 cells/μL may be seen.

ELECTROMYOGRAPHIC FINDINGS

Nerve conduction velocities are reduced and are usually less than 60% of normal. Distal latencies may be prolonged as much as three times normal. However, the process is patchy (as the segmental demyelination of the nerves is patchy), and therefore not all the nerves are involved. Sometimes when the proximal parts of the nerves are involved, the distal parts may display normal conduction velocities but F-wave conduction velocities are slowed.

Needle electrode examination shows evidence of denervation only if axonal damage has taken place. Nerve conduction abnormalities may persist for several months or even up to years after clinical recovery.

The severity of nerve conduction abnormality does not correlate well with the severity of the deficits or the degree of recovery.[2] However, when there is early evidence of denervation on needle electrode examination, a long-standing weakness and a less smooth and even an incomplete recovery are to be expected.

CLINICAL FEATURES THAT STRONGLY SUPPORT A DIAGNOSIS OF GUILLAIN-BARRÉ SYNDROME

The following features are indicative of Guillain-Barré syndrome[6, 7]:

1. *Rapid progression* within a few weeks (2 weeks in 50% of cases, 3 weeks in 80%, and 4 weeks in 90%) and then a plateau stage (of 2 to 4 weeks) before recovery begins

2. Relative *symmetry of weakness* and *mildness of sensory manifestations*

3. *Absence of pain* at onset, *presence of autonomic dysfunction,* and *frequent involvement of cranial nerves* (the facial nerve is involved in about 50% of cases).

CLINICAL FEATURES THAT CAST DOUBT ON A DIAGNOSIS OF GUILLAIN-BARRÉ SYNDROME

Certain features cast doubt on the diagnosis:

1. Persistent and marked *asymmetry of weakness*
2. *Bowel and bladder dysfunction* that appears *at onset or is persistent*
3. Sharp sensory level
4. Presence of *polymorphonuclear cells* of *more than 50/μL* in the cerebrospinal fluid.

COURSE AND PROGNOSIS

The characteristic progression of paralysis often reaches its maximum in 1 to 3 weeks. The progression is usually steady but may be stepwise. The downhill course is usually followed by a plateau period of 2 to 4 weeks before improvement becomes evident. The rate of recovery may be quick (1 to 3 weeks) or slower (sometimes as long as several months to a year or longer depending on the extent of axonal degeneration). Recovery is complete in more than half of the patients. In about 10% of patients, the residual deficits are severe. In a small percentage of patients, a biphasic pattern or recurrence after complete recovery may occur. The prognosis is more favorable in children. Overall, the mortality rate is 5%. Most deaths result from respiratory failure, pulmonary embolism, autonomic dysfunction, or intercurrent infection.

MANAGEMENT

Hospitalization

The cause of death in most patients with Guillain-Barré syndrome is either respiratory failure or its related complications. Respiratory failure may come quickly.

There should be no hesitation about hospitalizing patients suspected of having Guillain-Barré syndrome in the phase of evolution. In about 30% of hospitalized patients, respiratory failure severe enough to require assisted ventilation develops. The hospital chosen for admission should have the staff and the facilities to deal with this complication.

In the hospital, the patient's neurologic status and respiratory function should be monitored by daily or more frequent neurologic examinations and by measurements of vital capacity or maximal inspiratory pressure every 4 to 6 hours. Recording of respiratory rate and measurement of arterial blood gas tensions also provide important information.[8, 9]

Intubation

Indications for intubation are 1) increasing respiratory failure due to increasing weakness of respiratory muscles (that is, when the vital capacity decreases to 25% to 30% of normal), 2) aspiration (pharyngeal muscle weakness), and 3) retention of secretions (ineffective cough). It is far more desirable to perform the intubation electively through careful monitoring rather than in an emergency and in a panic. With an appropriately selected and properly placed endotracheal tube, tracheostomy can be delayed for 2 to 3 weeks. Many patients may improve in the interim and be spared this procedure.

Clearance of Secretions

Chest physical therapy should be implemented very early. Frequent manual hyperinflation of the lungs and suction of secretions from the airways are very important. Sterile techniques should be used. Complications, including aspiration pneumonia, bacterial pneumonia, secretion retention, and lobar atelectasis, can be prevented or dealt with by frequent changes in position, frequent removal of secretions, chest physical therapy, and antibiotics (only as indicated by results of a sputum culture).

Weaning from Mechanical Ventilation

Weaning should begin when there is clinical evidence of return of muscle strength. The patient should be allowed to trigger the ventilator with minimal effort and should exercise the weakened respiratory muscles. The weaning process should be monitored by measurements of the respiratory rate and arterial blood gas tensions. If no complications are present, extubation can be done after 24 hours of spontaneous ventilation.

Corticosteroids

Although corticosteroids are useful for the treatment of chronic inflammatory demyelinating polyneuropathy, they are of no benefit in the treatment of acute inflammatory demyelinating neuropathy (Guillain-Barré syndrome) and may even be detrimental.[10, 11]

Plasma Exchange

Plasma exchange can shorten the duration of respirator dependence, lead to faster recovery, and reduce the duration of acute hospital care. It is probably most effective when it is commenced during the first week of the onset of weakness. It is not without complications (hypotension, cardiac arrhythmias) and therefore may not be appropriate for cases of moderate severity.[12]

PHYSICAL THERAPY AND REHABILITATION MEASURES

Bed rest is prescribed during the acute stage, and overexertion and fatigue are avoided at any stage.

Proper positioning and frequent change in position are important to prevent contractures and to avoid bed sores and compression neuropathies in paralyzed or significantly weak patients. A firm mattress with a soft covering such as "egg-crate" foam and synthetic sheepskin reduce pressure over bony prominences. A change in position is recommended every 2 hours during the waking hours and every 4 hours during the sleeping hours. The application of ankle or foot splints helps prevent contractures of the gastrocnemius muscle and Achilles tendon. Flexed positions for extended periods can promote contractures and should be avoided. Use of pillows under the knees is discouraged to avoid knee flexor contracture. Passive range-of-motion exercises help prevent soft tissue contractures and need to be done twice daily.

If contractures develop, they can be helped by application of mild heat and stretching combined with range-of-motion exercises.

The prevention and management of edema are very important because edema decreases the soft tissue resistance to trauma, pressure sores, necrosis, infection, and phlebitis. It results from lack of muscle tone in the paralyzed extremities. Intermittent elevation of the limb above the heart level and the application of elastic support can help reduce edema.

Constipation and fecal impaction should be prevented through an adequate fluid intake (1,600 to 1,800 mL/day), a high-fiber diet, stool softeners if needed, and, when necessary, bisacodyl suppositories every other day.

Arthralgias and myalgias can be decreased through the application of mild heat in the form of an infrared lamp, moist packs, hydrotherapy (Hubbard tank), or warm baths. After application of heat, range-of-motion exercises are recommended. Simple analgesics such as acetylsalicylic acid or acetaminophen are also helpful.

Prevention of thromboembolic complications in immobilized patients is important. Appropriate preventive measures include the following:

1. Prophylactic anticoagulant therapy in the form of heparin, 5,000 units every 12 hours, or coumadin (not needed in small children because they are mobilized easier)
2. Prevention of trauma
3. Passive range-of-motion exercises to the lower limbs (every 2 to 3 hours)
4. Application of elastic stockings and sequential compression device (Thromboguards).

After the acute stage and when recovery begins to take place, the patient's physical activity level should be reevaluated and reduced if more weakness develops. The goal is to achieve the development of maximal function. If independence and safety of gait can be favorably achieved with the use of a brace for the lower extremities, the lightest-weight orthosis that can substitute for the function of the ankle and foot dorsiflexors is recommended. In the presence of severe sensory deficits, custom-made braces are preferred to prevent pressure sores. The patient is instructed to check the skin periodically for pressure sores during application of the brace. Severe paresthesias may be helped by the use of transcutaneous electrical nerve stimulation and other pain management procedures. The presence of autonomic neuropathy and hypotension may interfere with ambulatory activity. If orthostatic hypotension is present, use of an elastic (Ace) wrap will help, as will a tilt table to rehabilitate the cardiovascular system. High abdominal-contact elastic leotards are also helpful for persistent orthostatic hypotension.

A rehabilitation program for various stages of Guillain-Barré syndrome is summarized in Table 11–1.

During every stage, occupational therapy can be of much help, from the utilization of proper splints to the facilitation of self-care at the later stages. Diversionary recreational activities are important to patients who go through slow recovery courses.

TABLE 11–1

Comprehensive Program for the Rehabilitation Stages of Guillain-Barré Syndrome, by Stage of Disease

Stage			
Progression	Plateau	Recovery	Home Care and Follow-up
Respiratory care	Respiratory care	Active ROM	Gradual increase in ADL
Prevention of DVT	Prevention of DVT	Muscle education	Wheelchair
Proper positioning (use of splints)	Active ROM for distal joints	Mild strengthening with increasing repetition	Braces
Passive ROM	Active-assisted ROM for proximal joints	Mat activities	Canes
Skin care	Stretching with ROM	Parallel bars, assisted ambulation	Crutches
Control of pain and dysesthesia (trial of TENS, moist heat)	Hubbard tank	Transfer activities	Regular follow-up (monthly for 3 mo after dismissal, then every 6 mo for 2 yr)
Bowel and bladder care	Tilt table (elastic wrap for LEs)	Hubbard tank	
	Nonstrenuous diversionary activities	Avoidance of exertional physical activities	
	Bowel and bladder care	Self-care	
		Nonstrenuous ADL	

Abbreviations: ADL, activities of daily living; DVT, deep venous thrombosis; LE, lower extremity; ROM, range of motion; TENS, transcutaneous electrical nerve stimulation.

REFERENCES

1. Arnason BGW. Acute inflammatory demyelinating polyradiculoneuropathies. In: Dyck PJ, Thomas PK, Lambert EH, Bunge R, eds. Peripheral neuropathy. Vol 2, 2nd ed. Philadelphia: WB Saunders, 1984:2050–2100.
2. Pleasure DE, Schotland DL. Guillain-Barré syndrome. In: Rowland LP, ed. Merritt's textbook of neurology. 8th ed. Philadelphia: Lea & Febiger, 1989:609-612.
3. Schaumburg HH, Spencer PS, Thomas PK. Disorders of peripheral nerves. Philadelphia: FA Davis, 1983:25–39.
4. Prineas JW. Pathology of the Guillain-Barré syndrome. Ann Neurol 1981; 9(suppl):6–19.
5. Fisher M. An unusual variant of acute idiopathic polyneuritis (syndrome of ophthalmoplegia, ataxia and areflexia). N Engl J Med 1956; 255:57–65.
6. Ad Hoc NINCDS Committee. Criteria for diagnosis of Guillain-Barré syndrome. Ann Neurol 1978; 3:565–566.
7. Asbury AK. Diagnostic considerations in Guillain-Barré syndrome. Ann Neurol 1981; 9(suppl):1–5.
8. Gracey DR, McMichan JC, Divertie MB, Howard FM Jr. Respiratory failure in Guillain-Barré syndrome: a 6-year experience. Mayo Clin Proc 1982; 57:742–746.
9. Samuels MA, ed. Manual of neurologic therapeutics. 3rd ed. Boston: Little Brown & Company, 1986:359–361.
10. Hughes RAC, Kadlubowski M, Hufschmidt A. Treatment of acute inflammatory polyneuropathy. Ann Neurol 1981; 9(suppl):125–133.
11. Hughes RAC, Newsom-Davis JM, Perkin GD, Pierce JM. Controlled trial of prednisolone in acute polyneuropathy. Lancet 1978; 2:750–753.
12. The Guillain-Barré Syndrome Study Group. Plasmapheresis and acute Guillain-Barré syndrome. Neurology 1985; 35:1096–1104.

12

Parkinsonism

Gail L. Gamble

Parkinson's disease is described as a progressive neurologic disturbance of motor function characterized by the presence of rigidity, resting
tremor, and bradykinesia. The common and progressive nature of this disease mandates that primary care and rehabilitation physicians be familiar
with the manifestations, consequences, and treatment options of this condition. Parkinson's disease has an estimated annual incidence of 20 per
100,000 population and a prevalence rate of 100 to 180 per 100,000 population.[1, 2] Although the incidence rate has been reported to be unchanged,[2] the increased age-specific incidence curves, with incidence
peaks among people in their 60s, will increase the prevalence as our population ages in the 21st century.[3, 4] The quality of life of both patient and
family is affected by this disease. When instituted early, rehabilitation
techniques can be effective for helping patients maintain maximal function.

PATHOPHYSIOLOGY

The symptoms of parkinsonism are known to occur in connection with
several different pathologic states (Table 12–1). The clinical manifestations
are ascribed to lesions that involve the substantia nigra and its efferent
pathways. Parkinson's disease (paralysis agitans) accounts for most cases of
parkinsonism. Of interest is a recently identified form of parkinsonism in
patients with an associated history of drug use. A neurotoxin in street drugs
(1-methyl-4-phenyl-1,2,3,6-tetrahydropyridine) has been found to cause
progressive signs of the disease and associated pathologic findings.[1]

The common abnormality is progressive degeneration of nerve cells of
pigmented nuclei of the brainstem, especially the substantia nigra. These
are dopamine-containing neurons whose cell bodies are primarily in the
substantia nigra and whose axons project to the putamen and globus pall-
idus.[1]

TABLE 12-1
Conditions That May Exhibit Parkinsonian Features

Degenerative diseases
   Parkinson's disease (paralysis agitans)
   Shy-Drager syndrome
   Progressive supranuclear palsy
Infections
   Postencephalitic parkinsonism
Drug- or toxin-induced diseases
   Neuroleptics (phenothiazines, haloperidol)
   Carbon monoxide poisoning
   Chronic manganese poisoning
   MPTP*-induced parkinsonism
Vascular conditions
   Lacunar infarcts
Other chronic neurologic disorders
   Alzheimer's disease
   Huntington's disease
   Wilson's disease
   Normal-pressure hydrocephalus

*1-Methyl-4-phenyl-1,2,3,6-tetrahydropyridine.

On gross examination, the substantia nigra appears pale and depigmented. Microscopically, neuronal dropout and gliosis are noted, as are intracytoplasmic inclusions called Lewy bodies. Thus, pharmacologically, there is dopamine deficiency as the result of degeneration of the dopaminergic neuronal system.[5] The greater the cell loss in the substantia nigra, the lower the concentration of dopamine in the striatum and the more marked the parkinsonian manifestations.[6]

CLINICAL PRESENTATION

Parkinson's original description in 1817 included tremor but not rigidity or bradykinesia. The clinical manifestations in parkinsonism may be variable, depending on the stage of the disease. Advanced Parkinson's disease is immediately recognizable clinically. However, cases in the early stage of the disease may not be so easily diagnosed, especially when the typical tremor is absent. Most constant among the manifestations of the disease is the classic triad of tremor, rigidity, and bradykinesia.

Tremor

One of the most visible symptoms, tremor is the most common reason affected patients present to a physician. It is a resting tremor that is increased with anxiety, emotion, tension, or fatigue. The tremor characteristically has a rate of 4 to 8 Hz, and it can and should be distinguished from the intention tremor of cerebellar dysfunction and from essential familial tremor. The tremor, which can be bilateral or unilateral, most often affects the distal parts of the limbs; however, it can also involve the face, jaw, and even the tongue.

Rigidity

One clinical sign found on examination of nearly all affected patients is rigidity.[7] It is described as a consistent resistance exhibited in both flexion and extension with attempted passive range of motion. It is present constantly and is interrupted only by the cogwheel phenomenon, which is thought to be the transmission of tremor through the rigidity.

Bradykinesia

This important feature, characterized by slowed movement, is manifested in many ways. It has been shown to be different from pure rigidity by specific surgical ablation and is associated with hypokinesia, which is a poverty of movement or lack of movement initiation. It is distinctly not muscle weakness (which is not a characteristic of this disease). Patients may exhibit the typical masked facies, with paucity of facial expression and facial movements. Blinking is usually infrequent. Speech is often hypokinetic and monotonous. Handwriting becomes small (micrographia). Automatic movements of the limbs are sparse and hard to initiate. In general, patients are unable to perform any movement that requires the quick reciprocal muscle contractions that are so important for the coordinated movements of normal living. Many of the activities of daily living can be affected by a significant bradykinesia (Table 12–2).

Posture

Associated with the difficulty of motor initiation is the loss of appropriate posturing. Patients tend to assume a stooped posture with flexed trunk, neck, hip, and knees (Fig. 12–1). The inability to maintain erect posture has a significant effect on balance and gait. Patients find walking difficult

---

TABLE 12–2
Functions Affected by Bradykinesia

Swallowing (dysphagia)
Communication (hypokinetic dysarthria)
Transfers ("freezing")
Gait (propulsion, retropulsion)
Balance (en bloc movements)
Self-care activities

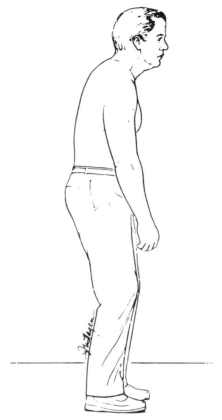

Figure 12–1
Flexed posturing of patient with parkinsonism.

to initiate because of the bradykinesia, and their forward-balanced posture makes gait extremely hard to control.[8] Arm swing is decreased or absent, and the postural and righting reflexes may also be affected. The tendency to fall is markedly increased; when this occurs, it is often without an attempt to protect oneself.

Autonomic Symptoms

Flushing of the skin may occur and is sometimes associated with increased sweating. Excretion from sebaceous glands may increase and the skin may feel greasy. Excessive salivation is common. Blood pressure may be low, and many patients have orthostatic hypotension, which in some cases can be severe and disabling. Urinary retention has been described, but in many cases this can be attributed to the effect of anticholinergic drugs. Constipation is common, and questions regarding bowel and bladder function should be included in the rehabilitation evaluation.

Neuropsychologic Changes

Various psychologic manifestations may also be exhibited, including depression and personality changes.[9] Patients with parkinsonism tend to isolate themselves from their normal social environment because of embarrassment about resting tremor, movement difficulty, impaired speech, or excessive drooling. This withdrawn behavior must be distinguished from a clear change in personality characteristics. Additionally, a mildly progressive dementia or other isolated cognitive deficits can be associated with this disease.[10-12] These findings are not present in all cases, however, and any suspected cognitive deficits need to be assessed in detail because frozen facial expression and poor ability to communicate may mask more normal cognitive function.

TREATMENT

Parkinson's disease is a gradually progressive degenerative disease, and a slow decline will occur despite adequate pharmacologic and physical management. However, the life expectancy of patients with this disease remains normal despite the considerable functional disability. The goals of any rehabilitation program, which include preservation of function and maintenance of independence, remain important in the care of patients with parkinsonism.

Various drugs have been used to treat Parkinson's disease (Table 12–3). A closely followed, well-adjusted dosage schedule for carbidopa-levodopa is the preferred method of pharmacologic management in most cases.[1] Levodopa combined with carbidopa (a peripheral decarboxylase

TABLE 12–3
Drugs Used for the Management
of Parkinson's Disease

Neurotransmitter replacement therapy
   Levodopa (Larodopa)
   Carbidopa-levodopa (Sinemet)
Receptor agonists
   Pergolide (Permax)
   Bromocriptine (Parlodel)
   Amantadine (Symmetrel)
Anticholinergics
   Trihexyphenidyl (Artane)
   Benztropine (Cogentin)
   Biperiden (Akineton)
Antihistamines
   Diphenydramine (Benadryl)
   Type B monoamine oxidase inhibitor
     Selegiline (Eldepryl, L-deprenyl)

inhibitor of dopa) has allowed for decreased dosages of levodopa, minimization of side effects, and improved levodopa concentrations in the central nervous system. With the use of carbidopa-levodopa in particular, an on-off effect may occur. Recent studies of the use of controlled-release levodopa have reported a prolonging of the "on" response—a benefit allowing increased function for a longer period.[13, 14] However, increased doses of this medication may cause dystonic movements.[15] Other classes of agents include receptor agonists,[16, 17] anticholinergics, antihistamines, and selective monoamine oxidase inhibitors.[18]

A recent pharmacologic advance in the treatment of Parkinson's disease has been the finding that selective monoamine oxidase inhibitors (selegiline) block the biologic effects induced by MTPT (1-methyl-4-phenyl-1,2,3,6-tetrahydropyridine).[18] Other studies report preliminary results showing that selegiline may delay the onset of disability, particularly in early cases of Parkinson's disease,[19] and may be useful in the treatment of more advanced Parkinson's disease.[20]

The rehabilitation physician should be aware of the effects and side effects of these medications and recognize that dosages do occasionally require adjustment and that the effects of the medications act over a period of hours. Physical therapy should be administered at a time when blood concentrations of these drugs, and therefore performance, are optimal. In some patients, particularly those who are elderly, antiparkinsonian drugs (especially anticholinergics) may cause hallucinations, disorientation, and confusion.

Other forms of treatment include investigations into surgical management, such as adrenal medullary transplantation, which currently is being studied with some caution.[21] Most recently, experimental data suggest that grafts of fetal dopamine neurons actually restore dopamine synthesis and improve motor function.[22] Further clinical evaluations are awaited.

PHYSICAL THERAPY

Patients who are even moderately affected with parkinsonism will benefit from a daily program of therapy. Speech therapy, if needed, may be helpful. At first, the intervention should be supervised, and then a daily home program can be developed.

The onset of disease is usually insidious, and family roles may have changed as discreetly as disease progression itself. Family members should be counseled to encourage the patient to assume the most active role possible in all areas of home life in order to preserve an inner sense of dignity. Efforts must be made to include the patient in decisions about family affairs and also the rehabilitation program. Enough time should be allowed for completion of daily tasks as long as the patient's independence can be maintained.

Exercises are particularly useful and should become part of a patient's daily routine.[23, 24] Exercises are more effective when they are used consistently and early in the course of disease to maintain a functional level

TABLE 12-4
Therapeutic Exercises for Parkinson's
Disease

Range of motion
Stretching
Posture
Coordination
Deep breathing
Facial
Transfers and gait

rather than to restore function in an unused contracted limb. Multiple types of exercises are used in a comprehensive therapy program (Table 12-4).

Range-of-Motion Exercises

These should be performed daily on all peripheral joints and may be done actively or on an active-assistive basis when a patient is unable to perform them independently. These simple movements will help minimize joint stiffness and will decrease the progressive tendency toward contracture.

Stretching

One of the major components of all exercise programs for parkinsonism is stretching. A gentle, prolonged, passive stretch program is frequently necessary to work against the effects of progressive rigidity in order to maintain full range of motion. Proper posture is the major goal, and stretching of multiple muscles, including pectoral and upper chest wall, neck flexors, abdominal flexors, and hip and knee flexors, should be included (see Fig. 19-3 and 19-4). Stretching the hamstring muscle is important because it affects the ability to assume an erect posture. The stretching program must become part of the patient's daily routine and should preferably be done twice a day. A simple gravity-assisted stretch may be done by merely having the patient lie supine without pillows for an extended time (Fig. 12-2).

Posture

Nearly all patients with parkinsonism have a tendency for stooped posturing, and avoidance of this posture is imperative. The patient should continually work toward avoiding downward gaze by learning correct cervical posture in sitting and standing positions. In addition to cervical flexor muscles, the pectorals frequently become contracted, and a program of pectoral stretch by doing pushups against a wall should be undertaken (see

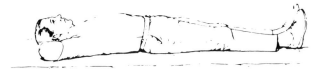

Figure 12–2
Supine stretch to avoid flexion.

Fig. 19–5). Extension exercises for the upper thoracic spine are also help-ful and can be done in either the prone or the erect sitting position (see Fig. 19–2). The patient should also be instructed to avoid both hip flexor and knee flexor posturing.

Coordination

The combined effects of rigidity and bradykinesia limit the ability to move in a smooth and well-controlled pattern. In an attempt to retain co-ordinated reciprocal movements, coordination exercises for both the upper and the lower extremities should become part of a daily regimen. Lower extremity coordination exercises should stress reciprocal movements and postural balance. Rhythmic exercises such as use of a stationary bicycle may improve ambulatory activities. Patients with parkinsonism live with an increased fear of falling, and exercises should be directed at overcoming this fear and insecurity. Upper extremity exercises should also be under-taken using reciprocal motions when possible.

Gait

The characteristic gait of rapid small steps, forward flexed posturing, and shuffling feet can be both socially embarrassing and unsafe. Gait me-chanics can be improved when attention is given to widening the gait base and directing the patient to take a longer stride. Because of the rigidity, patients are frequently unable to correct a minor imbalance with slight movement and, therefore, falls are frequent. As mentioned previously, righting reflexes can be impaired and the quick movement necessary to sustain balance is often lacking.

Truncal and rotational exercises are also important in gait reeducation. Rotatory movements are often impaired, and they are an essential compo-nent of independent gait and transfer activities. Rising from a chair can also be difficult. Attempts can be made to teach a "rocking" activity—leaning the body forward and backward until the patient can rise out of the chair.

An assistive device such as a cane is usually not helpful for gait stabi-lization because patients cannot use it in a coordinated fashion. Walkers can also tend to complicate gait patterns. However, a wheeled walker may be useful if it is spring loaded for a pressure stop on the two posterior feet. With this assistive device, the forward propulsion of gait is allowed with-out the necessity of picking up the walker with each step.

OCCUPATIONAL THERAPY

Early efforts with an intensive program of occupational therapy are important for patient and family. Patients should be taught skills that allow independent function, when possible.

An occupational therapy evaluation will document a patient's present level of functioning. Instruments such as the nine-hole peg test and bilateral upper extremity coordination tests and evaluation of hand strength, pinch, and grasp may prove helpful. Additionally, an evaluation of a patient's ability for self-care will identify areas in which improvements might be made (Table 12–5).

Occupational therapy activities include rhythmic prehension and coordination skills, both gross and fine. Upper extremity range-of-motion activities should be continued, with an emphasis on reciprocal rhythm. Exercises may be developed that specifically address a patient's handwriting abnormalities, because handwriting is usually an important vocational skill.

Training in activities of daily living is an important area of occupational therapy. Skills for dressing, including the small movements of buttoning, and the coordinated movements of feeding should be closely evaluated. Adaptive equipment options should be made available to patients. Items such as buttonhooks (see Fig. 17–10,C), feeding utensils, or a toilet-seat riser may allow patients to maintain independence (see Fig. 30–2). Periodic reevaluations should be scheduled because self-care abilities gradually change during the course of the disease. A relative may assume that a patient remains capable of performing daily activities, but a subtle decline in physical and intellectual capability may require an alteration of the home care plan.

SPEECH THERAPY

Altered speech can be an important and disabling effect of parkinsonism and, in many cases, it may have a significant effect on vocation. The characteristic speech pattern has a low volume with high monotonous pitch and a hurried unpunctuated rate. Loss of the ability to vary intonation

TABLE 12–5
Occupational Therapy for Parkinson's Disease

Activities of daily living
Adaptive equipment
Cognitive evaluation
Safety and judgment
Fine motor coordination
Handwriting

and cadence is defined as altered prosody.[25] These deficiencies were not thought to be amenable to speech therapy until recent years. Now, however, intensive efforts with speech therapy may help the patient vary intonation and control the rate of speech.[26]

In conjunction with speech therapy, patients should be taught deep-breathing exercises, which may help to add increased volume to speech. A form of dysarthria may be present if facial and tongue movements are poorly controlled. Facial, oral, and lingual exercises are also an important part of a speech therapy program. The ability to phonate may vary over the clinical course of the disease, and periodic evaluations are suggested.

REHABILITATION: AN INTEGRATED APPROACH

The rehabilitation needs for patients with parkinsonism vary widely, and an integrated program should be developed by the coordinator of care. The psychologic impact on patient and family may be a major disability factor, and the involvement of a psychologist or social worker can be important.[27] The physician coordinator or social worker should also provide educational information to patients and families regarding the disease, home management, and availability of local community resources and national support groups.[28-30] Parkinsonism is a chronically progressive disease, but independence and quality of life may be better maintained through appropriate pharmacologic management, specific rehabilitation interventions, and education and support of the patient and family.

REFERENCES

1. Adams RD, Victor M. Principles of neurology. 3rd ed. New York: McGraw-Hill, 1985:872–881.
2. Rajput AH, Offord KP, Beard CM, Kurland LT. Epidemiology of parkinsonism: incidence, classification, and mortality. Ann Neurol 1984; 16:278–282.
3. Diamond SG, Markham CH, Hoehn MM, McDowell FH, Muenter MD. Effect of age at onset on progression and mortality in Parkinson's disease. Neurology 1989; 39:1187–1190.
4. Koller W, O'Hara R, Weiner W, et al. Relationship of aging to Parkinson's disease. Adv Neurol 1986; 45:317–321.
5. Wolters EC, Calne DB. Parkinson's disease. Can Med Assoc J 1989; 140:507–513.
6. Yahr MD. Parkinsonism. In: Rowland LP, ed. Merritt's textbook of neurology. 7th ed. Philadelphia: Lea & Febiger, 1984:526–537.
7. Selby G. The Graeme Robertson Memorial Lecture, 1983: the long-term prognosis of Parkinson's disease. Clin Exp Neurol 1984; 20:1–25.
8. Cailliet R. Rehabilitation in parkinsonism. In: Licht S, ed. Rehabilitation and medicine. Baltimore: Waverly Press, 1968:430–445.
9. Mayeux R, Stern Y, Williams JBW, Sano M, Cote L. Depression and Parkinson's disease. Adv Neurol 1986; 45:451–455.
10. Dakof GA, Mendelsohn GA. Parkinson's disease: psychological aspects of a chronic illness. Psychol Bull 1986; 99:375–387.

11. Growdon JH, Corkin S. Cognitive impairments in Parkinson's disease. Adv Neurol 1986; 45:383–392.
12. Stern Y, Mayeux R. Intellectual impairment in Parkinson's disease. Adv Neurol 1986; 45:405–408.
13. Ahlskog JE, Muenter MD, McManis PG, Bell GN, Bailey PA. Controlled-release sinemet (CR-4): a double-blind crossover study in patients with fluctuating Parkinson's disease. Mayo Clin Proc 1988; 63:876–886.
14. Hutton JT, Morris JL, Román GC, Imke SC, Elias JW. Treatment of chronic Parkinson's disease with controlled-release carbidopa/levodopa. Arch Neurol 1988; 45:861–864.
15. Bergmann KJ, Mendoza MR, Yahr MD. Parkinson's disease and long-term levodopa therapy. Adv Neurol 1986; 45:463–467.
16. Ahlskog JE, Muenter MD. Treatment of Parkinson's disease with pergolide: a double-blind study. Mayo Clin Proc 1988; 63:969–978.
17. Robin DW. Pergolide in the treatment of Parkinson's disease. Am J Med Sci 1991; 301:277–280.
18. Tetrud JW, Langston JW. The effect of deprenyl (selegiline) on the natural history of Parkinson's disease. Science 1989; 245:519–522.
19. The Parkinson Study Group. Effect of deprenyl on the progression of disability in early Parkinson's disease. N Engl J Med 1989; 321:1364–1371.
20. Golbe LI. Long-term efficacy and safety of deprenyl (selegiline) in advanced Parkinson's disease. Neurology 1989; 39:1109–1111.
21. Goetz CG, Olanow CW, Koller WC, et al. Multicenter study of autologous adrenal medullary transplantation to the corpus striatum in patients with advanced Parkinson's disease. N Engl J Med 1989; 320:337–341.
22. Lindvall O, Brundin P, Widner H, et al. Grafts of fetal dopamine neurons survive and improve motor function in Parkinson's disease. Science 1990; 247:574–577.
23. Palmer SS, Mortimer JA, Webster DD, Bistevins R, Dickinson GL. Exercise therapy for Parkinson's disease. Arch Phys Med Rehabil 1986; 67:741–745.
24. Hurwitz A. The benefit of a home exercise regimen for ambulatory Parkinson's disease patients. J Neurosci Nurs 1989; 21:180–184.
25. Ross ED, Mesulam M-M. Dominant language functions of the right hemisphere? Prosody and emotional gesturing. Arch Neurol 1979; 36:144–148.
26. Robertson SJ, Thomson F. Speech therapy in Parkinson's disease: a study of the efficacy and long term effects of intensive treatment. Br J Disord Commun 1984; 19:213–224.
27. Brown RG, MacCarthy B, Gotham A-M, Der GJ, Marsden CD. Depression and disability in Parkinson's disease: a follow-up of 132 cases. Psychol Med 1988; 18:49–55.
28. Duvoisin RC. Parkinson's disease: a guide for patient and family. 3rd ed. New York: Raven Press, 1991.
29. Hutton JT, Dippel R. Caring for the Parkinson patient: a practical guide. Buffalo, New York: Prometheus Books, 1989.
30. McGoon DC. The Parkinson's handbook. New York: WW Norton & Company, 1990.

13

Movement Disorders

Joseph Y. Matsumoto
Mehrsheed Sinaki

Movement disorders encompass a wide range of neurologic problems in which the normal processes of motor control are disrupted, and affected patients have too much or too little movement. Too little movement is termed "akinesia" and generally occurs in the setting of Parkinson's disease (see Chapter 12). Too much movement occurs in various involuntary movement disorders such as tremor, chorea, tics, athetosis, and dystonia.[1] Physical medicine has been most useful in the treatment of dystonia.

DEFINITIONS

Tremor is a rhythmic oscillation of a body part. Tremor that occurs at rest is most often seen in Parkinson's disease or other extrapyramidal disorders. Essential tremor, in contrast, is maximal when the affected body part is placed into action, such as when holding a fork or writing. Cerebellar tremor or terminal tremor occurs at the end of a voluntary movement when the need for fine coordination is maximal. *Chorea* describes rapid, involuntary movements that occur randomly in different parts of the body. A typical movement might be a grimace or a sudden lifting of the leg. In children, Sydenham's chorea is a late complication of a streptococcal infection. A family history of chorea or mental deterioration generally indicates Huntington's disease. Senile chorea in the elderly seldom has a clear cause. *Athetosis* describes writhing involuntary movements that often are continuous, but which may be punctuated by chorea (chorea-athetosis). This movement disorder is frequent in childhood as a manifestation of perinatal anoxic brain injury. Violent, uncontrollable, flinging movements are termed *ballism,* and most often only one side of the body is affected in a disorder termed *hemiballismus.* This disorder is associated with infarction, trauma, or other disorders affecting the contralateral subthalamic nucleus.

Myoclonus refers to extremely brief and violent muscle jerks that can affect any part of the body. The jerks are more rapid than the involuntary movements of chorea. Myoclonus can be generated from the cortex, brainstem, or spinal cord and can have various causes. Cerebral myoclonus is often associated with a seizure disorder. *Tics* are complex movements such as vocal sounds, head shaking, or shrugging. There is often a certain amount of voluntary control over tics, although patients feel a mental tension during such suppression. The most common tic disorder is Tourette's syndrome, in which vocal tics occur in combination with various other motor tics.

DYSTONIA

Dystonia is a sustained abnormal posture of a body part maintained by prolonged involuntary muscle contractions. Dystonia can be focal and involve only one body area or it can be generalized. The most common focal dystonias affect the neck or the cranial muscles of the face, jaw, or tongue. Generalized dystonias can occur as a manifestation of various neurodegenerative disorders, but most often they occur as an isolated hereditary disorder termed "idiopathic torsion dystonia." The pathophysiology of all dystonias is unknown. Clinicopathologic studies have implicated disorders of the basal ganglia, especially the putamen, for cases in which dystonia was associated with a known lesion such as a stroke. In the vast majority of cases, however, no lesion can be detected, even by sophisticated imaging studies such as magnetic resonance imaging or positron emission tomography. As in all movement disorders, when no clear cause for dystonia is evident, a careful search for Wilson's disease should be undertaken because this is a protean and treatable disease. Physiologically, dystonic muscle contractions are characterized by excessive cocontraction of agonist and antagonist muscles. Currently, basal ganglia dysfunction is assumed to be responsible for the abnormal motor commands observed in all forms of dystonia.

SPASMODIC TORTICOLLIS

Cervical dystonias are the most common form of focal dystonia. Sustained muscle contractions can cause the head to rotate (torticollis) or to tip forward (antecollis), backward (retrocollis), or sideways (laterocollis) (Fig. 13–1). Most commonly, however, the head position is a complex combination of these abnormal postures. In infants and young children, torticollis may be the initial manifestation of an abnormality in the posterior fossa or upper cervical region such as a congenital malformation or tumor. In adults, in contrast, no cause is generally found, and the disorder is termed "idiopathic spasmodic torticollis."

The initial symptoms of spasmodic torticollis may be a sense of tight-

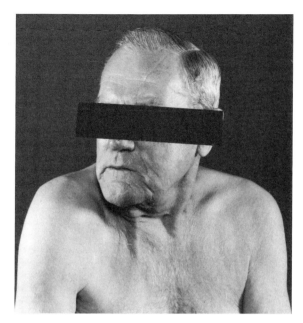

Figure 13–1
Patient with spasmodic torticollis. (From Davis et al.[4] By permission of Mayo Foundation.)

ness in the neck or head tremor. Over weeks to months, head deviation becomes evident. When the condition is severe, patients may be unable to drive or perform other simple activities of daily living because of the extreme tonic head deviation. Standing and walking worsen the symptoms, and torticollis is generally lessened in the supine position. Many patients learn simple tricks, such as touching the cheek or scalp ("geste antagonique"), that straighten the head for brief periods. Chronic, severe torticollis may be complicated by musculoskeletal neck pain, cervical radiculopathy, or thoracic scoliosis.

The cause of idiopathic spasmodic torticollis is unknown. Positron emission tomography has suggested abnormalities within the basal ganglia, but the abnormalities are not striking. The few autopsy studies that have been performed have been unrevealing. A psychologic cause has been considered, but patients seldom respond to psychotherapy, and no clear pattern of psychopathology is evident in affected patients.

Approximately 12% of patients with spasmodic torticollis undergo spontaneous remission; however, for most patients it is a lifelong condition. Medical therapy includes pharmacologic agents such as anticholinergic drugs,[2] baclofen, or clonazepam. The response to these agents is seldom gratifying. Recently, local injections of botulinum toxin, which can cause temporary weakness in selected muscles, has been used with success. A reduction in pain or improvement in head position has been reported in 90% of patients who received this treatment.[3] Currently, injections of botulinum toxin in combination with a comprehensive physical therapy program offer the greatest hope to patients with spasmodic torticollis. Surgical therapy may be indicated in severe cases or refractory cases.

In general, medical treatments are not usually effective unless a correctable pathologic process in the neck or head is present. Physical therapeutic measures are especially effective when implemented in conjunction with pharmacologic interventions in the management of nuchal myalgia secondary to dystonic muscle spasm.

Rehabilitation (Table 13–1) consists of the use of heat and analgesic techniques, such as friction massage, to decrease ischemia of the affected muscles caused by spasm and to decrease pain. The patient is positioned in a gravity-eliminated posture to decrease muscle contraction (head weight is supported), passive, gentle stretch is applied to the spastic muscles, and the intensity of current is increased until an uncomfortable sensation is produced. Cervical traction usually increases the involuntary movement. A cervical collar is not indicated, and it may even cause pressure sores and rub against the chin. Relaxation exercises in combination with biofeedback techniques and mirror imaging feedback are used to promote relaxation of the nuchal muscles. Strengthening of antagonistic muscles is recommended. Functional electrical stimulation may be used to strengthen and cause hypertrophy of the weakened muscles. Functional electrical stimulation must be applied for 30 minutes, 4 times a day.

If all forms of therapy fail and dystonic movement continues, the patient benefits from moral support and reassurance that dystonic movements are unlikely to develop in other areas of the body. A torticollis support group also benefits patients and reinforces the fact that they are not alone.

TABLE 13–1
Treatment of Spasmodic Torticollis

1. Application of ultrasound to the contracted muscles
2. Friction massage to the contracted muscles and painful areas
3. Range of motion to cervical spine with the head supported or dangling
4. Gentle stretch to the spastic muscles along with range of motion
5. Isometric strengthening of antagonistic muscles (contralateral noninvolved sternocleidomastoid)
6. Reciprocal relaxation to the involved sternocleidomastoid and synergistic muscles
7. Mirror imaging and biofeedback reeducation for postural alignment
8. Relaxation exercises to the trapezius and shoulder girdle muscles

CRANIAL DYSTONIAS

Blepharospasm describes dystonic contractions of both orbicularis oculi causing the eyes to be tightly squeezed shut. *Oromandibular* or *lingual dystonias* cause various movement abnormalities such as facial grimacing, jaw opening or closure, or tongue deviation. Such movements may follow exposure to antidopaminergic agents such as the antipsychotic drugs or metoclopramide. *Spasmodic dysphonia* is due to dystonic contractions of the laryngeal musculature. Most often the vocal cords are pulled into adduction, resulting in a tense, strained voice quality. Pharmacologic therapy is usually unhelpful in these disorders. Local injections of botulinum toxin have been particularly effective in the treatment of blepharospasm and spasmodic dysphonia.

LIMB DYSTONIAS

Most commonly, limb dystonias affect the hand and forearm and occur during tasks that require skill and are frequently repeated. These dystonias, which are often referred to as *occupational cramps,* may occur during writing, typing, or playing a musical instrument. During the dystonia, the fingers may flex into a useless posture or may extend off the pencil or instrument. Forearm pain or tightness accompanies the dystonia. Despite the obvious suspicion of secondary gain raised by these movement disorders, psychopathology is not found in affected patients. Drug therapy is similar to that for spasmodic torticollis, and the results are similarly disappointing. Injections of botulinum toxin are difficult, given the complex interaction of muscles involved in the dystonia. Physical therapy programs may help the patient learn new techniques for performing old tasks and so lessen the disability from these disorders. Physical therapy for writer's or occupational cramps is directed at reeducation for movement patterns; this induces periodic relaxation and improvement of posture. Physical therapy consists of maintenance of normal range of motion. Occupational therapy can provide splints that allow relaxation while the extremity is not in use. Periodic relaxation during use is helpful and prevents overuse contractures and pain.

GENERALIZED DYSTONIA

Generalized dystonia results in severe disability. The arms often are in a position of internal rotation, elbow extension, and wrist flexion. The legs are extended and inverted. The trunk and neck are twisted into extreme contorted postures. Standing is often impossible, and patients become bedbound and often have contractures.

Generalized dystonia most often begins in childhood. It may be the secondary manifestation of a neurodegenerative process or perinatal injury. When no cause is found, the disease is termed "idiopathic torsion dystonia." This disorder has an autosomal dominant inheritance and occurs most commonly in the Ashkenazi Jewish population.

Management of generalized dystonia combines drug therapy with an aggressive physical therapy program to avoid contractures. High-dose anticholinergic regimens often have a dramatic benefit, especially in children. Baclofen may provide further improvement. A small subset of patients with generalized dystonia may respond to small doses of levodopa.

REFERENCES

1. Lang AE. Movement disorder symptomatology. In: Bradley WG, Daroff RB, Fenichel GM, Marsden CD, eds. Neurology in clinical practice: principles of diagnosis and management. Boston: Butterworth-Heinemann, 1991;315–336.
2. Burke RE, Fahn S, Marsden CD. Torsion dystonia: a double-blind, prospective trial of high-dosage trihexyphenidyl. Neurology 1986; 36:160–164.
3. Jankovic J, Schwartz K, Donovan DT. Botulinum toxin treatment of cranial-cervical dystonia, spasmodic dysphonia, other focal dystonias and hemifacial spasm. J Neurol Neurosurg Psychiatry 1990; 53:633–639.
4. Davis DH, Ahlskog JE, Litchy WJ, Root LM. Selective peripheral denervation for torticollis: preliminary results. Mayo Clin Proc 1991; 66:365–371.

PART IV

Rehabilitation in Spinal Cord Injuries

14

Spinal Cord Injury

Carl W. Chan

The causes of spinal cord injuries are many. Approximately 70% of cases are due to *trauma*.[1] Frequent traumatic causes of spinal cord injuries include vehicular accidents, falls, sports accidents, and gunshot or stabbing wounds. Although the ages of patients with traumatic spinal cord injury range from birth to the oldest of the general population, about 80% are younger than 40 years; their mean age is 29 years.[2] Eighty percent of the patients are male.[2] The 30% of spinal cord injuries that are *nontraumatic* result from many possible causes: vascular insufficiencies or malformations, infectious processes, mechanical processes such as disk prolapse or bony spinal stenosis, multiple sclerosis, metastatic or primary cancer, and aftereffects of radiation. The mean age of patients at onset of nontraumatic spinal cord injury is about 55 years. The male:female ratio in the population with nontraumatic spinal cord injury is about 1:1.

TERMINOLOGY

The spinal cord is organized in a rostral to caudal manner such that there is a segmental representation of neuronal function. Each segment is referred to as a *"level"* of the spinal cord. Each level has a characteristic distribution of sensory function (a *dermatome*) and motor function (a *myotome*) (Fig. 14–1 and Table 14–1).

At the Mayo Clinic spinal cord injury center, the level of the spinal cord injury is defined as the last completely normally functioning motor and sensory level of the spinal cord. The level of injury does not refer to the level of bony injury (if there is any in a given patient). The term *"zone of injury"* refers to the up to three neurologic levels at the point of damage to the spinal cord where there is frequently some preservation, to various degrees, of motor or sensory function or both.[3] This zone may represent a

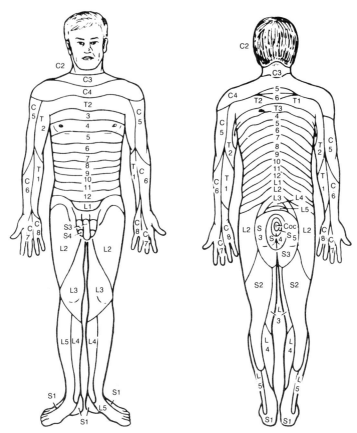

Figure 14–1

Sensory dermatomes. *Left*, Front view. *Right*, Back view. (From Standards for neurological classification of spinal injury patients. Chicago: American Spinal Cord Injury Association, October 1992. By permission of the publisher.)

gradation of damage that would be clinically manifested as a gradual decrease in, for instance, sensory function across several dermatomes.

A *complete* injury is one in which there is no voluntary motor or sensory function below the zone of injury. This results in either *paraplegia* or *tetraplegia*. An *incomplete* injury is one in which there is some sparing of useful motor or sensory function below the zone of injury. Some useful voluntary motor function throughout the entire remaining spinal cord below the zone of injury is referred to as paraparesis or tetraparesis.

Paraplegia or *paraparesis* results from injury in the thoracic (below T-1), lumbar, or sacral spinal segments. Arm function is normal.

Tetraplegia or *tetraparesis* results from injury in the cervical spinal segments (or uppermost thoracic level); therefore, arm function is involved to varying degrees, in addition to involvement of the trunk and legs.

TABLE 14–1
Key Muscles for Motor Level Classification

C–5 Elbow flexors (biceps, brachialis)	L–2 Hip flexors (iliopsoas)
C–6 Wrist extensors (extensor carpi radialis longus and brevis)	L–3 Knee extensors (quadriceps)
	L–4 Ankle dorsiflexors (tibialis anterior)
C–7 Elbow extensors (triceps)	L–5 Long toe extensors (extensor hallucis longus)
C–8 Flexors to the middle finger (flexor digitorum profundus)	
T–1 Small finger abductors (abductor digiti minimi)	S–1 Ankle plantar flexors (gastrocnemius, soleus)

From Standards for neurological classification of spinal injury patients.[3] By permission of the publisher.

ACUTE MANAGEMENT

An integrated multispecialty team approach is essential in order to provide appropriate care for the many problems (surgical, medical, psychologic, social, and vocational) of persons with spinal cord injuries.

Emergency medical technicians are specially trained in the proper methods to identify persons with actual or potential bony spinal or spinal cord injuries, their extrication, and their transport.

Typically, a trauma surgeon cares for the abdominal, thoracic, or vascular injuries and continues as the primary physician until these conditions are stable. A neurosurgeon takes primary responsibility when there is a spinal cord deficit or when it is presumed that a spinal cord deficit is imminent and no polytrauma exists. The patient is initially in the intensive care unit and is followed regularly by the orthopedic surgery and rehabilitation medicine services. A physiatrist, in association with other members of the spinal cord injury rehabilitation team, introduces the concept of rehabilitation to the patient, family, and significant others. The physiatrist coordinates the rehabilitation efforts throughout the hospitalization and during subsequent outpatient follow-up. The physiatrist also reviews the acute medical management of the patient and places special emphasis on preventive medical care in the areas in which the patient is at especially high risk. As part of the acute management of patients with new spinal cord injuries, it is customary that patients who are seen in the emergency room within the first 8 hours of injury be given methylprednisolone in high doses because it reportedly reduces motor deficits in these patients.[4] Typical doses are 30 mg/kg in an intravenous bolus over 15 minutes followed by intravenous infusion of 5.4 mg/kg per hour for 23 hours.

The orthopedic surgeon, in association with the neurosurgeon, provides for reduction of the spinal fracture by external or internal fixation and for management of other fracture sites. In cases of cervical injury, temporary stability is often provided first by halo traction and later by halo vest to provide firm fixation until the skeletal lesion is healed. The indications for open reduction and internal fixation of spinal fractures or management of significant soft tissue injuries that render the cervical spine unstable have been increasing during the past 10 years. The advantages of early open reduction and internal fixation include fewer physical and psychologic complications from prolonged immobilization and greater success within less time for reintegrating the patient into society.

In the thoracic and lumbar regions of the spine, temporary stability is usually achieved by placing the patient on a rigid frame. The frame allows for early turning of the patient. In the thoracolumbar area of the spine, skeletal disruption and partial neurologic deficit are common. In thoracolumbar fractures, early open reduction and internal fixation of the spine with Harrington rods and fusion allow early mobilization with the use of a molded body jacket, which allows early participation in intensive rehabilitation.

After the spinal fracture or soft tissue injuries have been managed to provide stability (or at least managed to provide eventual spinal stability), associated polytrauma has been treated, and markedly unstable medical conditions have stabilized sufficiently to allow transfer from the intensive care unit, the patient is transferred to the care of the physical medicine and rehabilitation service on the rehabilitation unit. A physiatrist serves as the primary physician during the remainder of the hospitalization. After dismissal from the hospital, the patient's general medical care is coordinated by the home physician. Subsequent follow-up visits for rehabilitation concerns are coordinated by the physiatrist. Guidelines for preventive care have been developed,[5] some of which are outlined below.

AREAS OF INCREASED RISK IN SPINAL CORD INJURIES

Pulmonary

Early mortality after acute traumatic tetraplegia is primarily due to retention of bronchial secretions and subsequent development of atelectasis and pneumonia. Other sources of pulmonary morbidity and mortality include respiratory failure secondary to impaired function of the diaphragm and intercostal and abdominal muscles and to pulmonary embolism.

Pulmonary assessment, in addition to a history and physical examination, includes a chest roentgenogram and measurement of arterial blood gases, vital capacity, and maximal inspiratory and expiratory pressures. Management includes (1) oxygen supplementation with humidification to maintain $P_{O_2} > 70$ mm Hg; (2) placement of a nasogastric tube for relief of gastric distention, prevention of aspiration of gastric contents, and easier movement of the diaphragm (adynamic ileus is often present initially); (3) for the prevention of secretion retention and atelectasis, turning the patient regularly, performing deep breathing, incentive spirometry, assisted coughing, and chest wall percussion and vibration, and externally rotating the humeri (unless contraindicated by shoulder injuries); (4) not allowing smoking; and (5) measuring pulmonary function twice weekly in the early stages and immediately before and after the application of potentially constrictive body casts or vests.

For the treatment of secretion retention and atelectasis, the following measures are used: (1) intermittent positive-pressure breathing with a bronchodilator solution (Bronkosol) and assisted coughing immediately before pronation, (2) bronchoscopy in the presence of radiologic evidence of lobar collapse, and (3) microbiologic examination of sputum and appropriate antibiotic management.

Eventually, the pulmonary regimen can be reduced in midthoracic paraplegia to a minimum of assisted coughing and incentive spirometry three times a day.

Vascular

Patients with acute spinal cord injury are at a significantly increased risk for deep venous thromboses and pulmonary emboli. The following methods of prevention are instituted in all patients with spinal cord injury who have weakness that does not allow for antigravity mobility of the lower extremities.

(1) Passive range-of-motion exercises for joints below the level of injury are performed twice a day. (2) Passive ankle dorsiflexion and plantar flexion maneuvers are performed, 10 repetitions every 2 hours. (3) Meticulous care is used to avoid trauma to the lower extremities and, therefore, avoid damage to the endothelial lining of the blood vessels. (4) Antithrombotic stockings are applied; they are removed three times a day to examine the skin. (5) The crossed-leg position is avoided. (6) Intermittent pneumatic compression devices are used. (7) Plethysmography is performed every other day. If it indicates deep thrombus formation of the popliteal and femoral veins, full therapeutic anticoagulation is indicated. Doppler studies or venography may be helpful to confirm and define the extent of the deep venous thrombosis. If anticoagulation is specifically contraindicated, a venous filter or umbrella may be used. If a deep venous thrombosis is present above the calf, bed rest for 7 to 10 days, leg elevation, Ace wraps (rewrapped every 3 hours to prevent sequential swellings and to inspect the skin) for the affected leg, and full-dose anticoagulation are prescribed; during this time, no range-of-motion exercises are applied to this leg. Administration of full-dose anticoagulation is then continued for 6 months.

For patients with no evidence of deep venous thrombosis or pulmonary embolus, low-dose subcutaneously administered heparin may be instituted as early as deemed safe after injury or after 2 weeks of negative impedence plethysmography or Doppler ultrasonography monitoring— unless contraindicated by bleeding or a history of bleeding diatheses. Therapy with low-dose heparin should be continued through the initial rehabilitation stay. Recent literature would suggest that low-molecular-weight heparin may provide even better prophylaxis and therapy.

Skin

Because of the lack of pain sensation, patients with spinal cord injury are at high risk for developing pressure sores. Measures used to prevent these sores are as follows. (1) While the patient is on a Foster frame, sheepskin is kept beneath the shoulder area and the sacrum. When the patient is placed on a regular bed, a full-length sheepskin is placed over a water mattress or an alternating air mattress. (2) When the patient is supine, whether on a frame, a water mattress, or a regular bed, a pillow should be placed under the calves to remove pressure from the heels ("bunny boots" or similar padding is not adequate for heel protection). (3) Until the patient can be turned, nursing personnel should reach under the patient and massage the bony prominences every 2 hours. (4) Once the patient is able to be turned, a schedule of turning every 2 hours should be initiated and continued 24 hours a day. (5) The skin should be inspected each time the patient is turned. (6) Bony prominences should be especially diligently monitored. (7) If the patient is wearing a halo vest, a flashlight should be used to assist in inspecting the skin beneath the vest. (8) Care of the halo pin site involves swabbing with hydrogen peroxide and applying an antibiotic ointment (Neosporin) twice a day. (9) When the patient is sitting, a proper wheelchair cushion should be used (for example, a ROHO cushion or a "Bye Bye Decubiti Cushion"). Regular pillows do not provide adequate protection.

Urinary Tract

The goals of urinary tract management are (1) to avoid urinary retention in excess of 500 mL, (2) to prevent upper and lower urinary tract infection, (3) to avoid noxious stimuli to the spinal cord from urinary tract complications, and (4) in 65% of patients, to achieve catheter-free voiding.

As long as intravenously administered fluids are necessary, continuous urinary drainage is maintained with an indwelling catheter and a closed system of urine collection. When an indwelling catheter is used, the following measures apply. (1) In male patients the catheter should be taped to the abdomen to avoid pressure ulcers within the urethra that may lead to penoscrotal fistulas. (2) In female patients the catheter should be taped to the inner aspect of the thigh to prevent pulling on the tube that may damage the bladder or urethra. (3) Fluid intake should be maintained between 2,500 and 3,000 mL per 24 hours, an amount that will allow adequate washout of rapidly multiplying bacteria from the bladder. (4) Because bacteriuria cannot be prevented and occurs within 6 to 10 days after catheterization, antibiotics are not indicated unless the patient is symptomatic or has sepsis. (5) The Silastic Foley catheter (16-F) should be changed every 2 weeks. (6) Urine specimens should be obtained weekly for culture and determination of susceptibilities. If relatively resistant organisms are present, proper isolation procedures should be instituted.

Intermittent catheterization should be started once the intravenous infusions have been discontinued, the urine is sterile, and urine output is approximately 1,400 mL per 24 hours. A urine specimen should be obtained for a Gram stain and a specimen for culture should be obtained from a newly inserted (within 3 days) Silastic Foley catheter (16-F) to determine whether urine is sterile. If either test result is positive, appropriate antibiotic full-dose treatment is initiated before the catheter is removed. If the result of a subsequent Gram stain is negative, intermittent catheterization may be initiated. Weekly urine specimens for culture are obtained during the remainder of hospitalization.

The routine 1,800-mL daily fluid intake schedule is instituted when intermittent catheterization is begun. Preventive measures during intermittent catheterization include bacteriostatic medications such as trimethoprim-sulfamethoxazole (Septra or Bactrim, 1 single-strength tablet orally at bedtime), which has been shown to be more effective than methenamine mandelate (Mandelamine, 1 g four times a day) or methenamine hippurate (Hiprex, 1 g twice a day). (See Chapter 15 for more information on the management of neurogenic bladder.)

Bowel

Once bowel sounds return and the patient is able to tolerate regular foods, the patient should receive a high-fiber diet and docusate sodium (Colace, 100 mg orally once or twice daily). At the same time every day or every other day, a glycerin or bisacodyl (Dulcolax) suppository is used 30 minutes after a meal (this schedule maximizes the use of the gastrocolic reflex). The suppository is not used as a laxative, but rather as a response regulator. If the patient does not expel stool within 20 to 30 minutes, a lubricated gloved finger may be inserted into the rectum for digital stimulation. If there are no results, the program should be repeated the following day at the established time.

Autonomic Hyperreflexia

Autonomic hyperreflexia is a potentially life-threatening syndrome of severe paroxysmal hypertension that can occur after spinal shock has ended in patients who have injuries with lesions above T6-8.[1] It occurs to various extents in upwards of 80% of such patients. Noxious stimulation below the level of the lesion produces massive sympathetic discharges (as part of cord spasticity) that result in marked arteriolar constriction. The result is a marked elevation of blood pressure that cannot be adequately counter regulated because of the interruption of inhibitory neuronal pathways by the spinal lesion.

Typical inciting factors include bladder distention, rectal distention or manipulation, decubital ulcers, urinary tract infection, urinary calculi, a surgical procedure, tight-fitting clothes, pressure on the testicles or glans penis, sexual intercourse, braces, acute abdominal conditions, labor in pregnant women, voiding and bowel movements, or any noxious input to the markedly hyperreflexic cord.

The patient usually experiences sudden marked hypertension, a pounding headache, anxiety, sweating, piloerection, and bradycardia (which results from strong vagal attempts at counterregulation). Other manifestations may include blurred vision, a feeling of impending doom, chest pain, nausea, and respiratory distress.

Immediate management includes elevation of the head of the bed to decrease intracranial pressure, monitoring of blood pressure and pulse every 5 minutes, removal of all tight clothing, braces, or leg bags, and checking for bladder and bowel distention. Because a distended bladder is frequently the cause, the urinary catheter should be routinely irrigated immediately; if the catheter is plugged, it should be changed immediately. If these procedures do not produce a satisfactory response, the patient should be checked for rectal impaction by applying an anesthetic ointment (Nupercainal) into the anal canal and to the perianal skin. Then, a well-lubricated gloved finger may be inserted slowly to check for a fecal impaction. Blood pressure should be monitored during the rectal examination. If an impaction is present and the blood pressure increases to 200/130 mm Hg, ganglionic blockage should be obtained before removal of the impaction.

If the patient does not respond to the above measures, drug treatment should be initiated while a primary cause is being identified. This could include nifedipine, mecamylamine (Inversine), hydralazine, or diazoxide, depending on the circumstances. Admission to the intensive care unit for monitoring and intravenous administration of nitroprusside may be necessary.

Orthostatic Hypotension

Not infrequently, patients with spinal cord injury are subject to precipitous drops in blood pressure, often without premonition. The patient may suddenly lose consciousness. Activities associated with the falls in blood pressure are usually related to postural changes such as going from supine to sitting or exceeding sitting tolerance, with a drop in blood pressure being the limiting factor. Blood pressure must be carefully monitored, especially in the earliest attempts to sit a newly injured patient. Other associated activities may include eating and drinking. The mechanism seems to be pooling of blood in the abdomen and the dependent extremities associated with the absence of reflex vasoconstriction with lesions above the sympathetic outflow (T-5 to T-8).[1]

If the patient complains of light-headedness, dizziness, or a feeling of faintness, he or she should be placed in a recumbent position with the lower extremities elevated. If the patient is in a wheelchair, the brakes should be locked and the chair should be tipped backward immediately to lower the patient's head and elevate the lower extremities.

Preventive measures include (1) the use of thigh-length support garments or Ace wraps (the skin is inspected and the wraps are reapplied every 3 hours), (2) the use of a lumbosacral corset with sheepskin lining, designed for spinal cord injuries, (3) gradual changes from the supine to the upright position, and (4) judicious increments in the time spent "up."

Spasticity

Spasticity is a condition of excessive reflex activity of the spinal cord below the level of the lesion, often associated with involuntary movements. In patients who are unable to initiate voluntary movement, marked involuntary movement sometimes evolves. Spasticity develops in most patients with injury above the sacral aspect of the spinal cord. The type and magnitude may vary greatly from patient to patient.

Spasticity is not present at the onset of spinal cord injury. The period immediately after injury is termed "spinal shock." It is characterized by diminished muscle tone and absent stretch reflexes. The duration of spinal shock varies from a few days to several months. As spinal shock subsides, the activity of the stretch reflexes and muscle tone gradually increase. Spasticity may cause discomfort, may interfere with daily functioning (for example, by interfering with stability during transfers), or may result in secondary complications such as contractures, decubital ulcers, bladder hypertrophy with vesicoureteral reflux, and fractures.

Identification, elimination, and diligent prevention of nociceptive input to the spinal cord and participation in a reasonable twice-daily stretching program are the basics of therapy. A hierarchy of treatment methods may be used. In addition to stretching, medications, intramuscular neurolysis of key muscle groups, intrathecal and peripheral neurolysis, tenotomies, neurectomies, rhizotomies, myelotomies, cordotomies, and cordectomies may be used.

Heterotopic Ossification

The deposition of para-articular bone occurs in from 10% to 50% of patients with newly acquired spinal cord injuries.[1] This bone formation typically appears within the first 6 months after injury and usually affects the hips, but other joints below the level of the spinal lesion may be involved. The clinical presentation is often a slight decrease in hip range of motion that may progress to severe loss of motion about the affected joints. The early clinical appearance may mimic that of a deep venous thrombosis with warmth and swelling in one or both lower extremities. Early roentgenograms may not demonstrate the calcium deposition, but a bone scan may be diagnostic. Typically, the bone fraction of alkaline phosphatase is elevated.

Vigorous passive range-of-motion exercises are necessary to maintain range. Etidronate (Didronel) may retard the development of this condition, but it is generally thought to be of little value once calcium deposition is evident roentgenographically. For cases in which the loss of range of motion has become so severe that it limits daily functioning (for example, an inability to flex the hips sufficiently to sit), surgical resection followed by radiation therapy may become necessary. Wedge resection of the heterotopic ossification should not be done until the bone has ceased to grow. An indication of cessation of bone growth is reduction of the bone fraction of serum alkaline phosphatase.

TABLE 14–2

Functional Goals for Patients With Spinal Cord Injury, by Level

Goal	Level of Injury*							
	C-4	C-5	C-6	C-7	C-8 to T-1	T-2 to T-12	L-1 to L-3	L-4 to S-1
Self-care								
Feeding	O	P	P	I	I	I	I	I
Dressing	O	D	D	P/I	I	I	I	I
Grooming	O	D/P	P	P/I	I	I	I	I
Bladder, bowel	O	D	D/P	I	I	I	I	I
Bathing	O	D	P	P	I	I	I	I
Wheelchair activity								
Special control, powered	I	I	I	I	I	I	I	I
Manual propulsion	O	P	P/I	I	I	I	I	I
Transfers to and from	O	D	P	I	I	I	I	I
Bed mobility	O	D	P	I	I	I	I	I
Communications								
Telephone	P	P	I	I	I	I	I	I
Writing	O	D/P	P	P	I	I	I	I
Typing	P	P	P	P	I	I	I	I
Ambulation	O	O	O	O	O	D	P	P
Orthoses	ECU	UEO	UEO	UEO		KAFO	KAFO	AFO
Transportation								
Driving with hand controls	O	D/P	P	I	I	I	I	I
Public (train, plane)	O	D	D	P/I	I	I	I	I
Public (bus without lift)	O	O	O	O	O	O	O	P

*AFO, ankle-foot orthosis; D, dependent, but can assist; ECU, environmental control unit; I, full independence; KAFO, knee-ankle-foot orthosis; O, not possible; P, partial or full independence with special equipment; UEO, upper extremity orthosis.
From Stover et al.[2] By permission of the publisher.

RESIDUAL FUNCTIONAL CAPACITIES

The level of spinal cord injury has implications for the expected level of functioning in daily life (Table 14–2).

PATIENT EDUCATION

Major emphasis is placed on patient education throughout rehabilitation. The person with a spinal cord injury must learn to function with a substantially reduced physical capacity in a society that retains many physical and attitudinal barriers for persons with disability. The person with a spinal cord injury must learn to practice new preventive living habits and must learn to educate persons who come in contact with him or her as to

TABLE 14–3

Guidelines for Annual Follow-up of Persons With Spinal Cord Injury

History and physical examination, with special emphasis on
1. the status of the spine, spinal cord, and brain
2. the function of the genitourinary, musculoskeletal, gastrointestinal, vascular, and respiratory systems and skin
3. nutritional, psychosocial, and vocational aspects of independent living and healthy living habits

Laboratory studies, to screen the overall state of health, including complete blood count, chemistry group, sedimentation rate, urinalysis, urine Gram stain, urine culture and susceptibilities, residual urine volume(s), iothalamate short renal clearance, roentgenograms of kidneys, ureters, and bladder, excretory urogram with 20-minute film (or diethylenetriamine pentaacetic acid short renal scan), cystometrogram-electromyogram with urethral pressure profile, cystoscopy, and spine roentgenograms as appropriate

Physical therapy review for mobility, transfers, range-of-motion exercises and stretching exercises, wheelchair and wheelchair mobility, braces, possible upper extremity reconstruction or tendon transfers

Occupational therapy review for activities of daily living, adaptive equipment, driving, possible upper extremity reconstruction

As appropriate, review by social services, psychologist, recreational therapist, orthopedist, neurologist or neurosurgeon, urologist, internist

In general,
1. patients with uncomplicated courses who have paraplegia or low tetraplegia (C-6 to C-8 lesions) may be reviewed on an outpatient basis
2. patients with mid- to high-level tetraplegia (weak C-5 and above) are better served in the hospital

proper care. The injured person must redevelop a positive self-image and learn to project in a constructive and self-assertive manner toward able-bodied persons who do not have experience in interacting with persons who have spinal cord injuries.[6]

DURATION OF INITIAL HOSPITALIZATION

A patient with mid- to low-level complete paraplegia may expect a 2- to 3-month initial hospital stay. A patient with tetraplegia may expect a 3- to 5-month stay if he or she has a relatively uncomplicated course.

FOLLOW-UP

Because many of the acute-care concerns remain significant risks for the rest of a patient's life, and many of the social, emotional, and vocational goals are pursued after the initial hospitalization, regular, life-long follow-up visits are essential for redeveloping and maintaining health and maximal functional capacities.

A typical follow-up schedule includes a return visit at 1 and 4 months after dismissal and at yearly intervals thereafter for a complete review. Additional follow-up contacts are made as necessary (Table 14–3).

REFERENCES

1. Ruskin AP, ed. Spinal cord injury. In: Current therapy in physiatry: physical medicine and rehabilitation. Philadelphia: WB Saunders, 1984:379–456.
2. Stover SL, Donovan WH, Freed MM, et al. Rehabilitation in spinal cord disorders. In: Self-directed medical knowledge program in physical medicine and rehabilitation—syllabus. 2nd ed. Chicago: American Academy of Physical Medicine and Rehabilitation, 1985:K1–22.
3. Standards for neurological and functional classification of spinal cord injury, Revised 1992. Chicago: American Paralysis Association, 1992.
4. Young W, DeGrescito V, Flamm ES, et al. Pharmacological therapy of acute spinal cord injury: studies of high dose methylprednisolone and naloxone. Clin Neurosurg 1988; 34:675–697.
5. Mayo Clinic Spinal Cord Injury Committee. Spinal cord injury preventive care guidelines. Rochester, Minnesota: Mayo Foundation, 1991.
6. SCI patient manual. Department of Physical Medicine and Rehabilitation, Mayo Clinic and Nursing Service, Rehabilitation Nursing, Saint Mary's Hospital, Rochester, Minnesota, 1979.

15

Bladder Retraining

Karen L. Andrews
Joachim L. Opitz

Bladder retraining has become an integral part of the rehabilitation of patients with spinal cord injury,[1-8] in selected brain-injured patients, and in patients who have atonic myogenic detrusor insufficiency (underactive bladder and normoactive outlet[9]) associated with habit contraction of the external urethral sphincter.[10] Bladder retraining can be effective with an organized training program[4] utilizing urodynamic diagnostic procedures, biofeedback, neuropharmacology, and appropriate urologic surgical procedures.[3, 5] The purpose of this chapter is to discuss the indications, contraindications, procedural guidelines, and results of bladder retraining.

GOALS

The goals of bladder retraining are (1) to ensure free flow of urine from the kidneys without overloading the ureteral work capacity, (2) to keep outflow resistance and bladder spasticity at acceptably low levels, (3) to empty the bladder regularly (generally every 3 hours) and adequately (consistently less than 100 mL of residual urine volume) for the maintenance of abacteriuria, and (4) to reestablish urinary continence.

INDICATIONS

Patients must be motivated to learn the motor skills that are necessary to regain efficient, catheter-free voiding (within safe voiding pressures) while permanently maintaining a regular voiding and drinking schedule to maintain continence. Bladder retraining is indicated in patients who have neurogenic hyperreflexic (overactive[9]) bladder dysfunction with or without

external sphincter dyssynergia, neurogenic hyporeflexic or areflexic bladder (underactive bladder[9]) dysfunctions with or without dyssynergia, or
atonic myogenic detrusor insufficiency. Patients with uninhibited bladder
dysfunction due to brain injury may also benefit from parts of the bladder
retraining program.

CONTRAINDICATIONS

Bladder retraining may be contraindicated in patients with decompen-
sating renal function, especially when paired with incompetent vesicoureteral junctions. It is also contraindicated in patients with severe cysti-
tis, bladder calculi, or major structural changes of either the bladder or the
urethra; in patients who cannot adhere to the necessary training procedures and record keeping; in the very young; in debilitated elderly patients; in unmotivated or undisciplined patients; and in patients who are
unable to do the necessary activities for voiding, such as transferring to the
toilet or dressing and undressing.

TEAM APPROACH

A team approach is necessary because bladder retraining requires (1)
regular intermittent catheterization, (2) urodynamic testing and retesting,
(3) acquisition of knowledge, (4) learning of new psychomotor skills and
living habits, and at times (5) neurourologic surgical procedures.

The team is headed by the physiatrist and includes the patient, the
neurourologist, the bladder therapist, the primary rehabilitation nurse, and,
when available, members of the catheterization team. The team is also
supported by diagnostic and therapeutic facilities of a major medical center.

The participation of a knowledgeable primary physician (frequently a
physiatrist) who has the proper understanding of (1) the urodynamics of the
various bladder and urethral dysfunctions, (2) control of infection of the
impaired urinary tract, (3) the effects of neurourologic medications, and (4)
the indications for neurourologic procedures is indispensable for successful
bladder retraining.

The physician must analyze the voiding data with the patient and
associated staff daily to determine optimal actions (such as voiding
technique, drug therapy, and urologic surgical procedures) for bladder retraining.

THE WORKUP

The success of bladder retraining depends on the correct urodynamic
diagnosis, psychosocial factors, and the exclusion of contraindications.

Bladder retraining should not be started until a stable neurourologic condition is established, the workup has been completed, the lower urinary tract is free of foreign bodies and infection, and intermittent catheterization yields acceptable volumes of retained urine (less than 400 mL).

Excretory urography (intravenous pyelography), [^{125}I]iothalamate short renal clearance test of renal function, and urine culture and sensitivity studies may be performed while the patient is still using an indwelling catheter. A complete blood cell count, serum electrolyte levels, serum creatinine value, and blood urea nitrogen value should also be determined. After the patient has received specific antibiotics for 24 to 48 hours for any existing bacteriuria and fluid output is reduced to less than 1,800 mL per 24 hours, intermittent catheterization may be started.

With intermittent catheterization, concomitant bacteriostatic medications should be used, such as trimethoprim-sulfamethoxazole (Septra or Bactrim, 1 single-strength tablet orally at bedtime) or methenamine salts (Mandelamine, 1 g four times a day, or Hiprex, 1 g twice a day). The patient is monitored with weekly Gram stain, urinalysis, or urine cultures as indicated while in the hospital. In 85% of patients, the lower urinary tract can be kept free of infection during hospitalization. With weekly monitoring, recurrent bacteriuria can be treated promptly and specifically. Further, intermittent catheterization rids both the bladder and the urethra of the ongoing irritation of an indwelling catheter, which is especially detrimental in patients with hyperreflexic bladders. After several days of intermittent catheterization, the bladder becomes less irritated.

If abacteriuria is demonstrated by a negative Gram stain on the day of the planned studies, a urodynamic evaluation is done with cystometrography/sphincter electromyography (CMG/EMG) and a urethral pressure profile (UPP). Cystoscopy, when indicated, should be performed thereafter because it interferes with the urodynamic testing. If bladder stones are suspected, cystoscopy may have to precede urodynamic studies.

CMG/EMG may be done with the patient in the lithotomy or sitting position. An indwelling Foley catheter is placed in the bladder and two EMG recording leads are placed at the 2 and 10 o'clock positions perianally to record the electrical activity of the pelvic floor musculature. The muscles of the pelvic floor receive innervation from the same sacral root levels as the external urethral sphincter. Therefore, increased electrical activity in these muscles is used as an indirect measure of the electrical activity of the external urethral sphincter—the greater the electrical activity, the tighter the sphincter closes about the urethra to obstruct urine flow.

Initially, the absence or presence of voluntary control of the pelvic floor musculature is documented. Then the presence or absence of the bulbocavernosus reflex, mediated by the S2–4 nerve root, is determined by tugging on the indwelling catheter and observing a momentary reflex increase in the activity of the pelvic floor musculature. Subsequently, warm normal saline or CO_2 is introduced into the bladder through the catheter at a rate of 25 mL per minute. The intravesicular (within the bladder) pressure is monitored during filling. The presence or absence of a sensation of fullness and of a need to void is monitored. Then, the quality, degree, control, or absence of a detrusor (bladder muscle) contraction is determined by observing the intravesicular pressure changes over time. The various voiding techniques (tapping, Credé maneuver, straining, massage, or perineal stimulation) are evaluated by observing the resulting pressure changes. It is important to observe whether the normal quieting of electrical activity in the pelvic floor musculature occurs with the contractions of the detrusor during attempted voiding. Incoordination may exist between the expulsive pressure (detrusor) and retentive pressure (external sphincter) when the detrusor and pelvic floor muscles cocontract. Such incoordination is called "detrusor-sphincter dyssynergia."

The internal urethral sphincter mechanism (bladder neck) is actually the base of the bladder, which normally forms a funnel shape when voiding is attempted. In certain types of bladder dysfunction, this funneling may not occur, resulting in an inability to empty the bladder properly without the use of a catheter. The function of this funneling can be tested with the use of a modified CMG/EMG technique called cinecystourethrography, or "video CMG/EMG." For this test, a radiopaque liquid is used instead of carbon dioxide or normal saline, and real-time fluoroscopy can be used to visualize the anatomic function of the bladder outlet (simultaneously, all the previously described factors are also recorded). Visualization of the bladder outlet and proximal urethra may also be accomplished with bladder ultrasonography using a rectal probe.[11]

CMG/EMG may be difficult. Patients may be unable to void while they are on the table or in the highly unfamiliar and populated diagnostic operating room.

Routinely, after the initial excretory urogram (intravenous pyelogram) has been obtained, a neurourologist is asked to evaluate the urologic data, participate in the urologic workup, and determine the need for possible surgical intervention before bladder retraining. At the Mayo Clinic, the initial "diagnostic" CMG/EMG is performed immediately before cystoscopy in the operating room. Subsequent CMG/EMG studies, known as "therapeutic" CMG/EMG, are performed in a special procedures room of the rehabilitation unit.

THE TRAINING PROGRAM

Once the team members and the patient decide to pursue bladder retraining, the patient is instructed by a bladder therapist or rehabilitation nurse in the basic urologic anatomy, the specific data recording required of the patient, the purpose and technique of therapeutic CMG/EMG, and the rationale of the retraining procedures as they relate to the specific bladder dysfunction present.

Because the team members can only assist the patient in his or her own efforts at bladder retraining, the patient is made fully responsible for adhering to a drinking, voiding, and catheterization schedule. The drinking schedule usually consists of a well-timed fluid intake of 1,800 mL per 24 hours (400 mL at meal times and 200 mL at 10 A.M., 2 P.M., and 4 P.M.). Attempts at voiding, by use of the specific techniques that gave the best response during CMG/EMG, should be made and promptly recorded by the patient at least every 3 hours while the patient is awake. The schedule of intermittent catheterization (every 6 hours) allows careful daily monitoring of residual urine volume.

The patient is responsible for recording the following data as soon as they become available: intake, intentional voiding (amount in milliliters), unintentional voiding (in relative degrees), and the amount of residual urine volume obtained every 6 hours (by intermittent catheterization, after attempted voiding). The residual urine volume is particularly helpful to determine the efficiency of voiding. The patient records the data on a daily record sheet (Fig. 15–1), which is kept on a clipboard at the bedside.

For an overview of the data that accumulate day by day, the patient also records the values of the 24-hour fluid volumes of the preceding day in the form of a graph, which indicates an increase, a leveling off, or a decrease in the efficiency of voiding (Fig. 15–2). This graph sheet is also

RECORD OF BLADDER RETRAINING

Date _____ Name _____ MC No _____

TIME	FLUID INTAKE — All beverages, also include soup, ice cream, jello, fruit	INTENTIONAL — VOLITIONAL (NOT triggered, strained or manually expressed)	INTENTIONAL — TRIGGERED, STRAINED or MANUALLY EXPRESSED	UNINTENTIONAL — INCONTINENCE— or SPONTANEOUS voidings	CATHETERIZATION — RESIDUAL CHECKS or RETENTIONS — SELF - TEAM
1:00 AM					
2:00					
3:00					
4:00					
5:00					
6:00					
7:00					
8:00					
9:00					
10:00					
11:00					
12:00 N					
1:00 PM					
2:00					
3:00					
4:00					
5:00					
6:00					
7:00					
8:00					
9:00					
10:00					
11:00					
12:00 MN					
SUBTOTAL					
TOTAL IN:		TOTAL OUT:			

Figure 15–1
Daily record sheet on which patients receiving bladder retraining record time and volumes of fluid intake, intentional and unintentional voidings, and residual urine volumes. (From Opitz.[10] By permission of the publisher.)

kept on a clipboard at the bedside. Initially, the 24-hour volumes of urine intentionally voided are much lower than the 24-hour volumes of residual urine. As success in bladder retraining evolves, a crossover occurs between the volumes of intentionally voided urine and those of residual urine, but the 24-hour fluid intake remains unchanged at about 1,800 mL. The graphic representation of the efficiency of voiding is a strong motivating factor for the patient. It also serves as an important instrument for quick orientation of the members of the rehabilitation team.

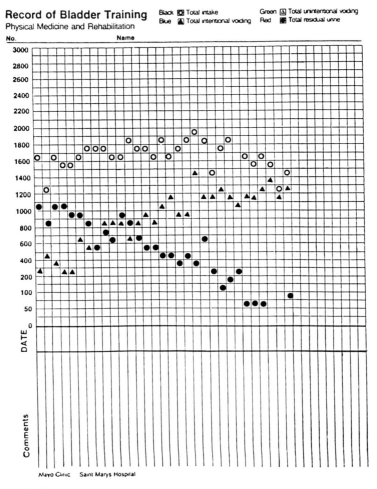

Figure 15–2
Data from woman with complete flaccid detrusor and external urethral sphincter paralysis after central disk compression of sacral cord. (From Opitz.[10] By permission of the publisher.)

GUIDELINES TO RETRAINING FOR SPECIFIC BLADDER AND URETHRAL SPHINCTER DYSFUNCTIONS

Uninhibited Neurogenic Bladder Dysfunction

Patients with brain injury in which a lesion exists between the cerebral cortex and the pontine micturition center have uninhibited neurogenic bladder dysfunction. Because the pontine micturition center, which remains intact, is responsible for the coordinated function of the spinal micturition center (S-2 to S-4), the normal kinesiology of micturition is undisturbed. However, because the patient lacks awareness of the urge to void and does not adequately suppress the pontine-spinal loops of micturition, incontinence by reflex voiding occurs. This incontinence is usually frequent and complete.

Patients with brain injury (cerebrovascular accident, trauma, or tumor) in whom either urinary retention or incontinence persists after removal of the catheter need to have a detailed urologic workup (as previously described) to determine whether the cause is structural or functional or both.

If the lower urinary tract is normal, bladder retraining consists of regular attempts at voiding, concentrating on the patient's early, conscious awareness of bladder fullness. These regular attempts at voiding should be coordinated with a balanced intake of liquids (the fluid schedule outlined previously). Light suprapubic tapping may be helpful as an initial sensory cue. When such a stimulus is consciously perceived, it can be associated with the sensation of a full bladder and the urge to void. Appropriate suppression of the urge to void then follows as the patient is able to suppress the micturition centers until it is socially acceptable to void.

Occasionally, the use of low-dose anticholinergic medications, such as propantheline bromide (Pro-Banthine) or oxybutynin (Ditropan), may lessen the resting tone of the bladder and inhibit the voiding reflex. Because these medications lessen the expulsive force of the detrusor, they may result in urinary retention—especially in elderly men.

Hyperreflexic, Dyssynergic (Upper Motor Neuron) Bladder Dysfunction

A neurologic lesion between the pons and the sacrum disturbs the relationship between and the pontine and sacral micturition centers, rendering the function of the sacral micturition center dyssynergic. Dyssynergia is characterized by various degrees of cocontractions of the detrusor and external sphincter muscles causing high voiding pressures and incomplete emptying of the bladder.' In bladder retraining the emphasis has to be placed on developing a spinal micturition reflex that favors detrusor contraction of adequate strength with minimal external sphincter cocontraction (dyssynergia).

Usually, the reflex is best developed by the use of rapid, yet light, suprapubic tapping (Fig. 15–3) at a place where the highest degree of reflex response is obtained. Performing heavy and slow suprapubic tapping—on the basis that if a little works, more is better—is a misconception to which uninformed staff and patients frequently succumb. Heavy tapping usually leads to increasing degrees of dyssynergia, which give rise to a vicious cycle of increased dyssynergia, increased detrusor contractions, increased residual urine volumes, increased incidence of bladder infection, and further increase of dyssynergia. Progressive bladder hypertrophy associated with dyssynergia will eventually result in vesicoureteral reflux and upper tract complications.

Anticholinergic medications such as propantheline, oxybutynin, or imipramine are often useful for the management of upper motor neuron bladder dysfunction by decreasing detrusor reflexivity and force of contraction. Occasionally, an α-sympathetic blocking agent such as phenoxybenzamine can be helpful by decreasing the tone of the bladder neck and proximal urethral smooth muscle. To a lesser degree, the spasticity of the striated muscle of the external urethral sphincter may be relaxed by antispasticity medications such as baclofen, diazepam (Valium), or dantrolene (Dantrium).

At times, all of these methods fail and a surgical procedure may be beneficial. A limited external sphincterotomy may be required to reduce the outlet resistance to urine flow.

Areflexic Detrusor and External Sphincter (Lower Motor Neuron) Bladder Dysfunction

A neurologic lesion involving either the sacral micturition center or its connections to the bladder and pelvic floor muscles gives rise to an

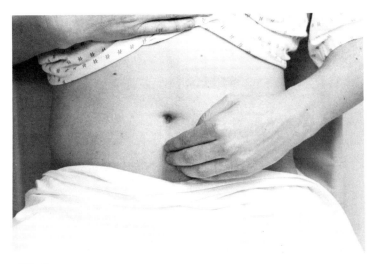

Figure 15–3
Method of catheter-free voiding for upper motor neuron bladder dysfunction: light tapping.

areflexic detrusor and external sphincter or lower motor neuron type of bladder dysfunction (underactive bladder and underactive outlet[9]). Because the bladder lacks expulsive force, such force needs to be supplied by straining (Valsalva maneuver) (Fig. 15–4) or by the open-hand or closed-hand Credé maneuver (manual compression of the bladder) (Fig. 15–5) so that the bladder neck is adequately pulled open for efficient emptying.

Initial use of an α-sympathetic blocking agent such as phenoxybenzamine (10 to 20 mg daily) reduces the resistance to opening of the bladder outlet as the intrabladder pressure is increased by either straining or the Credé maneuver. Once the tissue resistance of the bladder outlet has decreased with frequently practiced voiding, use of phenoxybenzamine can usually be discontinued before the patient is dismissed.

The technique of straining (Valsalva maneuver) involves sitting and resting the abdomen forward on the thighs for both men and women. During straining in this position, hugging of the knees and legs may prevent any bulging of the abdomen. In this manner, all of the increase in intraabdominal pressure is transferred to the bladder and the pelvic floor.

The open-hand Credé method involves placing the thumb of each hand over the area of the left and right anterosuperior iliac spine and the digits over the suprapubic area with slight overlapping of the tips. The slightly overlapped digits are then pressed into the abdomen. When they have gotten well behind the symphysis, the pressure is directed downward to compress the fundus of the bladder. Both hands are then pressed as deeply as possible downward into the pelvic cavity. At times, the bladder can be compressed more efficiently by using the fist of one hand (closed-hand method) (Fig. 15–5) or a rolled-up towel.

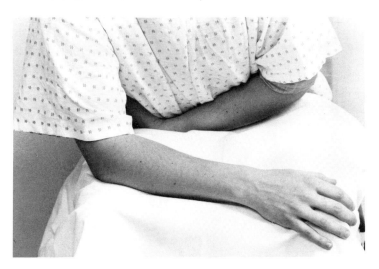

Figure 15–4
Method of catheter-free voiding for lower motor neuron bladder dysfunction: straining (Valsalva maneuver).

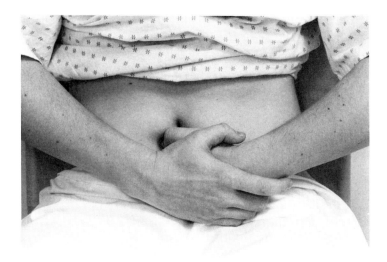

Figure 15–5
Method of catheter-free voiding for lower motor neuron bladder dysfunction: Credé maneuver.

Administering the cholinergic medication bethanechol 45 minutes before voiding may augment mechanical stimulation of the detrusor. This medication usually causes increased muscle tone of the bladder. A previously flaccid bladder can then be palpated suprapubically as a round organ with a definite tone. The Credé maneuvers can then generate higher transmural pressure and more efficient opening of the proximal urethra.

Straining (Valsalva maneuver) at the time the Credé maneuver is applied should be avoided because it increases the intra-abdominal pressure, causes bulging of the abdominal wall, and tends to lift the compressing hands off the fundus of the bladder. Instead, patients are asked to attempt voiding by one method first and then, after a period of relaxation, by the other method to determine whether it causes further voiding. In this way, both methods are tried and the more efficient method can be determined. In our experience, the duration of bladder retraining is about the same in patients with hyperreflexic as in those with areflexic neurogenic dysfunction of the bladder.

Others

The management of mixed neurogenic bladder dysfunctions (overactive bladder and underactive outlet or underactive bladder and overactive outlet, according to the International Continence Society classification[9]) and areflexic myogenic detrusor insufficiency (end-organ failure) is beyond the scope of this chapter. A detailed description of them, the optimal voiding techniques, and helpful neurologic medications has been published.[10]

TABLE 15–1

Success Rate of Bladder Retraining in Patients With Spinal Cord Injury

Reference	No. of Patients	Residual Urine (mL*)	Mean Time of Training (Days)	Retraining Successful (%)	Abacteriuric Patients (%†)
Bors[1]	36	—	—	78	—
Comarr[2]	109	Balanced bladder‡	—	87	—
Stover et al.[8]	33	150	21	57	32
Opitz[4]	120	65	62	78	91
Gjone and Ween[12]	116	150	59	80	65
Merritt and Ilstrup (unpublished data)	58	100	—	69	91
Sperling[6]	41	100	17	46	84
Perkash[5]	104	100	—	56	—
Fam et al.[3]	120	50	35	98	—
Total or average	737	102	39	72	73

*Acceptable maximal volume for catheter-free voiding.
†Colony counts were $\leq 10^5$/mL.
‡Residual urine volume was usually ≤ 100 mL.
Modified from Opitz.[9]

RESULTS

Data from nine studies comprising 737 patients who underwent bladder retraining between 1967 and 1978 (Table 15–1) indicated that the average acceptable residual urine volume after catheter-free voiding at the end of bladder retraining (mean duration, 39 days) was 102 mL. The success rate of bladder retraining was 72%. An average of 73% of 265 patients were free of catheter and urinary tract infection ($\leq 10^5$ colonies/mL) at dismissal.

Gjone and Ween[12] reported the follow-up data from 71 of their 116 patients (average duration of follow-up, 4½ years). Of these 71 patients, 63% had residual urine volumes of 150 mL or less at their follow-up visits. Episodes of recurrent bacteriuria occurred after dismissal in 42% of these patients. Positive findings on excretory urography were noted in 14% of the patients initially and in 11% at dismissal.

Viera et al.[13] analyzed the follow-up data from 99 patients. Of these 99 patients, 56 had their last follow-up examination more than 15 months after bladder retraining. The residual urine volume was 100 mL or less in 58%. The overall incidence of bacteriuria was 24% (colony count, $\leq 10^4$/mL).

SUMMARY

With the use of modern urodynamic evaluations (which may include exploration of the optimal voiding techniques for an individual patient), neurourologically active medications, a well-structured program of bladder retraining, and carefully selected urologic operations, the success rate of bladder retraining has been increasing. With the normalization of voiding pressures during catheter-free voiding, careful eradication of bacteriuria, regular and careful voiding habits, and regular follow-up surveillance of persons with neurogenic bladder dysfunction after successful bladder retraining, the incidence of serious complications of the urinary tract can be expected to decrease further. A need exists for carefully conducted, prospective follow-up studies.

REFERENCES

1. Bors E. Intermittent catheterization in paraplegic patients. Urol Int 1967; 22:236–249.
2. Comarr AE. Follow-up on intermittent catheterization among spinal cord injury patients. Proc Vet Admin Spinal Cord Injury Conf 1969; 17:133–139.
3. Fam BA, Rossier AB, Blunt K, et al. Experience in the urologic management of 120 early spinal cord injury patients. J Urol 1978; 119:485–487.
4. Opitz JL. Bladder retraining: an organized program. Mayo Clin Proc 1976; 51:367–372.
5. Perkash I. Intermittent catheterization failure and an approach to bladder rehabilitation in spinal cord injury patients. Arch Phys Med Rehabil 1978; 59:9–17.
6. Sperling KB. Intermittent catheterization to obtain catheter-free bladder function in spinal cord injury. Arch Phys Med Rehabil 1978; 59:4–8.
7. Stolov WC. Rehabilitation of the bladder in injuries of the spinal cord. Arch Phys Med Rehabil 1959; 40:467–474.
8. Stover SL, Miller JM III, Nepomuceno CS. Intermittent catheterization in patients previously on indwelling catheter drainage. Arch Phys Med Rehabil 1973; 54:25–30.
9. The International Continence Society. Fourth report on the standardization of terminology of lower urinary tract function. Br J Urol 1981; 53:330–335.
10. Opitz JL. Treatment of voiding dysfunction in spinal-cord-injured patients: bladder retraining. In: Barrett DM, Wein AJ, eds. Controversies in neurourology. New York: Churchill Livingstone, 1984:437–451.
11. Perkash I, Friedland GW. Transrectal ultrasonography of the lower urinary tract: evaluation of bladder neck problems. Neurourol Urodynamics 1986; 5:299–306.
12. Gjone RN, Ween E. Results of bladder training 1966–1974. Paraplegia 1977–1978; 15:47–54.
13. Viera A, Merritt JL, Erickson RP. Renal function in spinal cord injury: a preliminary report. Arch Phys Med Rehabil 1986; 67:257–259.

PART V

Rehabilitation in Metabolic Bone Disease

16

Metabolic Bone Disease

Mehrsheed Sinaki

Bone has three functions: 1) to make the mechanical framework for the body, 2) to be the body's major store of calcium, and 3) to protect the internal organs. The skeleton must be strong enough to withstand mechanical stress, and it also has to be available for the maintenance of homeostasis by yielding a part of its mineral content on demand.[1]

Metabolic and age-related bone loss syndromes create a significant health care problem. Because of an increasing geriatric population, the number of patients who will have musculoskeletal problems will increase (Fig. 16–1). These disorders not only cause pain and disability but also result in 1.2 million fractures in the United States each year.[2] A hip fracture will prove fatal in 12% to 20% of cases, and its overall economic impact on the health care system is about $6.1 billion annually.[3]

Osteoporosis is the most prevalent metabolic bone disease in the United States. It consists of a heterogeneous group of syndromes in which there is reduced bone mass per unit volume in otherwise normal bone, which results in more fragile bone. The increment in bone porosity results in architectural instability of bone and increases the likelihood of fracture. In osteoporosis, the ratio of mineral to matrix is normal, whereas in osteomalacia, mineral is significantly reduced. Osteoporosis becomes clinically significant only when the bone fractures. Osteopenia is the generalized reduction of bone mass.

PATHOGENESIS: BONE REMODELING

The cells of bone consist of osteoclasts, osteoblasts, and osteocytes. Multinucleated osteoclasts, bone-resorbing cells that originate in the monocyte-macrophage cell line, resorb an apparently predetermined volume of bone. After this process, the osteoclasts disappear and are replaced by osteoblasts, which lay down osteoid, refilling the cavity. After the osteoid is mineralized, the repair process is completed. Osteoblasts emerge

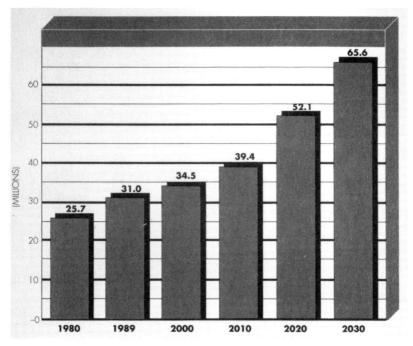

Figure 16–1
Number of persons in the United States age 65 years or older, 1980–2030. (From the American Geriatrics Society. Advertising pamphlet for Beck JC, ed. Geriatrics review syllabus: a core curriculum in geriatric medicine. 2nd ed. Chicago: The American Geriatrics Society, 1992. By permission of the Society.)

from the complex structure of the marrow cavity. These cells are separated from osteoclasts through lineage. Cell types in bone other than osteoclasts, such as macrophages, osteocytes, and perhaps even osteoblasts, may be capable of bone dissolution under highly selective circumstances. However, osteoblasts are not responsible for bulk resorption of bone under usual physiologic conditions.[4] Some osteoblasts are internalized in the newly formed matrix and become osteocytes. Osteocytes maintain contact with each other and with surface osteoblasts through cell processes that make up the microcanalicular system of bone.

Peak bone mass in the human skeleton is achieved in the third decade of life. The adult skeleton undergoes a continual process of remodeling in which bone resorption is coupled with bone formation.

The entire remodeling cycle, from activation to complete repair, takes about 100 days. Bone resorption and formation are coupled. In ideal homeostasis, the amount of bone at the initiation of a remodeling cycle is expected to be equal to the bone at the completion of the same cycle. At any one time, about 2 million remodeling units are active throughout the human skeleton.[5] Whenever bone resorption exceeds bone formation, osteopenia or osteoporosis occurs. Therefore, factors that increase bone turnover in favor of resorption decrease bone volume. The complex cellular system that preserves the bone mass consists of a heterogeneous group of cells forming the basic multicellular unit.[6] At each remodeling cycle, a stereotyped sequence of events occurs.

In humans, parathyroid hormone, 1,25-dihydroxyvitamin D_3, and possibly calcitonin are known regulators of calcium homeostasis,[7, 8] and their imbalance can contribute to bone loss. Changes in hormone levels can be associated with an increased risk of osteoporosis. Among these are changes in serum parathyroid hormone with age. Decreased renal function decreases plasma 1,25-dihydroxyvitamin D_3, and this decrease may stimulate the secretion of parathyroid hormone indirectly or directly. Parathyroid hormone stimulates osteoclastic activity and through this phenomenon increases bone resorption and the serum calcium concentration. It also increases distal tubular reabsorption of calcium in the kidneys. Parathyroid hormone, by stimulating osteoclastic activity, increases bone remodeling. In normal bone, the resorption and formation are coupled, and when there is an imbalance in the ratio of formation to resorption, an increment in the rate of remodeling bone can result in bone loss. In thyrotoxicosis, bone remodeling and loss of bone mass are increased, and these changes are associated with an increased incidence of osteoporosis.

The major determinant of calcium absorption is 1,25-dihydroxyvitamin D_3 (Fig. 16–2).[9] Vitamin D increases calcium and phosphorus absorption from the intestines and reabsorption from the kidneys.[10] Vitamin D at supraphysiologic levels can stimulate bone resorption.[11] Shortage of vitamin D can result in poorly mineralized bone or osteomalacia. Calcitonin is a 32-amino acid protein produced by thyroid C cells in higher mammals. Calcitonin inhibits osteoclast-mediated bone resorption. It is known

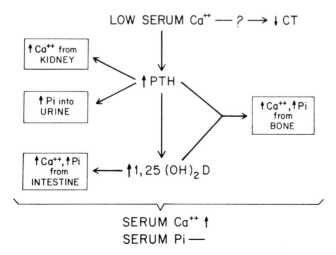

Figure 16–2
Sequence of events initiated in response to hypocalcemia. Ca^{++}, serum calcium; CT, calcitonin; $1,25(OH)_2D$, 1,25-dihydroxyvitamin D; PTH, parathyroid hormone; Pi, serum phosphorus. (From Stewart and Broadus.[9] By permission of the publisher.)

to block the stimulatory effects of parathyroid hormone and other humoral agents on bone resorption. Corticosteroids can cause osteoporosis by a direct inhibition of osteoblastic activity and inhibition of calcium absorption from the gastrointestinal tract.[12]

There are several types of clinical osteoporosis. The two most recognized clinical categories are primary and secondary (Table 16–1).[13] The most common form is primary osteoporosis, which includes involutional postmenopausal (type I) and age-associated (type II) forms.[14] Bone loss with deficiency of estrogen can significantly increase after menopause. In the axial trabecular bone, as in vertebral bone, the rates of loss are 5% to 10% per year for the first 2 years of menopause.[15] In contrast, the loss of cortical bone in the radius averages 2% to 3% per year.[16]

The difference in the rate of loss between cortical and trabecular bone may be due to the fact that trabecular bone has a larger surface area available for the metabolic activity, including resorption. Rates of bone loss after menopause are more rapid during the first 5 to 7 years, and then they gradually plateau, as in an exponential curve.[17]

Another form of primary osteoporosis is idiopathic osteoporosis in premenopausal women and young or middle-aged men or idiopathic juvenile osteoporosis. Secondary osteoporosis (type III)[13] results from an identifiable cause, such as early oophorectomy (in women), hypogonadism (in men), immobilization, pharmacologic doses of glucocorticoids or thyroid hormones, subtotal gastrectomy, vitamin D deficiency, and a diet deficient in

TABLE 16–1

Classification of Types of Osteoporosis

	Type I (Postmenopausal)	Type II (Senile)	Type III (Secondary)
Age, yr	55–70	75–90	Any age
Years after menopause	5–15	25–40	Any age
Sex ratio (F:M)	20:1	2:1	1:1
Fracture site	Spine	Hip, spine, pelvis, humerus	Spine, hip, peripheral
Bone loss			
Trabecular	+++	++	+++
Cortical	+	++	+++
Contributing factor			
Menopause	+++	++	++
Age	+	+++	++
Biochemistry			
PTH	↓	↑	↓ ↑
1,25(OH)$_2$D$_3$	↓	↓	↓ ↑
Calcium absorption	↓	↓	↓
1α-Hydroxylase response to PTH	↑	→	?

Abbreviations and symbols: 1,25(OH)$_2$D$_3$, 1,25-dihydroxyvitamin D$_3$; PTH, parathyroid hormone; +++, severe; ++, moderate; +, mild.
From Gallagher.[13] By permission of Elselvier Science Publishers B.V. (Biomedical Division).

calcium. Osteopenia and osteoporosis associated with multiple myeloma, disseminated carcinoma, or a long history of alcohol abuse are among some of the commonly missed diagnoses (Table 16–2).

Other factors that can contribute to a loss of calcium from bones include a high-protein dietary intake, which increases urinary excretion of calcium, and this effect may increase the dietary calcium required to maintain balance.[18] Furthermore, secondary loss of bone can result from changes in physical activity—either lack of activity or overactivity—and

TABLE 16–2
Some Common Causes of Osteoporosis

Hereditary, congenital: osteogenesis imperfecta, neurologic disturbances (myotonia congenita, Werdnig-Hoffmann disease), gonadal dysgenesis
Acquired (primary and secondary)
  Generalized
    Idiopathic (premenopausal women and middle-aged or young men; juvenile osteoporosis)
    Postmenopausal (type I)
    Senile (type II)
    Secondary (type III)
      Nutrition
        Malnutrition, anorexia nervosa
        Vitamin deficiency (C or D)
        Vitamin overuse (D or A)
        Calcium deficiency
        High sodium intake
        High caffeine intake
        High protein intake
        High phosphate intake
        Chronic alcoholism
        Sedentary life-style
      Gastrointestinal diseases (liver disease, malabsorption syndromes, alactasia, subtotal gastrectomy)
      Nephropathies
      Chronic obstructive pulmonary disease
      Malignancy (multiple myeloma, disseminated carcinoma)
      Immobility
      Drugs: phenytoin, barbiturates, cholestyramine, heparin
      Endocrine disorders
        Acromegaly
        Hyperthyroidism
        Cushing's syndrome (iatrogenic or endogenous)
        Hyperparathyroidism
        Diabetes mellitus (?)
        Hypogonadism
  Localized
    Inflammatory arthritis
    Fractures and immobilization in cast
    Limb dystrophies
    Muscular paralysis

these could be conducive to osteoporosis.[19] In 1892, Wolff[20] postulated that when a bone is bent under a mechanical load, it modifies its structure by bony apposition in the concavity and by resorption in the convexity, a principle known as Wolff's law. Since the early 1900s, studies of animals and humans have shown that mechanical stress and strain on bones as a result of muscle tension and pressure help prevent osteopenia.[21, 22] Jansen,[19] in an extensive study of the structure of bone, concluded that mechanical pressure rather than tension had a bone-forming effect. Several etiologic factors are related to osteoporosis, and, indeed, osteoporosis is a multifactorial disease (Table 16-2). It is not known to what extent any of these factors contributes to the development of osteoporosis.

CLINICAL PRESENTATION

Symptoms

The main clinical presentation is fracture as a result of minimal trauma. Vertebral compression fractures may be sudden and due to trauma beyond bone endurance and resilience, or microfractures of vertebral trabeculae may occur during normal daily activities. Significant loss of height in a short amount of time may indicate development of compression fractures (Fig. 16-3). The loads that occur with normal daily activity can be surprisingly large. When the trunk is bent, lumbar vertebrae are subjected to forces exceeding body weight.[23]

Lifting an object in a forward bending position can produce pressures

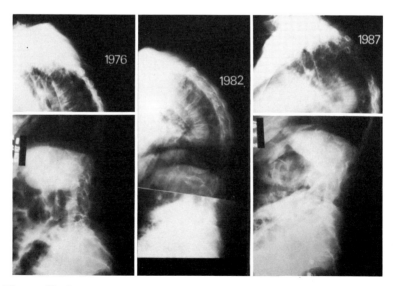

Figure 16-3
Progression of Kyphosis in a woman with osteoporosis vertebral compression fractures and reduction of height secondary to osteoporosis.

on the lumbar spine that are 10 to 20 times greater than the weight lifted.[24] Coughing and laughing are associated with compression loads that are 50% to 70% greater than the load associated with quiet standing.[25, 26]

Vertebral crush fracture and Colles' fracture are the most common in postmenopausal osteoporosis before age 65 years. Femoral neck fracture occurs in an older age group.

Back pain is usually a patient's main complaint. Vertebral compression fractures often occur in the low thoracic and upper lumbar bones, followed (in decreasing order of frequency) by the middle thoracic and lower lumbar bones.[27] The cervical and upper thoracic vertebrae are rarely, if ever, involved. The compression fractures are manifested by pain in the involved level of the spine. The pain related to compression fractures may develop gradually or occur suddenly after a heavy object has been lifted or after strenuous activity. Back pain secondary to compression fracture is self-limiting and usually resolves after 4 to 6 weeks. Persistent back pain necessitates further evaluation to rule out conditions such as multiple myeloma or other malignancies.

Diagnostic Evaluation

Diagnostic evaluation for osteoporosis consists of a thorough history and physical examination. Recommended tests consist of radiographs of the chest to look for lymphomas and rib fractures; radiographs of the lumbar and thoracic spine; complete blood cell count to rule out anemias associated with malignancy; chemistry group tests to assess the level of alkaline phosphatase, which can increase in osteomalacia, bony metastasis, and new fracture (these tests will also demonstrate an increase in calcium in hyperparathyroidism); determination of the erythrocyte sedimentation rate; and serum protein electrophoresis to determine changes indicative of multiple myeloma. Increased total thyroxine concentration may be a cause of osteoporosis because of increased bone turnover. Urinalysis is done to check for proteinuria secondary to nephrotic syndrome and for low pH secondary to renal tubular acidosis as causes of osteopenia; a 24-hour urine test can exclude hypercalciuria (normal calcium value: in men, 25 to 300 mg/specimen; in women, 20 to 275 mg/specimen).[28]

An objective evaluation of bone mass is not possible on conventional radiographs until at least 25% to 30% of bone mineral has been lost. Therefore, evaluation of bone mineral density through absorptiometry techniques is recommended. Calculated reduction of bone loss or gain is required in therapeutic trials of agents affecting bone remodeling.

Optional procedures for further confirmation of the diagnosis of osteoporosis are dual-energy absorptiometry and quantitative computed tomography to determine the bone density of the lumbar spine[29] and evaluate the risk of fracture, iliac crest biopsy (after tetracycline double labeling for bone histomorphometry) to evaluate high-turnover bone loss and determine therapeutic decisions, and bone marrow examination to exclude multiple myeloma and metastatic malignancy.[30]

TREATMENT

Treatment programs for osteoporosis are designed to decrease the rate of bone resorption and to improve bone endurance and the patient's quality of life. Currently, few options are available to restore lost bone density. Various medical therapeutic measures are applied in the management of osteoporosis and some have had promising results. Until a cure is found, however, symptomatic treatment will continue to be of utmost importance. Back pain is usually the patient's main complaint and can be manifested in the acute or chronic form.

Acute Pain

Management of acute pain requires implementation of sedative measures and proper positioning principles.[31] Strong analgesics (codeine sulfate or its derivatives) result in constipation; thus, if adequate, simple analgesics are preferred. Therapeutic exercise programs, preferably spinal extension exercises, and proper posture principles for activities of daily living are recommended (Table 16−3).[27]

Chronic Pain

Chronic pain may be a result of compression fractures and kyphotic or scoliotic changes in the spine with inappropriate stretch of ligaments. Sometimes pressure of the lower rib cage over the pelvic rim in patients with severe kyphosis causes significant pain and tenderness in the loin area. Measures that improve a patient's posture are needed. Modification of activities of daily living and facilitation of self-care can decrease the compressive force on the spine. Certain assistive devices have been shown to be helpful in facilitating self-care activities (Figs. 16−4 through 16−6). Occupational therapists can be of great help to patients with a fragile skeleton. Gait training for use of a cane or wheeled walker can enhance the

TABLE 16−3
Management of Acute Pain in Patients
With Osteoporosis

Bed rest (less than 1 week). Significant aggravation of bone loss is not likely to occur during 1 week of bed rest
Analgesics
Avoidance of constipation
Avoidance of exertional exercises
Proper positioning principles to avoid undue strain on spine
Physical therapy: mild heat and stroking massage

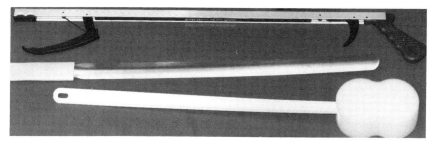

Figure 16–4

From top: Reacher, serves as an extension to reach items without straining in cases of pain or limited range of motion; useful for dressing and routine home management tasks. Long shoe horn, provides for ease in donning of shoes and eliminates the need to bend over. Long-handled bath sponge, allows individual to wash the back, legs, and feet with minimal bending, twisting, and reaching.

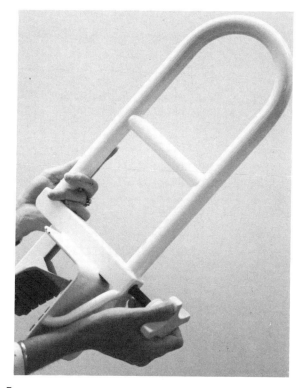

Figure 16–5

Bathtub grab bar: designed to fasten to the edge of the bathtub; provides stability while transferring in and out of the bathtub.

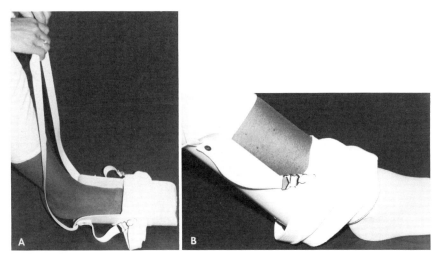

Figure 16–6
A and *B*, Stocking aid: allows donning of stocking without the need to bend over.

patient's safety (Fig. 16–7). For cases of severe osteoporosis in which ky-photic posturing results in poor balance and orthopnea, a wheelchair should be used for long-distance ambulation. Physical therapy instructions for safe ambulation are invaluable. These measures include the use of a back support and proper back extension exercises. In cases of severe os-teoporosis, these exercises should be nonstrenuous (Fig. 16–8). As the pa-tient progresses with the exercise program, more advanced exercises (such as those in Fig. 16–9) can be tried. Semirigid or rigid back supports are used, depending on the severity of spinal osteoporosis and the patient's tolerance. Flexion exercises are not recommended[32] because they can in-crease the vertical compression forces on the body of vertebral bones and may increase the possibility of compression fractures and further increase the kyphosis (Table 16–4).[23]

TABLE 16–4
Management of Chronic Pain in Patients
with Osteoporosis

Improve faulty posture, if possible
If beyond correction, apply a back support
  to decrease inappropriate stretch of
  ligaments
Avoid physical activities that increase
  vertical compression forces on body of
  vertebral bones
Prescribe a sound therapeutic exercise
  program
Start appropriate medical treatment, as
  indicated

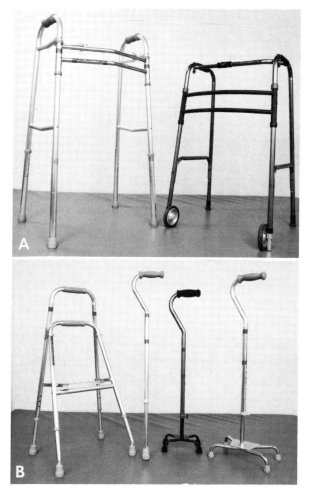

Figure 16–7
Gait-assistive devices for patients with osteoporosis. *A*, Walker *(left)* and wheeled walker *(right)*. *B (from the left)*, Walkane, cane, and two broad-based canes, for stability. (From Sinaki.[41] By permission of Mayo Foundation.)

Indications for Bracing

In order to minimize the incidence of kyphosis in at-risk populations, preventive measures that decrease anterior wedging and compression of vertebral bodies are highly desirable.[33] Erector spinae muscles are the anatomic support of the back, and if they are weak, extrinsic supports are used to substitute for or assist with their function.

The principles of back supports are based on three-point contact. If the objective is prevention of further flexion of the spine, the three points of contact are the base of the sternum, lumbar spine, and symphysis pubis, as

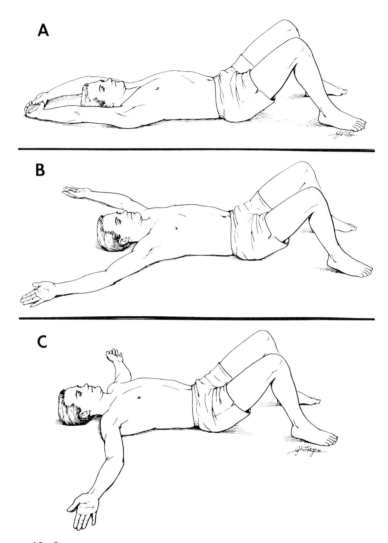

Figure 16-8

Nonstrenuous exercises for patients with severe osteoporosis. *A* through *C*, Upper back and shoulder extension exercise performed with spine supported. *D* and *E*, Flexibility of shoulder joint may contribute to improvement of upper back posture. To avoid upper back and neck strain in a fragile skeleton, shoulder rotation exercises can be performed in supine position. *F* and *G*, Pectoral stretching exercise performed in sitting position. This is used to reduce kyphotic posturing.

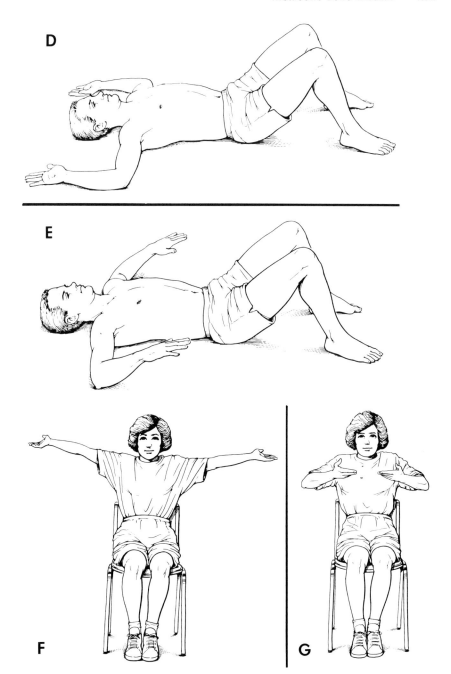

Figure 16-9 (cont.)

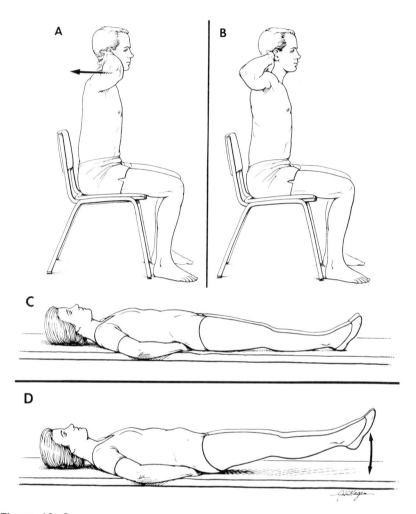

Figure 16–9
Advanced exercises for patients with severe osteoporosis. *A* and *B*, Deep-breathing exercise combined with pectoral stretching and back extension exercise. Patient sits on a chair, places hands at the level of head, and inhales deeply while gently extending the elbows backward. While exhaling, patient returns arms to the starting position. This is repeated 10 to 15 times. *C* and *D*, Isometric exercise to strengthen abdominal muscles. *E* and *F*, Technique of isometric exercise to strengthen abdominal muscles. *G*, Exercise to decrease lumbar lordosis with isometric contraction of lumbar flexors. *H* and *I*, Exercises for improving strength in lumbar extensors and gluteus maximus muscles (*H*, in cat-stretch position). *J* and *K*, Back extension exercise, in prone position. *L* and *M*, Back extension exercise, in sitting position. This position avoids or minimizes pain in patients with severe osteoporosis. (*C* through *G*, *J*, and *K*, From Sinaki.[41] By permission of Mayo Foundation.)

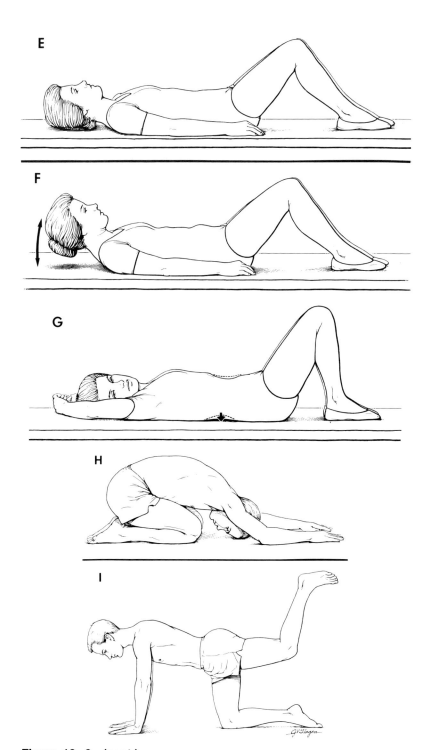

Figure 16-9   (cont.)

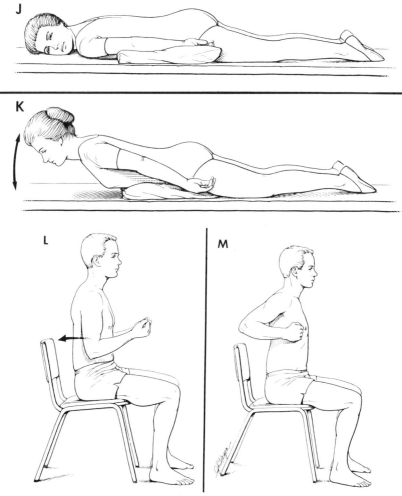

Figure 16–9 (cont.)

in a Jewett brace (Fig. 16–10). The conventional thoracolumbar supports assist spine extension through shoulder straps and paraspinal bars and increase intra-abdominal pressure (Fig. 16–11). When back supports function through increasing the intra-abdominal pressure, certain contraindications such as hiatal hernia or inguinal hernia, orthopenia secondary to chronic obstructive pulmonary disease, and obesity will limit their use.

The weight of the head and upper trunk in forward flexion of the spine may contribute to the progression of kyphotic posturing. Most activities of daily living require repetitive or sustained bent posture of the thoracic spine. Reduction of bone mineral density of vertebral bodies along with compression of the anterior portion of vertebral bodies may result in gradual anterior wedging of these structures.

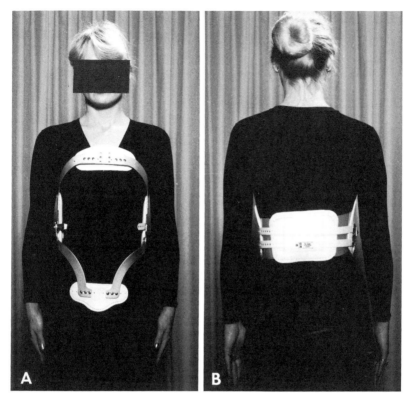

Figure 16-10
Jewett brace—used to prevent lumbar and thoracic flexion when patient has acute pain due to recent compression fracture of spine. Proper fitting requires proper contact at base of sternum and over pubic bone. *A*, Anterior view. *B*, Posterior view. (From Sinaki.[41] By permission of Mayo Foundation.)

Back supports that decrease kyphotic posture through counteracting the anterior compressive forces that are exerted on the vertebral bodies can be helpful. Improvement of body mechanics, which includes proper static and dynamic posturing and prevention of kyphosis, is a major component of treatment. A slight posterior shift of the weight of the upper trunk through the application of weight below the scapulae can significantly decrease the compressive forces exerted on the lower thoracic spine. To balance the weight of the upper trunk, minimal effective weight can be added to the support (Fig. 16-12). This weight can vary from 1.5 to 1.75 lb, according to patient's tolerance correction.

Bracing may be considered in three stages of management of osteoporotic patients.

1. Acute Stage. The objectives of bracing during this stage are to decrease the acute pain resulting from muscle spasm secondary to subperiosteum edema, which is due to fractured bone. Movement of the spine in-

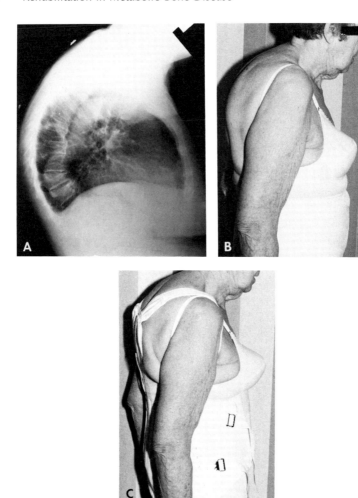

Figure 16–11

Patient with spinal osteoporosis. *A,* Lateral radiograph of thoracic spine demonstrates osteoporosis and compression fractures of several mid and lower thoracic vertebral bodies. *B,* Kyphotic posture resulting from osteoporosis and compression fractures. *C,* Patient fitted with thoracolumbar semirigid support with shoulder straps, which decreased back pain significantly. Stays in support are semirigid; if they are replaced with rigid stays, support is transformed into rigid back support. (From Sinaki.[27] By permission of Mayo Foundation.)

creases pain, and pain induces further secondary muscle overuse for protecting and immobilizing the painful area. To break this vicious cycle, bracing becomes helpful and decreases the duration of the patient's confinement to bed because of pain. Braces vary from bivalved shields (Fig. 16–13) to Jewett (Fig. 16–10), CASH, and thoracolumbar braces (Fig.

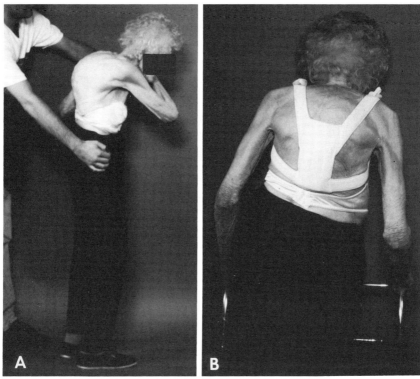

Figure 16–12

A, Woman with severe osteoporosis and compression fractures who was unable to walk independently without the newly developed support. *B*, Posture Training Support consists of a weight fitted below inferior angles of scapulae which rests above waistline. (*A*, From Sinaki.[33] By permission of the publisher.)

16–11). The principle of bracing at this stage is to provide spine extension through necessary trunk contact to achieve improvement in extrinsic support and immobilization.

2. Chronic Stage. The main objective of bracing during this stage is to substitute the function of weak supportive muscles of the spine. Bracing may also be considered when severe loss of bone exists and when further compression fractures may develop during conventional daily activities. In patients who have severe kyphotic posturing, pain is induced with any physical activity that exerts strain on the spine and ligamentous structures. Therefore, bracing decreases the undue strain on these structures and allows the patient to be more independent and physically active (Table 16–4). For patients who need proper back extension posturing but do not tolerate increased intra-abdominal pressure or need a reminder to avoid kyphotic posturing during activities of daily living, an alternative to con-

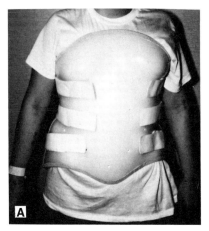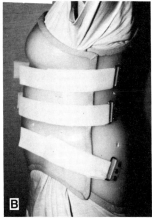

Figure 16–13
Left and right, Anterior (left) and lateral (right) views of rigid back support or bivalved body jacket. This brace, made of polypropylene, is custom fitted. (From Sinaki.[27] By permission of Mayo Foundation.)

ventional bracing, such as a Posture Training Support, can be considered (Fig. 16–12, *B*). Bracing can decrease back strength as a result of reduction in muscle contraction. Posture Training Support does not result in reduction of back strength.[34]

3. Back Supports for Activities of Daily Living or Recreational Activities. To achieve independence and promote mobility in osteoporotic patients, the use of back supports is recommended to a limited extent. Extensive and unnecessary supports are discouraged because they may contribute to the patient's discomfort or disuse of the patient's erector spinae muscles. Therefore, bracing should be decreased to the minimal effective level. We have found a few limiting factors with the conventional supports: 1) shorter stature (< 147 cm [58 in.]), 2) presence of dyspnea or chronic obstructive pulmonary disease, 3) presence of hiatal or inguinal hernia, 4) moderate to severe obesity, and 5) scoliosis secondary to osteoporosis and compression fractures.[33]

Pharmacologic Interventions

Certain progestogens and anabolic agents produce effects similar to those of estrogen.[35] For years, anabolic steroids or androgens have been known as potential therapeutic agents for osteoporosis.[36] Approximately 10% to 20% of men with osteoporosis have partial or complete hypogonadism of various causes.[37] Patients with low plasma testosterone levels should receive replacement therapy, such as testosterone enanthate, under the supervision of an endocrinologist. However, androgens are not well tolerated by women because of their virilizing effects. Chestnut et al.[38] examined the effects of stanozolol and found a small but significant increase in total body calcium value during 2 years of treatment.

Estrogen and calcitonin are known as bone antiresorptive agents and have been approved by the Food and Drug Administration for use in osteoporosis. Calcitonin inhibits osteoclastic activity, but about 20% of patients fail to respond to this treatment. Bisphosphonates can also inhibit osteoclastic activity and recently have been advocated for research trials. Proper use of bisphosphonates is extremely important because impaired bone mineralization and osteomalacia-type syndrome can develop with high doses. Short courses of use with 12 weeks between trial periods are being assessed in research protocols. Fluoride stimulates osteoblastic activity. However, its use results in increased thickening of trabecular bone but reduction of cortical bone. It may also result in impaired mineralization and an increased fracture rate. Recent controlled trials indicate an increased incidence of hip fracture in patients treated with sodium fluoride. Thiazides decrease renal calcium excretion, and this effect may be helpful for reduction of bone loss.

Estrogen, calcitonin, and calcium are among the most commonly advocated pharmacologic treatments for involutional osteoporosis. These medications act by inhibiting or decreasing bone resorption.

Effect of Estrogen

The mode of effect of estrogen on the skeleton has been under much discussion and investigation. A search for estrogen receptors in bone has recently demonstrated that cultured human osteoblast-like cells possess the properties of target cells for estrogen. The presence of specific estrogen receptors in osteoblasts could indicate a direct effect of estrogen on these cells.[39]

Estrogens have been shown to diminish the rate of bone loss and fractures in postmenopausal women, whether the menopause is natural or surgically induced.

Vitamin D

Vitamin D deficiency decreases the intestinal absorption of dietary calcium. The recommended daily intake of vitamin D is 400 IU. Although higher levels of supplementation increase the risk of vitamin D intoxication, elderly people may tolerate two to three times the recommended daily allowance of vitamin D if cutaneous generation of vitamin D, mediated through exposure to the sun, is reduced.

Calcium

Calcium performs several different functions in the body. These functions can be simplified into two principal effects: 1) structuring of human skeleton along with collagenous fibers and 2) regulation of many cellular activities. The serum calcium concentration is one of the most accurately regulated biologic factors (Fig. 16−2).

Estrogen contributes to the intestinal absorption of calcium. Therefore, there is a need for an increase in the dietary intake of calcium in estrogen-deficient women. Aging is also associated with a reduction in the intestinal absorption of calcium. The recommended intake of calcium is 800 to 1,000 mg per day at premenopausal stage and 1,500 mg per day at post-menopausal stage.

An adequate calcium intake is required to permit normal bone development and potentially to decrease excessive loss of bone tissue with advancing age. One of the risk factors for osteopenia is inadequate calcium intake. Adequate calcium intake, assumed from the data of Heaney et al.,[40] is a total of 1.5 g/day of elemental calcium for postmenopausal women. If at all possible, this amount of calcium is better absorbed from nutritional sources. One 8-ounce glass of whole or skim milk yields about 300 mg of calcium. Table 16−5 shows the principal nutritional sources of calcium.[31] A nutritional diet rich in calcium reduces the risk of osteoporosis. Proper diets rich in calcium and low in cholesterol can improve the patient's intake of calcium without an increased risk of obesity.[31]

Exercise

Mechanical loading and exercise play a significant role in promoting bone growth and preventing osteopenia secondary to immobility.[41] Proper

TABLE 16−5

Foods High in Calcium

Food	Serving Size (oz)	Calcium Content (mg)
Milk		
Whole	8	290
Skim	8	300
Buttermilk	8	285
Yogurt		
Low-fat plain	8	415
Low-fat fruited	8	315
Frozen	8	200
Cheese		
Low-fat cottage (2%)	8	154
American	1	174
Cheddar	1	204
Swiss	1	272
Ice cream	8	176
Sardines (with bones)	3	372
Salmon	3	180
Shrimp	8	147
Tofu (bean curd)	4	154
Broccoli (cooked)	8	136
Turnip greens (cooked)	8	267

From Sinaki et al.[31] By permission of Mayo Foundation.

exercise and rehabilitative measures have the potential to build bone mass and decrease the rate of bone loss or decrease the frequency of falls. Therapeutic exercise programs that improve the natural extrinsic support of the spine have been demonstrated to contribute to the maintenance of posture.[42] Spinal extensor strength has been shown to correlate with the prevention of vertebral wedging or kyphosis.[42] The recommended therapeutic exercises for osteoporotic patients are shown in Figure 16–9.[41] Recreational physical activities that do not overstrain the spine, especially in flexion posturing, are desirable and recommended.[32] Further research to determine the proper dose of exercise and the most effective rehabilitation measures is needed.

PREVENTIVE MEASURES

Prevention of fall is as important as improvement of the patient's bone mineral density. Use of a cane provides better balance, reduces the possibility of falls, and decreases the low back pain resulting from weight bearing. Patients should be instructed to avoid heavy lifting and strenuous bending activities.

Measurement of Muscle Strength

Among the factors that contribute to the risk of fall and fracture in the osteoporotic patient are changes in muscle strength and development of severe kyphosis, which result in poor balance.

In a recent study, back strength was demonstrated to be significantly lower in osteoporotic women than normal women.[43] The same study demonstrated that upper extremity strength in the two groups was comparable. Therefore, measurement of muscle strength can contribute to the develop-

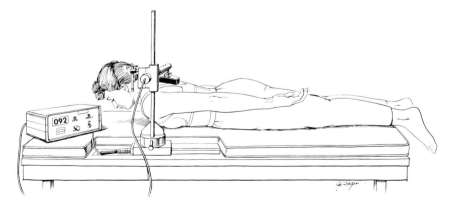

Figure 16–14
Proper positioning of subject for measurement of back extensor strength with strain-gauge dynamometer (BID-2000). (From Limburg et al.[44] By permission of Mayo Foundation for Medical Education and Research.)

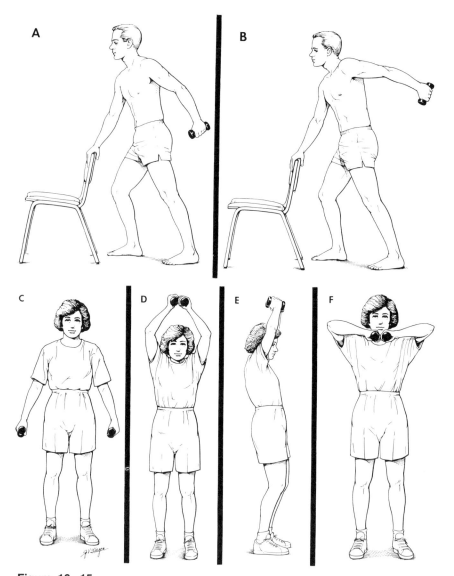

Figure 16–15

Muscle strengthening and weight-bearing exercises that may decrease bone loss. (These exercises were developed for the osteopenic spine by M. Sinaki through a grant from the Retirement Research Foundation. These techniques are designed to decrease strain on the spine despite weight bearing.) A and B, Shoulder extensors contribute to reduction of kyphotic posturing. Shoulder extensors can be strengthened with a proper combination of weight lifting and weight-bearing exercises while balance is maintained. One knee is bent to avoid lumbar strain. *Note:* The amount of weight lifted is about 1 to 2 lb in each hand, not to exceed 5 lb in each hand. The amount of weight needs to be prescribed according to the patient's bone mineral density (status of osteoporosis) and the condition of the upper extremities. C through E, Bilateral or unilateral spine and hip weight-bearing exercise. To avoid straining the spine and to maintain balance, leaning or holding onto a steady object for support is recommended. When weight is lifted above the head, knees should be bent slightly to avoid straining the lumbar spine. *Note:* The amount of weight lifted is about

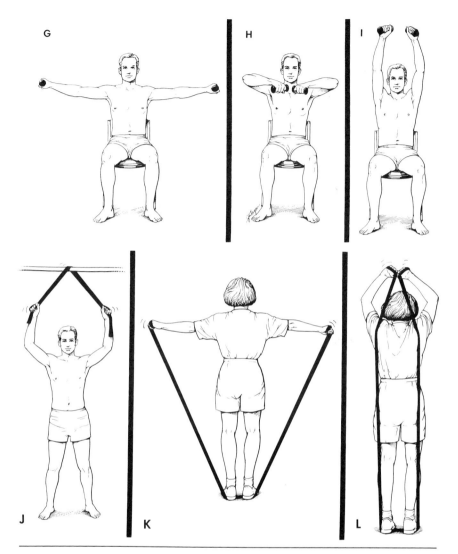

Figure 16–5 (cont.)
1 to 2 lb in each hand, not to exceed 5 lb in each hand. The amount of weight needs to be prescribed according to the patient's bone mineral density (status of osteoporosis) and the condition of the upper extremities. *F,* In cases of limited shoulder abduction, weight lifting *only* to the shoulder level is recommended. *Note:* The amount of weight lifted is about 1 to 2 lb in each hand, not to exceed 5 lb in each hand. The amount of weight needs to be prescribed according to the patient's bone mineral density (status of osteoporosis) and the condition of the upper extremities. *G* through *I,* Weight-bearing exercises can be performed in a sitting position by individuals with poor balance or lower-extremity arthritis. *Note:* The amount of weight lifted is about 1 to 2 lb in each hand, not to exceed 5 lb in each hand. The amount of weight needs to be prescribed according to the patient's bone mineral density (status of osteoporosis) and the condition of the upper extremities. *J* through *L,* Elastic bands of suitable resistance can be used for isodynamic strengthening of anatomically related back muscles. *J,* Latissimus dorsi and shoulder adductors. *K,* Shoulder abductors and extensors. *L,* Back extensors.

ment of an appropriate exercise program for the maintenance of posture. Measurement of back strength with techniques that do not induce compressive forces on the spine is desirable. Indeed, a technique that can be used for safely measuring back strength in most osteoporotic patients was developed[44] because most commercially available measuring techniques induce more than tolerable stress on the osteoporotic spine (Fig. 16–14).

Physical Activities and Diet

Patients should be instructed to try pectoral stretching, deep breathing, and back extension exercises and to avoid stooping. They should be encouraged to try swimming or bicycling as a means of keeping fit rather than exercises or recreational activities that could predispose them to vertebral compression. Weight-bearing exercises are more effective than swimming for improving bone mineral density (Fig. 16–15).[45] However, swimming is recommended when general conditioning and fitness are desired. Osteoporotic patients have to avoid flexion exercises because they seem to predispose the spine to compression fractures. Strenuous flexion of the spine that is beyond the biomechanical competence of vertebral bodies can result in compression fractures due to golfing have been reported in osteoporotic women.[46] Also, a balanced diet is important and should contain 1,000 mg of elemental calcium daily, which is contained in three glasses of whole or skim milk or its equivalent in ice cream or cheese (1,000 mg before menopause and 1,500 mg after menopause). The beneficial effects of a high-calcium intake on age-related bone loss are debated extensively.[18]

REFERENCES

1. Mazess RB, Cameron JR. Bone mineral content in normal U.S. whites. In: Mazess RB, ed. International Conference on Bone Mineral Measurement (DHEW Publication No. [NIH] 75-683). Washington DC: United States Department of Health, Education, and Welfare, 1973:228–237.
2. Riggs BL, Melton LJ III. Involutional osteoporosis. N Engl J Med 1986; 314:1676–1686.
3. Holbrook TL, Grazier K, Kelsey JL, Stauffer RN. The frequency of occurrence, impact and cost of selected musculoskeletal conditions in the United States. Chicago: American Academy of Orthopaedic Surgeons, 1984.
4. Peck WA, Woods WL. The cells of bone. In: Riggs BL, Melton LJ III, eds. Osteoporosis: etiology, diagnosis, and management. New York: Raven Press, 1988:1–44.
5. Parfitt AM. Quantum concept of bone remodeling and turnover: implications for the pathogenesis of osteoporosis (editorial). Calcif Tissue Int 1979; 28:1–5.
6. Frost HM. Treatment of osteoporosis by manipulation of coherent bone cell populations. Clin Orthop 1979; 143:227–244.
7. Eastell R, Heath H III, Kumar R, Riggs BL. Hormonal factors: PTH, vitamin D, and calcitonin. In: Riggs BL, Melton LJ III, eds. Osteoporosis: etiology, diagnosis, and management. New York: Raven Press, 1988:373–388.

8. Wallach S. Hormonal factors in osteoporosis. Clin Orthop 1979; 144:284–292.
9. Stewart AF, Broadus AE. Mineral metabolism. In: Felig P, Baxter JD, Broadus AE, Frohman LA, eds. Endocrinology and metabolism. 2nd ed. New York: McGraw-Hill Book Company, 1987:1317–1453.
10. Mayer E, Kadowaki S, Williams G, Norman AW. Mode of action of $1\alpha,25$-dihydroxyvitamin D. In: Kumar R, ed. Vitamin D: basic and clinical aspects. Boston: Martinus Nijhoff Publishing, 1984:259–302.
11. Maierhofer WJ, Gray RW, Cheung HS, Lemann J Jr. Bone resorption stimulated by elevated serum $1,25\text{-(OH)}_2$-vitamin D concentrations in healthy men. Kidney Int 1983; 24:555–560.
12. Adams JS, Wahl TO, Lukert BP. Effects of hydrochlorothiazide and dietary sodium restriction on calcium metabolism in corticosteroid treated patients. Metabolism 1981; 30:217–221.
13. Gallagher JC. The pathogenesis of osteoporosis. Bone Miner 1990; 9:215–227.
14. Riggs BL, Melton LJ III. Evidence for two distinct syndromes of involutional osteoporosis. Am J Med 1983; 75:899–901.
15. Cann CE, Genant HK, Ettinger B, Gordan GS. Spinal mineral loss in oophorectomized women: determination by quantitative computed tomography. JAMA 1980; 244:2056–2059.
16. Johnston CC Jr, Hui SL, Witt RM, Appledorn R, Baker RS, Longcope C. Early menopausal changes in bone mass and sex steroids. J Clin Endocrinol Metab 1985; 61:905–911.
17. Gallagher JC, Goldgar D, Moy A. Total bone calcium in normal women: effect of age and menopause status. J Bone Miner Res 1987; 2:491–496.
18. Heaney RP, Gallagher JC, Johnston CC, Near R, Parfitt AM, Whedon GD. Calcium nutrition and bone health in the elderly. Am J Clin Nutr 1982; 36:986–1013.
19. Jansen M. On bone formation, its relation to tension and pressure. London: Longmans Green & Co, 1920.
20. Wolff J, ed. Daz Gesetz der Transformation der Knochen. Berlin: A Hirschwald, 1892.
21. Gillespie JA. The nature of the bone changes associated with nerve injuries and disuse. J Bone Joint Surg [Br] 1954; 36:464–473.
22. Whedon GD, Deitrick JE, Shorr E. Modification of the effects of immobilization upon metabolic and physiologic functions of normal men by the use of an oscillating bed. Am J Med 1949; 6:684–711.
23. Schultz AB, Andersson GBJ, Haderspeck K, Örtengren R, Nordin M, Björk R. Analysis and measurement of lumbar trunk loads in tasks involving bends and twists. J Biomech 1982; 15:669–675.
24. Perey O. Fracture of the vertebral end-plate in the lumbar spine: an experimental biomechanical investigation. Acta Orthop Scand Suppl 1957; 25:3–101.
25. Nachemson A. Towards a better understanding of low-back pain: a review of the mechanics of the lumbar disc. Rheum Rehabil 1975; 14:129–143.
26. Sinaki M. Is the effect of exercise on bone measurable? In: Dequeker J, Geusens P, Wahner HW, eds. Bone mineral measurement by photon absorptiometry. Leuven, Belgium: Leuven University Press, 1988:322–335.
27. Sinaki M. Postmenopausal spinal osteoporosis: physical therapy and rehabilitation principles. Mayo Clin Proc 1982; 57:699–703.
28. Sinaki M. Exercise and osteoporosis. Arch Phys Med Rehabil 1989; 70:220–229.

29. Wahner HW, Riggs BL. Methods and application of bone densitometry in clinical diagnosis. Crit Rev Clin Lab Sci 1986; 24:217–233.
30. Riggs BL. Practical management of the patient with osteoporosis. In: Riggs BL, Melton LJ III, eds. Osteoporosis: etiology, diagnosis, and management. New York: Raven Press, 1988:481–490.
31. Sinaki M, Dale DA, Hurley DL. Living with osteoporosis: guidelines for women before and after diagnosis. Philadelphia: BC Decker, 1988.
32. Sinaki M, Mikkelsen BA. Postmenopausal spinal osteoporosis: flexion versus extension exercises. Arch Phys Med Rehabil 1984; 65:593–596.
33. Sinaki M. A new back support in rehabilitation of osteoporosis program-exercise: posture training support. In: Christiansen C, Overgaard K, eds. Osteoporosis 1990. Vol. 3. Copenhagen, Denmark: Osteopress ApS, 1990:1355–1357.
34. Kaplan RS, Sinaki M. The Posture Training Suport (PTS): report on a case series of patients with symptomatic improvement of osteoporotic complications. Mayo Clin Proc, in press.
35. Lindsay R, Hart DM, Purdie D, Ferguson MM, Clark AS, Kraszewski A. Comparative effects of oestrogen and a progestogen on bone loss in postmenopausal women. Clin Sci Mol Med 1978; 54:193–195.
36. Albright F. The effect of hormones on osteogenesis in man. Recent Prog Horm Res 1947; 1:293–345.
37. Seeman E, Melton LJ III, O'Fallon WM, Riggs BL. Risk factors for spinal osteoporosis in men. Am J Med 1983; 75:977–983.
38. Chestnut CH III, Ivey JL, Gruber HE, Matthews M, Nelp WB, Sisom K, Baylink DJ. Stanozolol in postmenopausal osteoporosis: therapeutic efficacy and possible mechanisms of action. Metabolism 1983; 32:571–580.
39. Eriksen EF, Colvard DS, Berg NJ, Graham ML, Mann KG, Spelsberg TC, Riggs BL. Evidence of estrogen receptors in normal human osteoblast-like cells. Science 1988; 241:84–86.
40. Heaney RP, Recker RR, Saville PD. Calcium balance and calcium requirements in middle-aged women. Am J Clin Nutr 1977; 30:1603–1611.
41. Sinaki M. Exercise and physical therapy. In: Riggs BL, Melton LJ III, eds. Osteoporosis: etiology, diagnosis, and management. New York: Raven Press, 1988:457–479.
42. Rogers J, Sinaki M, Bergstralh E, Limburg P, Wahner H. The effect of back extensor strength, physical activity, and vertebral bone density on postural change (abstract). Arthritis Rheum 1990; 33 suppl:S124.
43. Sinaki M, Limburg PJ, Rogers JW, Khosla S, Murtaugh PA. Back muscle strength in osteoporotic compared with normal women. In: Christiansen C, Overgaard K, eds. Osteoporosis 1990. Vol. 3. Copenhagen, Denmark: Osteopress ApS, 1990:1353–1354.
44. Limburg PJ, Sinaki M, Rogers JW, Caskey PE, Pierskalla BK. A useful technique for measurement of back strength in osteoporotic and elderly patients. Mayo Clin Proc 1991; 66:39–44.
45. Nilsson BE, Westlin NE. Bone density in athletes. Clin Orthop 1971; 77:179–182.
46. Ekin JA, Sinaki M. Vertebral compression fractures sustained during golfing: report of three cases. Mayo Clin Proc 1993; 68:566–570

PART VI

Rehabilitation in Connective Tissue Disorders

17

Physical Management of Arthritis

John L. Merritt

Terry H. Oh

Arthritis refers to a category of diseases and conditions that primarily affect the joints. Arthritis may, however, also have profound effects on associated musculoskeletal and other organ systems. There are several dozen types of arthritis, but the most common fall within six categories: (1) degenerative joint disease (osteoarthritis), (2) rheumatoid arthritis and its variants, (3) B27 arthropathies (such as ankylosing spondylitis), (4) scleroderma, (5) lupus erythematosus, and (6) other, mixed connective tissue diseases. Although arthritis, by definition, is associated with joint inflammation, the most common type, osteoarthritis (or degenerative joint disease), is primarily degenerative. The joint effects of scleroderma are secondary to noninflammatory changes in overlying and surrounding soft tissues. Rheumatoid arthritis and its variants, mixed connective tissue diseases, lupus erythematosus, and the B27 arthropathies all are associated with significant and readily detectable joint inflammation.

Joint evaluation (see Chapter 3) is essential for diagnosis and for establishing an effective program of management. The intent of this chapter is not to discuss in detail the differential diagnosis, or even the medical management, because excellent references are already readily available for those purposes. This chapter is instead intended to provide guidelines for formulating rational physical and rehabilitation management of two exemplary forms of arthritis. The physical management of arthritis, although generally recognized to be important, is much less discussed in the current literature.[1-4]

RHEUMATOID ARTHRITIS

Rheumatoid arthritis is a disease of unknown cause for which no curative treatment is known. Effective treatment is therefore limited to controlling the disease and minimizing its effects. Rheumatoid arthritis is the epitome of an inflammatory disease of multiple joints. Therefore, management exemplifies principles of control of joint inflammation. Successful management of inflammatory arthropathies primarily depends on control and reduction of joint inflammation. The early effects of joint inflammation (synovitis) are joint swelling, pain, stiffness, limitation of motion, and consequential loss of function. These are at first a result of intra-articular effusions and swelling of inflamed synovium. Both effusion and synovial swelling distend and stretch joint capsules and the surrounding soft tissues. As the disease progresses, the swollen hypertrophic synovium develops into an aggressively invasive tissue that erodes joint cartilage, subchondral bone, and adjacent tendons, bursae, and capsules. These effects result in further limitations of motion, with consequential development of joint contractures, muscle atrophy, and weakened capsules, tendons, and ligaments. The loss of joint and tendon motion in addition to muscular weakness and incoordination, pain and stiffness, and finally joint deformities result in progressive functional deterioration. Declining mobility and the psychological and social consequences contribute further to the generally decreasing functional independence.

Maintaining general body mobility, performing activities of daily living, and prevention of deformities are primary rehabilitation goals. To accomplish these goals, regional treatment needs to include reduction of pain and stiffness, preservation (or restoration) of joint motion and muscle strength, and preservation of endurance, balance, and coordination. Knowledge of the disease process and efficient use of joints and muscles are needed.

Several medications are available to reduce inflammation, but none are entirely effective alone. Salicylates remain the initial drug of choice, but other nonsteroidal anti-inflammatory drugs may be equally effective. Second-line drugs include antimalarials, gold salts, and penicillamine. Low-dose corticosteroids are used in combination with second-line drugs in patients who do not respond adequately to nonsteroidal anti-inflammatory drugs and in those with severe joint destruction during the first year of the disease. Cytotoxic medications are reserved for refractory and rapidly progressive synovitis. If inflamed joints are not protected physically, however, medications alone will inevitably be inadequate to control inflammation and its consequences. In addition, no medication can restore range of motion or increase strength, coordination, and endurance without physical adjuvants. Physical measures are therefore essential for comprehensive and effective management of arthritis. Physical measures include rest, exercise, heat, cold, joint protection, patient education, splinting, and assistive devices (Fig. 17–1).

Rest

Rest is a powerful anti-inflammatory instrument. Before corticosteroids and nonsteroidal anti-inflammatory drugs were available, rest was the only

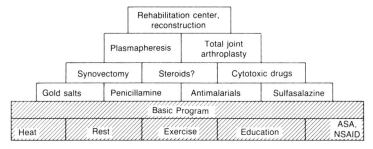

Figure 17–1
Management of rheumatoid arthritis. Items in lowest level, the basic program, are for all affected patients. Those who do not respond to this management are then treated with items in second level, in addition to items in first level. Note that four of the five first-level methods are physical, nonpharmacologic methods. ASA, acetylsalicylic acid; NSAID, nonsteroidal anti-inflammatory drug.

effective anti-inflammatory prescription. Although rest still has its strong advocates, it has taken a back seat to drug therapy.

Effective drugs and constraints on hospitalization or rest at home often result in neglect of rest as a therapeutic tool for arthritis. However, the effectiveness of rest as a primary or adjuvant therapy for inflammatory joint disease was well described by Smith and Polly,[5] Partridge and Duthie,[6] and Gault and Spyker.[7] Gault and Spyker showed a reduction in the indices of inflammation after local joint rest (splinting). Smith and Polly long advocated an additional systemic benefit from general body rest. In a controlled trial, Partridge and Duthie reported a benefit from both general rest and joint splinting. Further study of joint rest is needed.

Rheumatologists and physiatrists agree with the general principle that too much joint stress will increase joint inflammation, and most prescribe rest as a part of the management of rheumatoid arthritis. Defining how much rest is needed and in what manner it is achieved, however, still need individual refinement. The main principle is that the more inflammation that is present on examination, the more rest that is needed. Thus, the quantity of rest should be increased or decreased according to symptoms and signs.

A frequent general guideline for moderate, early rheumatoid arthritis may be 8 hours of rest at night, 1 hour of rest at noon, and 1 hour of rest before dinner. With this recommendation, many patients can continue employment or productive lives. Of course, heavy labor and strenuous or frequent repetitions of one motion should be avoided. Task modification, adaptive devices, and improved body and hand mechanics may further allow productive lives within a framework of joint protection and joint rest. Resting wrist-hand splints can add to joint rest at night and during daytime general rest periods (Fig. 17–2). These splints may also help to reduce deforming stresses by maintaining proper joint alignment, but this theory is at present unproven. A wrist splint (the "cock-up" splint) can keep the wrist in a functional position during daily activities while allowing the hand and fingers freedom of movement (Fig. 17–3). Maintaining the wrist or other

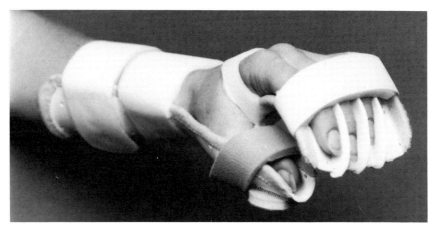

Figure 17-2
Resting wrist-hand splint with fins between fingers. It supports wrist, fingers, and thumb and keeps digits in alignment.

joints in a middle range or functional position will also help keep intra-articular pressures low and thus reduce joint pain when synovial swelling or effusion is present.

Too much rest can, however, have detrimental effects on joints (contractures), bones (osteoporosis), muscles, tendons, ligaments, and capsules (weakness and atrophy), the brain and spinal reflexes (neuromuscular incoordination), and the respiratory and cardiovascular systems (loss of endurance and aerobic capacity). Rest must, then, be coupled with a concomitant exercise program.

Exercise

An exercise prescription requires as much care and specification as a drug prescription, especially for inflammatory arthritis. Exercises may include: (1) range of motion (active, active-assisted, or passive), (2) stretch-

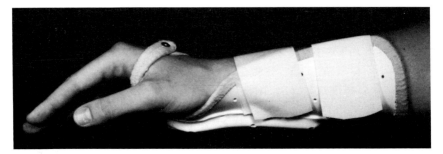

Figure 17-3
Volar wrist splint. It stabilizes wrist volarly, allowing free movement of finger and thumb joints.

ing (active or passive), (3) strengthening (isotonic, isometric, or isokinetic), (4) reeducation, (5) coordination, and (6) endurance and conditioning (aerobic). Each type may be useful in some patients but may be useless, inappropriate, or even contraindicated in others.

Range-of-motion exercises are the mainstay of an exercise program for arthritis. Active, low-repetition (5 to 10 repetitions) range-of-motion exercise is usually preferable to passive range-of-motion exercise, but the passive form may be needed to achieve full range for joints in which the patient cannot perform full arcs of motion. Before one prescribes a range-of-motion program, however, one should carefully consider, for each joint, why loss of motion is present or expected (Table 17–1).

Joint contractures can limit motion. Such a limitation is most commonly due to contractures of joint capsules. Joint capsules readily develop contractures because of the anatomy of their braid-like intersecting fibers, which tighten if they are not taken through a full arc of their potential motion frequently (daily). All joint capsules have large "redundancies" that allow the joint to move through a full arc without tightening the capsule until the full arc for that motion is achieved. If these capsular redundancies are reduced by contractures, the capsule will tighten before the full natural arc of motion is achieved, effectively limiting the motion of the joint (Fig. 17–4). This type of capsular contracture is readily recognized by the skilled examiner by the type of resistance encountered at the end of an arc of passive motion (a "soft-end" feel).

Tendons, unlike joint capsules, usually are not readily shortened. Most supposed tendon tightness (for example, "heel cord contractures") has in fact been shown to be contractures of the respective muscles. Once a contracture has developed, whether of a capsule or of a muscle, range-of-motion exercises are inadequate to reverse the contracture. Appropriate stretching exercises are then indicated to restore motion. Range-of-motion exercises are appropriate primarily to maintain a given arc of motion and to help prevent joint contractures.

In the early stages of inflammatory arthritis, loss of motion is first and foremost due to joint capsule distention. As mentioned above, if capsular

TABLE 17–1
Causes of Limitation of Joint Motion

Contracture
  Tendon
  Muscle
  Joint capsule
Capsular distention
  Effusion
  Synovial proliferation
Intra-articular free bodies
  Foreign body
  Meniscus tear
  Villonodular synovitis
  Synovial plica
Joint surface incongruity

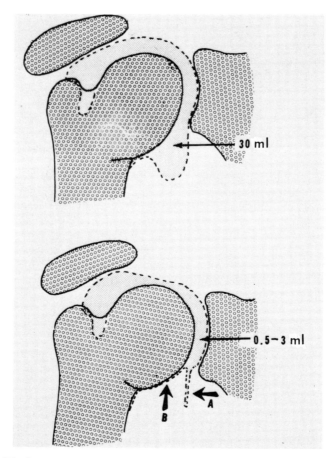

Figure 17–4

Upper, Normal shoulder capsule. *Lower,* Adhesive capsulitis, with contracted, adhered capsule (*A* and *B*); capsule volume is reduced markedly. Joint capsular "redundancies" allow joint motion. A contracted capsule limits range of motion, as does a distended capsule. (From Cailliet R. Shoulder pain. 2nd ed. Philadelphia: FA Davis, 1981. By permission of the publisher.)

redundancies are reduced by contracture, the capsule will tighten before the full potential arc of motion is achieved. If, however, the capsular redundancies are filled with fluid from an effusion or with proliferative synovium, the redundancies are already "stretched" at middle range and further motion is not possible without further stress on painful capsular fibers. Joint motion is then limited by the capsular distention from effusion or proliferative synovium or both. In such cases, range-of-motion exercises are ineffective for improving range of motion or even preventing limitation of motion, unless the effusion or synovial proliferation can be controlled or reduced. Likewise, stretching exercises are painful and ineffective and may even result in capsular disruption. Aggressive medical anti-inflammatory measures are indicated instead. These will, of course, include rest (local or systemic) to help reduce inflammation (that is, effusion and synovial proliferation). Rest may, in fact, be part of a prescription to improve range of motion. As inflammation ebbs, careful and painless range-of-motion and gentle stretching exercises can help restore the potential motion of each joint and thus help to prevent contractures from developing during this critical stage.

Loss of motion from intra-articular bodies or from joint surface incongruity (end-stage cartilage erosions) can be effectively resolved only with surgical intervention. Joint resurfacing (total joint arthroplasty) is the most effective procedure for joint surface incongruity.

In each patient, of course, different degrees and combinations of the factors that limit joint motion are present. Thus, range-of-motion and stretching exercises, rest, anti-inflammatory measures, and operation may be, and frequently are, combined and changed as the situation warrants, according to the principles outlined here.

Stiff joints and pain inevitably lead to muscle cocontraction and incoordination. Muscle reeducation is warranted for this frequent situation.

Patients who have been immobile for increasing durations often need general neuromuscular coordination and endurance training as disease, mobility, and strength permit. Individualized programs are necessary.

Strengthening exercises are indicated, in general, when weakness is present, when weakness is interfering with function, and when strengthening is possible and will not worsen the disease or cause damage. Weakness is common in patients with rheumatoid arthritis, due in part to a general decline in activities as well as a reduction in the intensity of activities. Generalized vasoconstriction, especially to major muscles, has also been implicated but not proved. Weakness of two major muscle groups—the hip and knee extensors (the glutei and quadriceps femoris)— has particular functional significance (Fig. 17–5). Weakness in these two groups results in increasing difficulty getting out of chairs and in climbing or safely descending stairs.

Strengthening exercises can be performed in patients with active arthritis, but not with traditional isotonic, weight-lifting methods. Isometric exercises can effectively strengthen muscles. Isometric exercises (weight holding) allow significant resistance to the muscle with minimal effects on joint inflammation. Clinical experience and animal studies have shown that isometric exercises cause the least adverse effects on inflammation.[8] However, allowing the slightest joint movement during a vigorous muscle contraction may increase joint inflammation. Thus, careful attention to correct technique is necessary to achieve selective muscle strengthening in rheumatoid arthritis. The Magnus belt exercise technique is one simple and effective method of accomplishing this (Fig. 17–6 A). Isometric strengthening of the quadriceps femoris with sandbags has an advantage in that quantification is possible, progression can be monitored, and patient feedback is present (Fig. 17–6 B).

Dynamic, repetitive, low-resistance isotonic exercises are appropriate after articular inflammation and pain are controlled and when sufficient

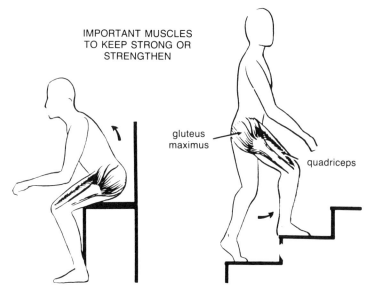

Figure 17–5
Hip and knee extensor muscles are important functionally.

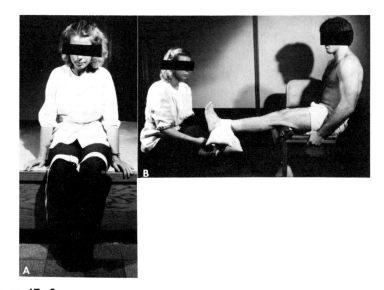

Figure 17–6
Two methods of isometric strengthening of hip and knee extensors. *A*, Magnus belt exercise. *B*, Progressive resistance exercise with sandbags.

isometric strength has been achieved. This type of exercise can be done by lifting light weights through a short arc of motion for a few repetitions.

Endurance and general fitness, in addition to selected strengthening, are also important and can be maintained or restored by low-resistance activities. Swimming is an ideal fitness program if a warm pool is available. Swimming and water exercises provide bouyancy, reduce gravity loading, and also provide a constant, low resistance. Range of motion of the joints is less painful in water. Bicycling and walking are alternatives, provided cycle resistance is kept low and proper footwear is available. Local chapters of the Arthritis Foundation often provide swimming and water programs in heated pools.

Isometric and isotonic exercises may, however, be painful during the muscle contraction and for a few moments afterward because of an increase in intra-articular pressure during the muscular contraction. Increased intra-articular pressure is present with isotonic and isometric contractions as well as, although to a lesser extent, with passive motion. This transient increase apparently is not, however, a stimulus for increased inflammation, at least with isometric exercises. A general rule of exercise is that pain may be allowed if it is transient, does not last for more than 1 hour, and is not associated with detectable increases in joint swelling, warmth, or tenderness. If these occur, the exercise should be modified or temporarily discontinued. A common problem is the performance of isotonic exercises at home, even when instructions have stressed an isometric technique. We have frequently encountered this, even in bright, well-motivated patients. On a recheck examination, the patient should always be asked to demonstrate the exercise he or she has or had been doing to identify this common error.

Exercises for the rheumatoid hand need special attention. The same principles applied to other joints for the prevention of loss of motion, for reduction of joint inflammation, and for restoration of function also apply to hand joints. However, the goals for maintaining hand function and preventing deformities require some special rules.

Rheumatoid hand deformities include digital ulnar deviation, "intrinsic plus" (or "seal flap") hands, boutonniere and swan-neck finger deformities, and various thumb deformities. Several factors contribute to ulnar deviation (Fig. 17–7): (1) the shape of the metacarpal head which tilts radially, (2) a relatively weaker metacarpal radial collateral ligament compared with the ulnar ligament, (3) the ulnar pull of the finger flexor tendons during power grip, (4) metacarpal subluxation, which is inevitably volar and radial, (5) radial and volar subluxation of the wrist, which adds to the ulnar pull of finger flexors, and (6) functional lengthening of the finger flexors when bony absorption of the carpal bones causes shortening of the wrist. Many of these factors relate to forces transmitted through finger flexors.[9] As a consequence, strengthening of finger flexors is undesirable in the rheumatoid hand because strong flexors increase ulnar deviating forces. Power grip is also discouraged. Squeezing a rubber ball is to be avoided. Motion and dexterity are instead emphasized. A general rule is to perform only low-stress exercises and activities for the upper extremities.

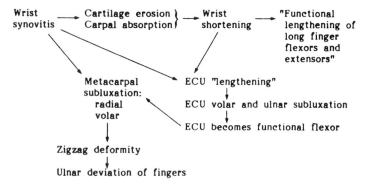

Figure 17-7
The role of the wrist in promoting ulnar deviation of fingers in rheumatoid arthritis. ECU, extensor carpi ulnaris.

Opening doors, jars, and other containers with counterclockwise resistance, if done with the right hand, as is most commonly done, stretches the radial collateral ligaments and promotes ulnar deformity. Jar and door openers can help with these tasks and thus spare the radial ligaments. Alternatively, containers can be opened (counterclockwise forces) with the left hand and closed (clockwise forces) with the right hand. The use of such assistive devices and joint protection procedures can potentially reduce subsequent hand deformities and help preserve function.

The "intrinsic plus" hand is due to a gradual tightening of the intrinsic muscles, secondary to pain and persistent spasm of these groups. Methods to reduce pain should thus be a part of a regular daily routine, as should regular intrinsic muscle stretching exercises. Intrinsic stretches are performed by actively flexing the proximal interphalangeal joints while the metacarpophalangeal joints are held in extension. These can often be performed simultaneously with warm soaks or during contrast baths.

Deformities of the wrist are reflected in "zigzag" deformities in the more distal aspects of the hand and fingers. Therefore, stabilization and early correction of volar and radial subluxation of the wrist with wrist splints are indicated.

Physical Methods

Heat, cold, massage, vibration, transcutaneous electrical nerve stimulation, and hydrotherapy are frequently prescribed for patients with rheumatoid arthritis. Each of these methods has unique physical properties, indications, and rationales. Heat is the most frequently prescribed physical method for rheumatoid arthritis. The local and systemic effects of heat are well known and described, but most of these effects are undesirable in inflamed joints. Heating of human tissue increases local blood flow, local metabolism, capillary pressure, and intracellular edema. Increased blood flow results in increases in local oxygen and nutrients, increases in leukocyte and antibody concentrations, and increases in the activity of collagenases. With this in mind, the application of cold packs to inflamed joints has been advocated. However, as has been well demonstrated, neither hot packs nor cold packs actually change the temperature of underlying large joints (shoulders, hips, or knees). Only ultrasound can effectively heat deep joints (Fig. 17−8). Heat and cold, as well as transcutaneous electrical nerve stimulation, vibration, massage, and a host of other physical methods, do relieve pain even though they do not directly heat or cool the joint. This nonspecific analgesia is apparently mediated through a neural mechanism (the "gate control" pain modulation theory). Pain relief may thus be achieved by local superficial heat, and adverse intra-articular heating effects are avoided. Even though cold packs can also relieve pain, they are not tolerated as well in patients with generalized vasoconstriction, such as those with active rheumatoid arthritis, and patients generally prefer heat for pain relief.

Warm water baths, showers, or soaks remain favorite and effective methods to reduce pain and stiffness and thus allow a more effective exercise program or increased function. Warm soaks can, however, cause hand or foot edema. An empiric system that combines the vasodilatation of warm water and the vasoconstriction of cool water was developed to minimize the formation of edema. This contrast bath consists of alternating warm (105° to 110°F) and cool (65° to 75°F) water soaks (Fig. 17−9). This is a popular and convenient method to reduce pain and stiffness in hands and feet without edema formation.

Education

Patients with rheumatoid arthritis, like those with other chronic diseases, need a thorough base of knowledge of the disease, its effects, and

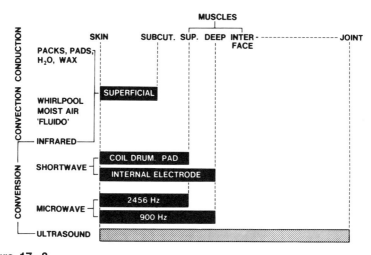

Figure 17−8
Methods of tissue heating and depth of heating. Note that only ultrasound therapy can effectively heat deep joints. Subcut., subcutaneous; Sup., superficial.

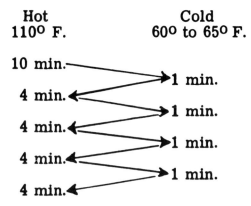

Figure 17–9
Program for contrast baths. Start and finish in warm water. Temperatures can be modified as needed and tolerated. (From Martin GM. Physical therapy in the general practitioner's office. Minn Med 1959; 42:235–239. By permission of the Minnesota Medical Association.)

its chronicity. They need to know that the cause of the disease is unknown, that there is no known cure, and that treatment is designed to prevent the effects of the incurable disease. They need thorough instruction in home therapy programs, in general health care, in hand care, and in joint protection measures. They need to be aware of possible adaptions to the home, for a hobby, and to their environment (Figs. 17–10 and 17–11).

A program of joint protection for arthritis patients includes avoiding use of the fingers in ways that might increase the potential for deformities, using good body mechanics to protect joints, using the strongest joint available for the job, avoiding the same joint position for prolonged times, respecting joint pain, and scheduling a balance of rest and activity during the day.[10]

Many rheumatic diseases are accompanied by systemic symptoms such as fatigue. Conserving energy to maximize functions becomes an important part of one's life-style. Energy conservation principles include setting priorities, pacing activities, planning for efficiency, and assuming proper positions of posture.

A knowledge of organizations such as social services, public health nursing, and therapy and vocational rehabilitation services can be valuable. Families are affected by the disease and may participate in its treatment, and therefore they also need to be included in the educational process. Finally, patients with rheumatoid arthritis, like those with cancer, need to be aware that quackery is widespread and aimed specifically at people with diseases such as theirs. Peer-oriented organizations such as the Arthritis Foundation can provide assistance and valuable advice.

Orthotics

Orthotics are used to stabilize joints, provide better positioning, reduce pain, prevent deformity, and improve function. An orthotic device

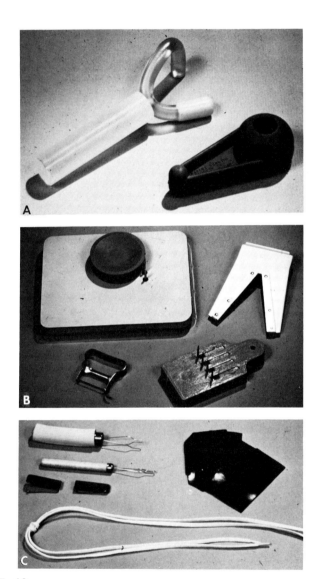

Figure 17–10
Assistive devices commonly used by patients with rheumatoid arthritis. *A,* Car door opener (left) and door knob turner (right). *B,* Jar openers and holders. *C,* Buttonhooks (left), friction rubber gripper (right), elastic shoe strings (bottom).

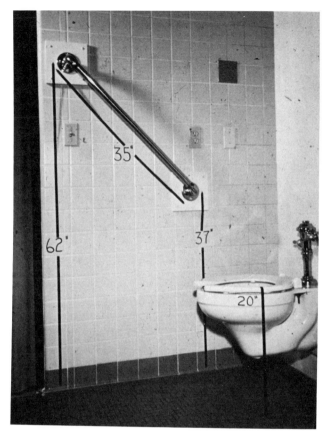

Figure 17–11
Dimensions for toilet and grab bar placement. If these cannot be remembered accurately, the patient should be sent to an occupational therapist who can provide this detailed information. (From Ellwood PM Jr. Transfers—methods, equipment, and preparation. In: Kattke FJ, Stillwell GK, Lehmann JK, eds. Krusen's handbook of physical medicine and rehabilitation. Philadelphia: WB Saunders, 1982:473–491. By permission of the publisher.)

may be needed temporarily to decrease an acute problem or may be used as a permanent device for a chronic problem.

Successful types of braces and splints include resting hand splints, wrist splints, thumb posts, and ring splints. Resting hand splints immobilize the entire hand and wrist but in doing so they interfere with function (Fig. 17–2). They are thus used at night and periodically during the day to support acutely inflamed joints. They are used primarily to decrease pain and synovitis, limit contractures, and maintain a position of optimal function during acute flares.

Static wrist splints stabilize the wrist in a functional position while allowing the fingers freedom of prehension, interfering only with power grip (Fig. 17–3). They provide wrist and ligament support when inflammation

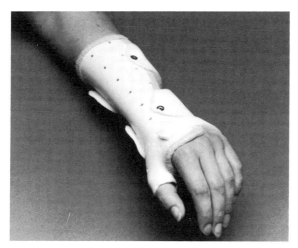

Figure 17–12
Thumb shell splint. It stabilizes the wrist and carpometacarpal and metacarpophalangeal joints of thumb. The interphalangeal joint may or may not be included.

or instability is present. This support has been shown to improve grip strength, ease the performance of the activities of daily living, and decrease pain.[11] Such a splint prevents flexion at the wrist and reduces strain and pain in associated carpal tunnel syndrome and de Quervain's tenosynovitis.

A thumb shell splint is useful for patients with a painful carpometacarpal joint (Fig. 17–12). It immobilizes the thumb in a functional, abducted position. Ring splints are useful for correctable swan-neck and boutonniere deformities (Fig. 17–13).[12]

Foot Problems

The foot may be the initial site of involvement of rheumatoid arthritis. Eventually, about 80% of patients with rheumatoid arthritis will have foot involvement.[12] Problems include pain, swelling, and deformities of the forefoot, cocked-up toes, hallus valgus, subluxed metatarsophalangeal heads, and hindfoot inflammation and deformities.

Properly fitted shoes are the first principle of management. Depth-inlay shoes are usually indicated. A wide toe box and soft deerskin upper leather help accommodate swelling and deformities (Fig. 17–14). Metatarsal pads, metatarsal bars placed proximal to the metatarsal heads, or metatarsal relief inlays can reduce metatarsalgia (Fig. 17–15). Plastozote is the material of choice because it conforms to deformities and provides shock absorption. Rocker-bottom shoes may help reduce pain due to limited motion of the first metatarsophalangeal joint, hallux rigidus, or limited ankle motion (Fig. 17–16). Athletic running and walking shoes have gained popularity and could be worn with or without modifications if foot involvement is minor.

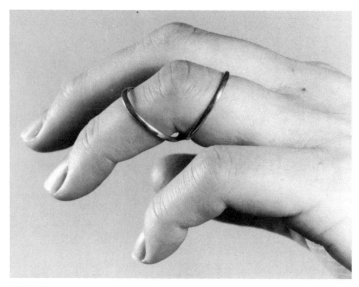

Figure 17–13
Ring splint for swan-neck deformity. It prevents hyperextension at the proximal interphalangeal joint of finger.

Mobility Aids

Various mobility aids are available to reduce lower extremity stress and to improve mobility in later stages of progressive arthritis. Canes, crutches, and walkers may be prescribed to reduce stress on inflamed hips, knees, ankles, or feet; but while doing so, they simply transfer that stress to the upper extremities, including the wrist and hand. One way to avoid this stress on the hand and wrist is to add platforms to the gait aids (see Chapter

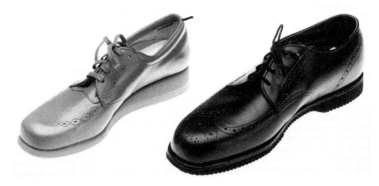

Figure 17–14
Extra-depth shoes. Wide toe box and soft deerskin upper help accommodate swelling and deformities.

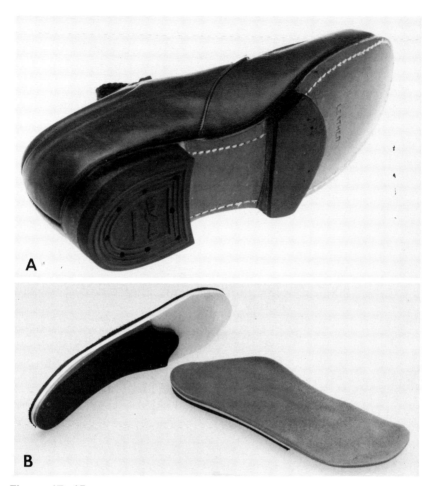

Figure 17–15
A, Extra-depth shoe with metatarsal bar. Metatarsal bar should be placed proximal to the metatarsal heads. *B,* Metatarsal relief inlays. They are placed inside extra-depth shoes to relieve metatarsalgia.

38). These devices, although still shifting stress to the upper extremities, eliminate weight-bearing stresses on the wrists and hands. Stair gliders enable one to ascend or descend stairs despite inflamed joints or weak muscles. Wheelchairs can provide an energy-efficient method for mobility, but the stress placed on the upper extremities from propelling a wheelchair is not any less than the stress placed on the lower extremities with walking. If a wheelchair is needed for mobility, an electric wheelchair should be considered. Vans with hydraulic lifts may allow improved mobility for the wheelchair-dependent patient.

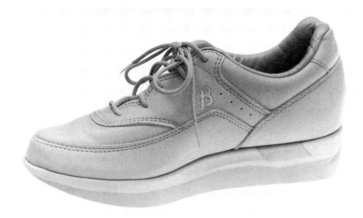

Figure 17–16
Rocker-bottom shoe. It facilitates toe-off.

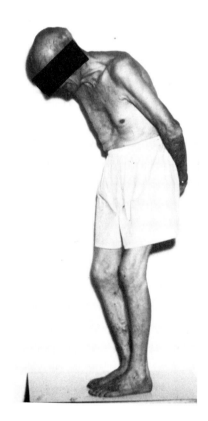

Figure 17–17
Flexed, ankylosed spine in ankylosing spondylitis. Note tight pectoral, hip, and knee flexor muscles, dorsal kyphosis, protracted shoulders, loss of cervical lordosis, and proximity of rib cage to iliac crest.

ANKYLOSING SPONDYLITIS

Ankylosing spondylitis is a unique disorder in that the synovitis associated with it is predominantly localized to the posterior joints of the spine, including the spinal facet joints, the costovertebral joints, and the sacroiliac joints. Loss of motion of the cervical, thoracic, and lumbar spine and loss of chest wall motion result. Ankylosis of the spine is not the final result because characteristic ankylosis in a flexed, stooped posture causes severe functional impairment (Fig. 17–17).

Regular physical examinations should include measurements of height, chest expansion, and the C-7 to S-1 spinal flexion (in centimeters).

If spinal fusion occurs in this flexed position, balance, ambulation, and respiration can be severely impaired. Although no cure is available and no treatment can necessarily prevent spinal ankylosis, efforts should be made to prevent fusion in a flexed position. It is necessary to understand that such a flexed posture is a result of one's attempt to reduce pain by flexing the spine and therefore unloading the inflamed facet joints. Exercises that stretch the chest flexors (pectoral stretches) and strengthen the spinal extensors are provided, as are range-of-motion exercises for the neck and shoulders, deep-breathing exercises, and posture principles. But these principles must be accompanied by pain relief, including heat, massage, and nonsteroidal anti-inflammatory medications.

Assistive devices such as prism glasses, wide-angle rear vision mirrors for the car, and reachers may be helpful to compensate for limited spine motion. Contact sports, diving, and motorcycle riding are high-risk activities and can result in vertebral fractures. Such fractures are frequently associated with spinal cord compression in ankylosing spondylitis.

REFERENCES

1. Swezey RL. Arthritis rehabilitation: staff, facilities, and evaluation. In: Ehrlich GE, ed. Rehabilitation management of rheumatic conditions. 2nd ed. Baltimore: Williams & Wilkins, 1986:1–23.
2. Downey JA. The physiatrist in rheumatoid arthritis management. In: Ehrlich GE, ed. Rehabilitation management of rheumatic conditions. 2nd ed. Baltimore: Williams & Wilkins, 1986:24–30.
3. McCarty DJ. Arthritis and allied conditions: a textbook of rheumatology. 11th ed. Philadelphia: Lea & Febiger, 1989:773–825.
4. Swezey RL. Arthritis: rational therapy and rehabilitation. Philadelphia: WB Saunders, 1978:1–192.
5. Smith RD, Polly HDF. Rest therapy for rheumatoid arthritis. Mayo Clin Proc 1978; 53:141–145.
6. Partridge REH, Duthie JJR. Controlled trial of the effect of complete immobilization of the joints in rheumatoid arthritis. Ann Rheum Dis 1963; 22:91–98.
7. Gault SJ, Spyker JM. Beneficial effect of immobilization of joints in rheumatoid and related arthritides: a splint study using sequential analysis. Arthritis Rheum 1969; 12:34–44.
8. Merritt JL, Hunder GG. Passive range of motion, not isometric exercise, amplifies acute urate synovitis. Arch Phys Med Rehabil 1983; 64:130–131.

9. Gramse RR. The rheumatoid hand, mechanism of deformity, and the rationale for using splints. Semin Phys Med Rehabil, Mayo Clinic, October 1977:25.
10. Joint protection for the arthritic person. Mayo Clinic: Occupational Therapy publication, 1985.
11. Merritt JL. Advances in orthotics for the patient with rheumatoid arthritis. J Rheum (Suppl 15) 1987; 14:62–67.
12. Hicks JE, Nicholas JJ, Swezey RL. Handbook of rehabilitative rheumatology. Atlanta: American Rheumatism Association, 1988.

18

Inflammatory Myopathies

Janet M. Cogoli
Mary L. Jurisson
Mehrsheed Sinaki

Inflammatory myopathies are characterized by muscle weakness and evidence of inflammation. There are several types of inflammatory myopathies; the most common of these are categorized in Table 18−1.[1] These categories are useful because the myopathies generally have different presentations, different courses, different pathologic features, and different responses to treatment.[1−3] Polymyositis and dermatomyositis are themselves heterogeneous diseases and may occur in several subtypes (Table 18−1). They may be associated with systemic autoimmune disorders such as rheumatoid arthritis, systemic lupus erythematosus, and scleroderma; they can also be associated with systemic malignancies. The childhood form of polymyositis can be associated with systemic vasculitis. Inclusion body myositis may characteristically involve distal muscles. Management of inflammatory myopathies requires accurate diagnosis, identification of associated functional problems, anticipation of complications, and timely use of appropriate medication and rehabilitative interventions. Although much has been written about these disorders, there is a dearth of literature concerning the application of physiotherapy for their management. They vary in severity; therefore, a rehabilitation program that addresses the variability of the illness needs to be established. This chapter discusses the essential components of a physiotherapy program directed at the physical and functional problems of these illnesses.

DIAGNOSIS

The diagnosis of an inflammatory myopathy may be suspected on the basis of clinical findings and evolution of the disease. Differentiating in-

TABLE 18–1

Types of Inflammatory Myopathies

Polymyositis and dermatomyositis
  Polymyositis of adults
  Dermatomyositis of adults
  Dermatomyositis of children
  Polymyositis and dermatomyositis
    associated with other rheumatic
    conditions
  Polymyositis and dermatomyositis
    associated with malignancy
Inclusion body myositis
Acute viral myositis
Miscellaneous

Modified from Banker and Engel.[1]

flammatory myopathies from other myopathies requires additional testing. Inflammation of muscles is suggested by an elevated concentration of serum creatine kinase; electromyogram showing increased insertional activity or myopathic motor unit potentials; and inflammatory cell infiltration in muscle tissue or vessels on biopsy. Quantitative muscle strength testing usually shows muscle weakness. Confirmatory evidence of the inflammatory nature of the myopathy is not always present in all tests in every case.

TREATMENT

Obviously, underlying diseases should be identified and treated. The treatment options are listed in Table 18–2.

TABLE 18–2

Treatment of Inflammatory Myopathies

Corticosteroids (prednisone)
Other immunosuppressive agents
  Methotrexate
  Azathioprine
  Cyclophosphamide
  Chlorambucil
Cyclosporine
Rehabilitation
  Physical therapy
  Occupational therapy
  Speech therapy
  Orthotics
  Vocational counseling
  Other

TABLE 18–3

Comprehensive Program for the Three Rehabilitation Phases of Acute Inflammatory Myopathy

Early Acute Phase	Middle Phase	Remission Phase
Proper positioning	Active or active-assisted	Active ROM†
Prevention of DVT*	ROM†	Strengthening exercises
Screening of swallowing	Mild strengthening	Assistive devices
function	exercises	(occupational therapy
Respiratory care	Progressive ambulation	evaluation)
Tilt table	Assistive devices	Vocational counseling
Skin care	(occupational therapy	Dismissal planning
Mild heat, hydrotherapy	evaluation)	
Stroking massage	Avoidance of exertional	
Passive ROM†	physical activities	
Assistive devices		
(occupational therapy		
evaluation)		

*DVT, deep vein thrombosis.
†ROM, range-of-motion exercises.

Glucocorticosteroids are the foundation of medical treatment and are ideally given early in high doses (1 to 1.5 mg/kg), sometimes in divided doses. Other immunosuppressive agents such as methotrexate, azathioprine, and cyclophosphamide may be given as steroid-sparing agents or when glucocorticosteroids are ineffective.[4]

Inclusion body myositis and the myositis associated with scleroderma are often less responsive to prednisone. If there is no clear improvement in activity and progression after 6 to 9 months of treatment, the complications of steroid administration may outweigh the benefits.

Rehabilitation measures are important in every patient with inflammatory myopathies. We have found that, for purposes of organizing our rehabilitation techniques for inflammatory myopathies, it is helpful to group patients according to the course of their illness; the three rehabilitation phases are early acute, middle, and remission (Table 18–3).

EARLY ACUTE PHASE

Polymyositis and dermatomyositis syndromes and occasionally inclusion body myositis may be responsive to glucocorticosteroids. Early use of glucocorticosteroids may improve the response to treatment.[5, 6] During this initial phase of diagnosis and initiation of treatment, bed rest or extremely limited activity is usually recommended. Although most of the inflammatory myopathies are not marked by pain, occasionally arthritis and myalgia may be prominent. Pain may be minimized by the application of mild heat; superficial heat can be applied with an infrared heat lamp. Hydrotherapy may also be used for the relief of pain; immersion in a Hubbard tank (temperature, 36.7°C to 37.2°C) or a warm tub bath for 20 to 30 minutes may be used. The alleviation of pain by these simple methods is effective for decreasing secondary muscle spasm. However, before and during the use of these methods, the cardiac status of the patient must be determined. Electrocardiographic abnormalities have been noted in polymyositis.[7-9] In the presence of cardiomyopathy, serious rhythm abnormalities, or heart block, these treatments are contraindicated. A gentle, stroking massage over the bony prominences of bedridden patients has a relaxing, sedative effect. Massage would be inappropriate in patients who manifest dermatomyositis because of the presence of fragile, atrophic skin.

To maintain the tone of the cardiovascular system in the early acute stage with severe weakness, we recommend the use of a tilt table once or twice daily, before which the lower extremities of the patient are wrapped in elastic bandages to provide support against venous pooling and resultant orthostatism.

In the presence of pharyngeal and laryngeal weakness, the patient should be referred for fluoroscopic swallowing evaluation of dysphagia, occupational therapy or speech therapy evaluation, and instruction in techniques to avoid aspiration of food during swallowing.

In patients with involvement of the respiratory muscles, respiratory function should be determined at least once daily. Some patients will need respiratory assistance with a positive-pressure respirator. The danger of pneumonia exists in debilitated patients with acute polymyositis,[10] and treatment should include adequate postural drainage and chest physical therapy.

Because remission of polymyositis and dermatomyositis may occur,[11, 12] patients should not be left with disabling residua that could have been avoided with proper daily care. Therefore, a major emphasis of the treatment program should be the maintenance of flexibility. Muscle contractures may develop as the weak muscles are unable to move the respective joints through their normal range of motion and as intrinsic changes within the muscle, such as fibrosis, occur.[13] Tightness occurs early in the two-joint muscle groups, such as the gastrocnemius-soleus muscles, the hip flexors, and the hamstrings. In the upper extremity, the forearm pronators and the elbow, wrist, and finger flexors are often tight. Examination for tightness should be a part of the evaluation of all patients with polymyositis during all stages.[13]

Gentle range-of-motion exercises that avoid the production of pain but gradually increase the arc of motion are a necessity. During the early acute stage, only passive range-of-motion exercises should be applied to the joints. They should be done by an experienced therapist once or twice daily, and care should be taken to avoid pain and fatigue. Active range-of-motion exercises performed by the patient are not recommended during the early acute stage because they may cause overuse of the muscles involved by an active inflammatory process. Properly performed range-of-motion exercises help to decrease myalgia and to protect against the early development of contractures. If allowed to develop, contractures are a painful, disabling, time-consuming, and expensive complication to correct. Other measures that should also be taken to prevent contractures are proper positioning of the joints when the patient is in bed and maintaining the joints in their functional positions to avoid ankylosis and deformities. This effort is greatly helped by splinting the wrists, digits, and ankles, as needed. The principles of proper positioning are discussed in Chapter 6.

A common problem with immobility is constipation or bowel impaction, which can be prevented with a proper fluid intake and use of stool softeners (docusate sodium, Colace), bulk formers, or suppositories (bisacodyl, Dulcolax) on an as-needed basis. Frequent use of laxatives should be avoided (see Chapter 6).

The skin must be scrupulously cared for in order to prevent the development of pressure sores. It should be inspected daily, and the patient should be provided with a water mattress or an alternating air mattress and synthetic sheepskin. If unable to turn himself or herself, the patient should be turned by the nursing staff every 2 hours during the day and every 4 hours while sleeping. The heels should be prevented from resting on the mattress by placing a pillow under the calves.

Deep vein thrombosis in the lower extremities of severely weakened patients must also be prevented. Subcutaneously administered low-dose heparin may be helpful toward this end, as in the treatment of patients with spinal cord injuries.[14, 15]

MIDDLE PHASE

Many patients with myositis respond well to glucocorticosteroids, as evidenced by a cessation of progression, normalization of the creatine kinase value, and improved muscle strength in several weeks to several months. This response marks the middle phase of the disease. In the presence of any significantly weakened proximal muscles, therapy should be aimed at transfers and gradual ambulation with the use of an appropriate gait aid, if needed. Involvement of the distal extremities has also been documented in both polymyositis[10] and dermatomyositis.[16] The use of lightweight ankle-foot orthoses may be beneficial because weakness of the distal extremities significantly interferes with gait. Bracing should be kept to a minimum to avoid limitation of the patient's functional ability.

During this stage, as serum enzyme levels improve, the range-of-motion exercises can be safely progressed to active-assisted and then to active, in which the patient performs the motions on his or her own power. Each session, at least once but preferably twice daily, should consist of three to five consecutive full-range movements of each joint. Initially, to avoid fatigue, we prefer to limit the patient's participation in the performance of range-of-motion exercises on the major peripheral joints (that is, the shoulders, hips, and knees). When the patient has adequate strength to perform independently without muscle fatigue, he or she may begin resuming normal activities.

REMISSION PHASE

As the patient continues to improve and serum enzyme levels decrease toward normal, active range-of-motion exercises may be performed. Mild strengthening exercises may also become a part of the treatment program. The exercise program may advance from simple isometric contraction to resistive exercises. Documenting muscle strength with quantitative muscle testing can be helpful for following the patient's outcome.[17] This can be done with free weights or isokinetic dynamometry using a few repetitions of representative muscles.

During all stages of acute inflammatory myopathy, occupational therapy is invaluable. Functional assessment by evaluating the patient's ability to perform activities of daily living is of vital importance. This information must be known to determine treatment goals and to help with the planning for dismissal. Adaptive equipment may be needed to help the patient translate motor residuals into practical function.

When dismissal is planned, the patient's occupation needs to be considered. Some modification may be needed to avoid overuse of the muscles in exertional activities. In some cases, a major change in career becomes necessary.

All patients with myositis should be carefully followed up for reactivation of the myositis.[11] Those receiving maintenance doses of corticosteroids[18] should also be watched for the development of side effects, which could include a steroid-induced myopathy and increased weakness or osteoporosis predisposing to compression fractures of the spine. If osteoporosis occurs, measures outlined in Chapter 16 and application of a back support during physical activities are recommended.

Steroid myopathy has been shown to respond well to isokinetic strengthening.[19]

Although the dose of glucocorticosteroids can be tapered and use of the agents can be discontinued, occasionally a patient suffers exacerbations with withdrawal of steroids. In these instances, steroid-sparing agents such as azathioprine or methotrexate may be instituted. Some of the inflammatory myopathies may be entirely self-limited. Some may become chronic and may be entirely unresponsive to medication; in these instances, it may become appropriate to attempt gentle strengthening and to optimize activities.[20]

REFERENCES

1. Banker BQ, Engel AG. The polymyositis and dermatomyositis syndromes. In: Engel AG, Banker BQ. Myology: basic and clinical. New York: McGraw-Hill Book Company, 1986:1385–1422.
2. Bunch TW. Polymyositis. In: Spittel JA Jr, ed. Clinical medicine. Vol. 4, Chapter 36, 2nd ed. Philadelphia: Harper & Row, 1980:1–8.
3. Bunch TW. Prednisone and azathioprine for polymyositis: long-term followup. Arthritis Rheum 1981; 24:45–48.

4. Bunch TW. The therapy of polymyositis. Mt Sinai J Med 1988; 55:483–486.
5. Henriksson KG, Sandstedt P. Polymyositis—treatment and prognosis: a study of 107 patients. Acta Neurol Scand 1982; 65:280–300.
6. Bohan A, Peter JB, Bowman RL, Pearson CM. A computer-assisted analysis of 153 patients with polymyositis and dermatomyositis. Medicine 1977; 56:255–286.
7. Bohan A, Peter JB. Polymyositis and dermatomyositis. N Engl J Med 1975; 292:344–347, 403–407.
8. Fernandez-Herlihy L. Heart block in polymyositis. N Engl J Med 1971; 284(Letter):1101.
9. Hill DL, Barrows HS. Identical skeletal and cardiac muscle involvement in a case of fatal polymyositis. Arch Neurol 1968;19:545–551.
10. Malpe RR, Lee MHM, Alba A. Rehabilitation technics in polymyositis. NY State J Med 1973; 73:1208–1210.
11. Winkelmann RK, Mulder DW, Lambert EH, Howard FM Jr, Diessner GR. Course of dermatomyositis-polymyositis: comparison of untreated and cortisone-treated patients. Mayo Clin Proc 1968; 43:545–556.
12. Pearson CM. Polymyositis and dermatomyositis. In: Hollander JL, ed. Arthritis and allied conditions: a textbook of rheumatology. 8th ed. Philadelphia: Lea & Febiger, 1972:940–961.
13. Kottke FJ, Stillwell GK, Lehmann JF. Krusen's handbook of physical medicine and rehabilitation. 3rd ed. Philadelphia: WB Saunders, 1982:334, 683.
14. Watson N. Anti-coagulant therapy in the prevention of venous thrombosis and pulmonary embolism in the spinal cord injury. Paraplegia 1978–1979; 16:265–269.
15. Cotton LT, Roberts VC. The prevention of deep vein thrombosis, with particular reference to mechanical methods of prevention. Surgery 1977; 81:228–235.
16. Resnick JS, Mammel M, Mundale M, Kottke FJ. Muscular strength as an index of response to therapy in childhood dermatomyositis. Arch Phys Med Rehabil 1981; 62:12–19.
17. Miller LC, Michael AF, Baxter TL, Kim Y. Quantitative muscle testing in childhood dermatomyositis. Arch Phys Med Rehabil 1988; 69:610–613.
18. Gilroy J, Meyer JS. Medical neurology. 3rd ed. New York: Macmillan Publishing Company, 1979:733–736.
19. Horber FF, Scheidegger JR, Grünig BE, Frey FJ. Evidence that prednisone-induced myopathy is reversed by physical training. J Clin Endocrinol Metab 1985; 61:83–88.
20. Jurisson ML. Rehabilitation in rheumatic diseases: what's new. West J Med 1991; 154:545–548.

PART VII

Geriatric Rehabilitation

19

Geriatric Rehabilitation: Basic Considerations

Kevin P. Murphy

Mehrsheed Sinaki

According to US census statistics, the number of Americans older than 65 years has been growing at a rate 3 times faster than that of the general population. In 1950, 12 million people older than 65 years were living in the United States.[1] Currently, approximately 25 million people older than 65 years are living in the United States, and this number will rise to approximately 55 million by the year 2030.[1] This increase is expected because persons born during the baby boom (following the end of World War II) will reach this age by the year 2030. At present, about 5% (1.3 million) of the nation's elderly population resides in nursing homes; by the year 2000, this number is expected to increase by approximately 50%.[1]

As the elderly population increases in number, it will require an increasing proportion of medical care. At present, this group uses more medical services than any other age group, being hospitalized twice as often and staying in the hospital twice as long.[1] Traditional medical care competently handles, in an increasingly professional manner, the life-and-death matters that contribute to the duration of life. It is a simple fact that sophisticated medical technology and profound medical knowledge have added years to the average human life span.

Rehabilitation medicine has been evolving rapidly since World War II and deals directly with the quality of life. To keep up with the estimated needs of the present and the future, the subspecialty of geriatric rehabilitation is beginning to define itself. This chapter attempts to portray some basic considerations of geriatric rehabilitation, which is generally defined as the rehabilitation of persons age 65 or older. Many of the basic physical medicine and rehabilitation principles for different disease states and for therapeutic exercise have been discussed in previous chapters or apply to patients of all ages and will not be discussed further here. Any rehabilitation plan must first establish the patient's overall general medical condition and subsequently optimize this condition toward obtaining maximal rehabilitation goals and potential.

MEDICAL CONSIDERATIONS

Certain *medical conditions* appear with high frequency in the elderly population and have a considerable effect on the outcomes of rehabilitation.[2] Anemia is prevalent in the elderly population and may explain why a patient is falling short of goals in mobility and therapeutic exercise. Other conditions that can contribute to suboptimal performance are myxedema, occult malignancy, cardiovascular disease, chronic infection, metabolic imbalance, and pulmonary dysfunction. With aging, maximal voluntary ventilation and vital capacity decrease, as do respiratory muscular strength and endurance. These effects contribute significantly to easy fatigue and lowered working capacity.

Nutritional deficits are of major concern also. The basic metabolic rate decreases about 2% per decade in adults, and the average protein requirement remains about 1 g/kg per day throughout life.[3] Calorie requirements remain essentially the same throughout adult life at approximately 1,800 to 2,000 calories per day.[4] Vitamin deficiency in elderly persons is relatively uncommon, probably because of the many over-the-counter supplements available and ample support by the media for increased vitamin intake.[5] Anorexia and subsequent cachexia are common, especially in the presence of chronic disease. Reasons for poor nutrition include restricted mobility and inconvenience for food preparation, loss of appetite, depression, decreased motivation, gastritis and gastroesophageal reflux, dysphagia, poor dentures, and excessive medications. *Polypharmacy* is a common problem in the elderly patient, and it is magnified when the patient does not have the cognitive ability to adhere to a therapeutic medication schedule. The side effects and toxicity of excessive medications are real, limiting, and, at times, deadly.

The effects of *immobility* need some basic consideration. About 3% of muscle strength can be lost per day during complete immobilization.[6] Therefore, an immobilized individual who has marginal mobility and self-care ability can quickly become totally dependent because of loss of muscle strength. Other effects of chronic immobility include contractures, osteoporosis, orthostatic hypotension, reduced cardiac performance and blood volume, negative nitrogen and calcium balance, electrolyte imbalance, urinary tract stones, deep venous thromboses and pulmonary emboli, skin pressure sores, and pulmonary hypoventilation syndromes.[7] No less disabling consequences are those that arise from severe sensory and emotional deprivation, which may lead to increased confusion, depression, and general disorientation.

Skin tolerance to pressure is decreased in the elderly population. This results from atrophy of subcutaneous adipose tissue with loss of skin resilience and turgor and from possible sensory motor neuropathies.[5] Peripheral edema and venous stasis syndromes also lead to decreased skin tolerance, and pressure sores develop easily along the hindfoot and medial and lateral malleolar areas. Capillary closing pressure in adults is estimated to be 25 mm Hg and is of consideration when prescribing elastic support garments.[2] In general, over-the-counter elastic stockings provide approximately 10 mm Hg of pressure and, in this capacity, have an optimal effect on the control of peripheral edema only when the patient is supine. The energy expenditure for donning high-pressure elastic garments can be tremendous, and a high level of manual dexterity and eye-hand coordination is required.

Visual and auditory impairment can be tremendously disabling to the elderly patient and is often mistaken for depression, poor cooperation, cognitive dysfunction, hostility, and speech impairment. A cataract in a patient with severe loss of distal proprioception can be exceptionally disabling because visual feedback to correct for the loss of joint position is inadequate. In such a patient, removal of the cataract may allow for a more functional and independent state. In an amputee who is visually impaired, a prosthetic lower extremity may provide more sensory-motor feedback, distal proprioception, and independence than if a wheelchair were used alone. Not uncommonly, a prescription for a hearing aid or new eyeglasses causes dramatic improvements in the overall course of rehabilitation.

Geriatric rehabilitation generally involves two medical divisions: healthy and frail. Healthy persons are usually vigorous, 65 years of age or older, retired or financially comfortable, relatively well-educated, and politically active. Those classified as frail generally have significant physical or mental deterioration. In addition, they commonly suffer from loss of social and financial support and require a network of public services (social, financial, avocational, and health care) to maintain any quality of life or semi-independence. Frail, elderly persons are generally older than 80 years, but the definition resides more on their present state of functioning.

NEUROMUSCULAR-SKELETAL CONSIDERATIONS

Therapeutic exercise in the elderly population has some special considerations. Both anaerobic and aerobic programs need assessment if physical and cardiopulmonary limitations are present. Stationary bicycling, swimming, or daily walking can be excellent aerobic and general mobility programs. An aerobic workout for 20 minutes three times a week that does not exceed 60% to 80% of the maximal heart rate, with appropriate warm-up and cool-down periods, may be optimal but certainly must be individualized carefully.[8] The Borg perceived scale of exertion can be helpful for discerning the limitations of the aerobic exercise program.[8, 9] Appropriate shoe modifications to allow comfort while walking may allow a patient to remain active and well conditioned. For less mobile, bedridden patients, bimanual activities can be used for both anaerobic and aerobic conditioning. Isometric exercises, in contrast to an isotonic strengthening program, seem to demand more from the cardiovascular system because a state of cardiovascular equilibrium is not achieved.[10]

According to Müller,[6] one 6-second isometric contraction per day per muscle group can be enough to ward off the daily 3% decline in muscle strength that results from complete immobilization. Deep-breathing exercises and postural drainage techniques may be especially important in a patient with chronic pulmonary disease. Contractures of intercostal muscles and early costochondral calcifications can occur with a decrease in chest wall compliance if range-of-motion exercises are not performed.

Daily range-of-motion exercises and stretching by simple techniques can be helpful for preventing contractures that would further limit mobility (Fig. 19–1 and 19–2). The simple knee or hip flexion-contracture can create a significant leg-length discrepancy or flexed posture during the gait cycle. This may increase the energy consumption of walking above the physiologic tolerance of the patient and result in falling, cessation of gait, and the subsequent sequelae of trauma and immobilization. Simple techniques

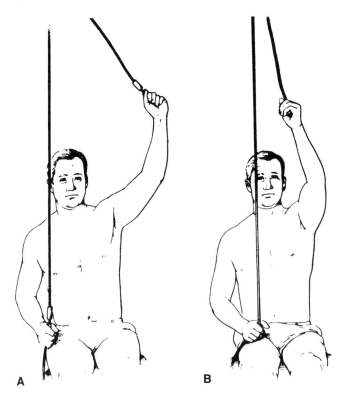

A   B

Figure 19–1
Range-of-motion exercises for shoulders, with pulley. *A*, Abduction. *B*, Flexion.

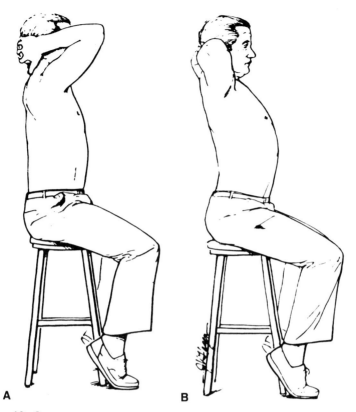

Figure 19–2
A, Shoulder abduction and external rotation combined with pectoral stretching. B, Deep-breathing combined with pectoral stretching to prevent stooped posture.

in the supine or upright posture for stretching hip and knee flexors and the pectoral muscles can be of great benefit for avoiding these problems (Fig. 19–3 through 19–5). In the presence of weakness and ataxia, stretching while in the supine position is preferred. More complex exercises involving neuromuscular reeducation and relaxation techniques, including biofeedback, may be limited in elderly patients with mild to moderate cognitive dysfunction. In any therapeutic exercise program, especially in elderly patients, the work-rest cycle needs to be optimal, preventing unwanted fatigue.

Use of physical methods in the elderly population demands appropriate understanding of the contraindications. In general, microwave and shortwave methods are contraindicated in the presence of joint arthroplasties, cardiac pacemakers, insensate regions of the body, areas of poor arterial perfusion, and areas of malignancy.[11] Therapeutic electricity can also be contraindicated in patients with cardiac disorders or pacemakers.[11] Use

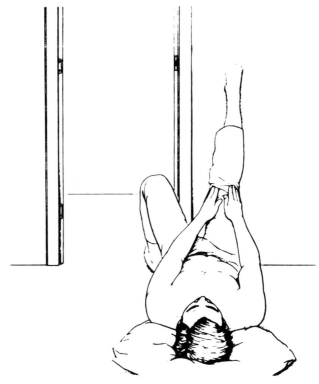

Figure 19–3
Stretching hamstrings while in supine (resting) position. This technique can be applied in the presence of ataxia and poor coordination.

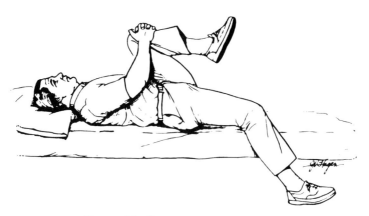

Figure 19–4
Simple technique for stretching hip flexors.

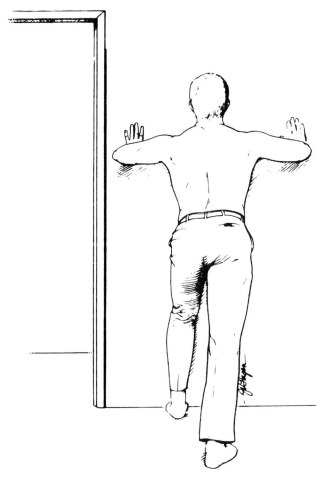

Figure 19–5
Method of stretching hamstring and pectoral muscles in ambulatory patients.

of cold therapy can trigger Raynaud's phenomenon and cryoglobuline-mia.[11]

Osteoporotic patients—particularly postmenopausal women—need special consideration for therapeutic exercise and protective spinal bracing. Vertebral compression fractures are common in osteoporosis and can be an extreme cause of limitation and chronic pain. Evidence suggests that spinal extension and isometric exercises are appropriate for patients with postmenopausal osteoporosis to ward off vertebral compression fractures.[12] If osteoporosis is severe, bone mineral density should be ascertained and medical treatments evaluated. Degenerative joint disease and rheumatoid arthritis are discussed in Chapter 17.

MOBILITY

Mobility in the geriatric population varies from playing tennis and mountain climbing to being wheelchair-dependent because of degenerative joint disease.

In general, approximately 70% of nursing home residents have some form of restricted mobility, which varies from needing a cane or a wheelchair to being bedridden.[1] Mobility is certainly one of the most important factors used to determine whether institutional care is needed for an elderly patient. A comprehensive rehabilitation program is probably the best way to assess and perpetuate functional mobility. An important part of this program is the therapeutic principles of exercise mentioned above, including contracture-free range of motion, strengthening, posture principles, coordination routines, appropriate footwear modification, gait-aid assessment, and a functional prescription for the amputee.

Significant consideration must be given to energy expenditure and the various forms of gait aids that are available. In general, crutch walking consumes about 70% more energy than the normal gait pattern.[13] According to most studies, wheelchair mobility on level ground increases the energy expenditure by only 7% to 10%.[13] Foremost in any consideration of mobility in the elderly population should be the idea of safety over function. This is of utmost importance to prevent trauma sequelae such as fractured hips and chronic subdural hematomas. Architectural barriers, such as stairs, curbs, carpet, and tile, need special consideration. Safe mobility in patients receiving anticoagulants is often overlooked, and the result can be a life-threatening situation. An individual with normal neuromuscular function but significant cognitive, visual, or perceptual dysfunctions may require mobility limitations to optimize safety. Approximately 30% to 40% of nursing home residents fall each year.[14, 15] Studies suggest that only 1% to 5% of these falls result in fracture, and 5% to 10% result in severe soft tissue injuries.[14, 16] Some studies suggest that those who are injured tend to be more independent in their self-care and are less likely depressed and more likely to have lower extremity weakness.[17] Factors associated with serious injury during falls by nursing home residents are presently an area of expanding study.

One basic and often forgotten consideration in all age groups, especially the elderly, is the value of transfer ability. The ability to perform independent transfers or transfers with minimal assistance may allow the patient to be placed in a low- rather than high-nursing-skill unit with subsequent improvement in the quality of life. The ability to transfer into and out of a chair or onto or off a commode is basic and simple, yet its importance is commonly overlooked in a patient's overall care.

ACTIVITIES OF DAILY LIVING

The activities of daily living are of prime importance in determining an independent living status in elderly patients. Dysphagia can be the result of multiple causes. Comprehensive swallowing evaluation with various liquids and food substances may be helpful in achieving a functional and nutritive swallow. Recent increased use of videofluoroscopy with barium-impregnated nourishments also seems helpful in this regard and adds more objectivity to dietary selections. For the evaluation of dressing ability, energy conservation techniques need attention, as do practical time limits for dressing and undressing. A metal razor blade may be too dangerous for shaving in some patients, especially those who have significant cognitive dysfunction or are receiving anticoagulant medications. A detailed occupational assessment must include household duties, vocational and avocational interests, and safety and judgment evaluations. A patient who leaves a burner ignited on a stove after finishing a meal shows poor safety habits and judgment ability, as does a senile, visually impaired carpenter who continues to use power tools and electric saws. A patient's ability to gain access to an emergency care system must also be assessed. This assessment often involves evaluating the ability to dial the "911" emergency telephone number or the telephone number of a hospital facility, neighbor, or friend.

Toileting ability is an important determinant of quality of life, regardless of age group. A good bowel program with a high-fiber diet, psyllium hydrophilic mucilloid (Metamucil) twice a day, adequate fluids, and every-other-day use of rectal suppositories may prevent unwanted intestinal ileus and provide for predictable bowel evacuation. Many nursing homes do not provide assistance with intermittent catheterization schedules; thus, long-term indwelling catheters are more common in nursing home residents. Antibiotic suppression is usually not advised with an indwelling catheter because of the possibility of developing resistant urinary tract infections.[18] Most therapy plans recommend changing the catheter every 2 to 3 weeks in addition to performing a urinalysis, Gram stain, and culture. If a positive colony count (more than 100,000 organisms) is present, symptoms of the urinary tract infection are generally required before institution of antibiotic medications. Such symptoms commonly include cloudy urine, fever, catheter leakage, dysuria, and an elevated leukocyte or erythrocyte count on a screening urinalysis.

PSYCHIATRIC CONSIDERATIONS

More than 50% of nursing home residents are estimated to have some form of senile dementia, mostly Alzheimer's type.[1] These persons need to be differentiated from delirious patients whose conditions may be secondary to medications or an abnormal metabolic state and usually follow a more acute to subacute time course. Depression can masquerade as several somatic complaints, including chronic pain, absentmindedness, anorexia with weight loss, and insomnia. Antidepressant medications may be of benefit in patients with strong vegetative symptoms, and their anticholinergic side effects need consideration. A patient with chronic pain behavior may respond better to an approach that involves controlled use of analgesics and measures of behavior modification. In a proper environment, one can decrease the use of analgesics in an organized fashion through substitution with other physical measures. Codeine should not be used as an analgesic in order to avoid the problem of constipation, which is common in elderly persons.

Communication disorders, including dyspraxias and dysphasias, can make it difficult to determine the degree of cognitive impairment that is present. Most psychometric evaluations demand some recognition of objects, symbols, or the written or spoken word. General orientation to place and person, memory from day to day of various activities, and the ability to follow one- or two-step simple commands are basic abilities first sought in any cognitive retraining program. Motivation,[19] a quality that transcends psychiatric doctrines, is certainly a key element in achieving rehabilitation goals and potential. Many times there is an organic explanation for a poorly motivated patient, and a change in medication or the establishment of hormonal, nutritional, or electrolyte balance may provide the needed impetus for progressive rehabilitation gains. A patient with mental confusion who also has an ataxic gait and incontinence should be evaluated for the possibility of normal-pressure hydrocephalus or for cerebral mass lesions.

Elderly patients can be difficult to teach because they may think they are "too old to learn." Some of them may be resistant to change or have a significant fear of failure. The role of a rehabilitation psychologist as a member of the rehabilitation team cannot be overemphasized. Further considerations include discussions about death and dying and the practice of sexuality. Many older people are sexually active, and almost all need and want some form of companionship. More centers are beginning to realize this need for companionship in the long-term care of elderly persons and are allowing for quiet areas where married couples can spend time with each other.

SOCIAL CONSIDERATIONS

The degree of family support may be the sole most important ingredient in determining whether an elderly patient can live safely outside of a nursing home.[20] Other factors in this decision process were mentioned above and have various degrees of importance. Community assistance and home health aids, including public health nurses, can be of major importance in providing a safe disposition for elderly patients. Numerous senior citizen living centers with a registered nurse on call 24 hours a day are providing a heightened quality of life for many elderly people throughout the United States. Further growth in these institutions is hoped for in order to accommodate the estimated needs of the 21st century.

Driving ability is of major importance when assessing the overall independence of an elderly patient, and it is often a most difficult area to discuss when the results of the evaluation are negative. Senior citizen bus passes, discount cab rates, and institutional shuttles can significantly relieve this transportation void. The feelings of loneliness, desperation, and isolation are heightened tremendously by the inability to operate a motor vehicle. Alternatively, the operation of a motor vehicle by an unsafe, cognitively impaired driver, regardless of age, is a major cause of morbidity and mortality throughout the world.

Disposition is a family decision in which the patient actively participates whenever reasonable cognitive capacity allows. Various forms of voluntary employment exist both within and outside institutional care homes and may fulfill a heightened need in some patients. Avocational considerations need to be addressed, and hobbies and various leisure activities need to be pursued for as long as is reasonably possible. At some point, modifications in past hobbies and leisure activities by a competent recreational therapist or concerned medical care provider can help patients find increased avocational satisfaction. Occasional trips outside the living environment and being part of the mainstream of society can be a most valuable therapeutic intervention. Variance in care, geographic location, and patient and family preference are important variables when choosing among various nursing home options.

CONCLUSION

The standard rehabilitation care is of benefit to the geriatric population when the patients to be treated show no significant degree of mental impairment. Such techniques seem less beneficial to those with a moderate degree of mental impairment and without benefit to those with a severe degree of mental impairment.[21] Other variables, as discussed above, must also be considered when deciding on a patient's rehabilitation potential and the optimal use of rehabilitation facilities and professionals. Almost all severely disabled persons can benefit in some small way from a comprehensive individualized rehabilitation program. Because of the limited time and resources available, selection of the most appropriate candidates for rehabilitation is a much needed and difficult area of decision making. As a part of this decision-making process, the trained medical professional must summate the "cumulative disability" of a patient in the hope of setting realistic goals and limitations. At the present time, the economic cost of chronic disability and dependency seems to be much higher than the monetary cost of a successful rehabilitation program.[22] Certainly of more importance than the monetary gains of rehabilitation are the heightened levels of satisfaction and quality of life that come with independence in living.

REFERENCES

1. DDHS Publication No. (OHDS) 81-20704. "The need for long term care: a chartbook on the federal council on aging." Section I (numbers), and Section III (utilization).

2. Petersdorf RG, Adams RD, Braunwald E, Isselbacher KJ, Martin JB, Wilson JD. Harrison's principles of internal medicine. 10th ed. New York: McGraw-Hill, 1983.
3. Robinson CH, Lawler MR, Chenoweth WL, Garwick AE. Normal and therapeutic nutrition. 17th ed. New York: Macmillan Publishing, 1986.
4. Blackburn GL, Bistrian BR, Maini BS, Schlamm HT, Smith MF. Nutritional and metabolic assessment of the hospitalized patient. JPEN J Parenter Enteral Nutr 1977; 1:11–22.
5. Andres R, Bierman EL, Hazzard WR. Principles of geriatric medicine. New York: McGraw-Hill, 1985.
6. Müller EA. Influence of training and of inactivity on muscle strength. Arch Phys Med Rehabil 1970; 51:449–462.
7. Kottke FJ. The effects of limitation of activity upon the human body. JAMA 1966; 196:825–830.
8. American Heart Association. The Committee on Exercise. Kattus AA, Chairman. Exercise testing and training of individuals with heart disease or at high risk for its development: a handbook for physicians, 1975.
9. American College of Sports Medicine. Guidelines for graded exercise testing and exercise prescription. 2nd ed. Philadelphia: Lea & Febiger, 1980.
10. Fardy PS. Isometric exercise and the cardiovascular system. Physician Sportsmedicine Sept 1981; 9:43–56.
11. Kottke FJ, Stillwell GK, Lehmann JF. Krusen's handbook of physical medicine and rehabilitation. 3rd ed. Philadelphia: WB Saunders, 1982.
12. Sinaki M, Mikkelsen BA. Postmenopausal spinal osteoporosis: flexion versus extension exercises. Arch Phys Med Rehabil 1984; 65:593—596.
13. Fisher SV, Gullickson G Jr. Energy cost of ambulation in health and disability: a literature review. Arch Phys Med Rehabil 1978:59:124-133.
14. Gryfe CI, Amies A, Ashley MJ. A longitudinal study of falls in an elderly population: I. Incidence and morbidity. Age Ageing 1977; 6:201–210.
15. Tinetti ME, Williams TF, Mayewski R. Fall risk index for elderly patients based on number of chronic disabilities. Am J Med 1986; 80:429–434.
16. Morris EV, Isaacs B. The prevention of falls in a geriatric hospital. Age Ageing 1980; 9:181–185.
17. Tinetti ME. Factors associated with serious injury during falls by ambulatory nursing home residents. J Am Geriatr Soc 1987; 35:644–648.
18. Merritt JL. Urinary tract infections, causes and management, with particular reference to the patient with spinal cord injury: a review. Arch Phys Med Rehabil 1976; 57:365–373.
19. Hesse KA, Campion EW. Motivating the geriatric patient for rehabilitation. J Am Geriatr Soc 1983; 31:586–589.
20. Lehmann JF, DeLateur BJ, Fowler RS Jr, et al. Stroke rehabilitation: outcome and prediction. Arch Phys Med Rehabil 1975; 56:383–389.
21. Schuman JE, Beattie EJ, Steed DA, Merry GM, Kraus AS. Geriatric patients with and without intellectual dysfunction: effectiveness of a standard rehabilitation program. Arch Phys Med Rehabil 1981; 62:612–618.
22. Lehmann JF, DeLateur BJ, Fowler RS Jr, et al. Stroke: does rehabilitation affect outcome? Arch Phys Med Rehabil 1975; 56:375–382.

PART VIII

Cardiopulmonary Rehabilitation

20

Pulmonary Considerations in Rehabilitation

Peter T. Dorsher

John C. McMichan

Pulmonary dysfunction is a common sequela of both acute and chronic neurologic and musculoskeletal disorders. Primary lung disorders are also an important cause of morbidity and mortality in patients undergoing rehabilitation for these disorders. Chronic obstructive pulmonary disease, which includes emphysema, bronchitis, and asthma, now ranks as the fifth leading cause of death in the United States.

This chapter provides an overview of the pathophysiology and treatment of the most common pulmonary disorders seen in the practice of physical medicine and rehabilitation.

PHYSIOLOGY

The primary function of the lung is to exchange gas between inspired air and venous blood, and normally more than 100 m^2 of alveolar membrane surface area is available for this purpose. Alveolar ventilation and pulmonary blood flow are closely matched. At rest, pulmonary ventilation is about 5 liters/min; but this may increase 20-fold during exercise.[1]

The diaphragm, the external intercostal muscles, and the accessory muscles of respiration are the important inspiratory muscles. The diaphragm is the most important of these, contributing approximately two-thirds of the tidal volume in normal circumstances during quiet breathing in the sitting or standing position. The diaphragm is innervated by the phrenic nerves (C-3, C-4, C-5). The 11 external intercostal muscles are also important inspiratory muscles; they draw the ribs upward and outward and thus further increase the diameter of the chest wall and, consequently, tidal volume. The intercostal muscles are innervated by the intercostal nerves (T-1 through T-11). The accessory muscles of respiration (sternocleidomastoid, scalene, serratus anterior, pectoralis major and minor, trapezius, and erector spinae) are the third set of inspiratory muscles; their contribution becomes important in various disease states and in normal circumstances during exercise.[2]

During normal quiet breathing, the passive elastic recoil of the lungs and chest wall accomplishes expiration. Forced expiration uses the abdominal muscles to force the diaphragm back to its resting position. The internal intercostal muscles actively reduce the diameter of the chest wall through rib inversion during forced respiration. Both the abdominal and internal intercostal muscles are important for generating the elevated intrathoracic pressures that are necessary to produce an effective cough for clearing pulmonary secretions.

Respiration is controlled in the pontine and upper medullary reticular formation respiratory centers.[3] The primary regulation of respiration is through the response of these chemoreceptors to the pH of the surrounding extracellular fluid, which in turn is dependent on the carbon dioxide partial pressure in arterial blood. Arterial hypoxemia also stimulates ventilation through its effect on the chemoreceptors of the carotid body, whose visceral afferent signals traverse the glossopharyngeal nerves to terminate in the pontomedullary reticular formation. This mechanism is a relatively weak contributor to respiratory drive in normal circumstances, but it may dominate during chronic hypoxemia.[4] Finally, lung stretch receptors, irritant receptors, and alveolar juxtacapillary receptors may affect the ventilatory drive under some conditions.[5]

PATHOPHYSIOLOGY

Figure 20-1 and Table 20-1 present a summary of some of the factors that can lead to dysfunction of ventilation. Strokes, especially brain stem strokes with cranial nerve deficits, may cause dysphagia and resultant aspiration pneumonitis. Disorders of ventilatory control are uncommon.

Injuries of the cervical spinal cord produce respiratory impairments, and early mortality in association with acute quadriplegia is primarily related to retention of pulmonary secretions, which leads to atelectasis and pneumonitis. Cord lesions above C-3 produce immediate respiratory failure, whereas lesions at the C-3 to C-5 levels may have more delayed onset of respiratory failure with progressive involvement of the diaphragm. In lesions of the lower cervical cord, the loss of function of the external intercostal musculature results in reliance on the function of the diaphragmatic and accessory musculature for inspiration, whereas paralysis of the internal intercostal muscles and abdominal musculature leads to loss of most expiratory effort with subsequent retention of pulmonary secretions and its attendant complications.[6] Lesions of the thoracic cord producing paraplegia usually do not result in the same degree of respiratory compromise, but the reduced expiratory effort and coughing ability predispose affected persons to the same pulmonary complications.

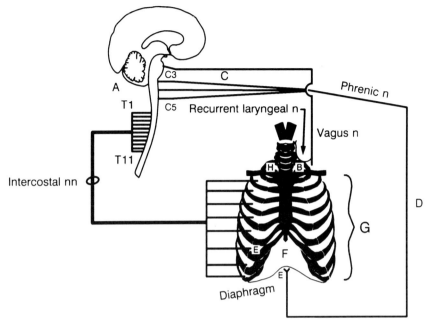

Figure 20–1
Anatomy of respiratory neural control. (See table 20–1 for an explanation of A through H.)

Individuals with quadriplegia have better lung ventilation when supine than when sitting. This difference is related to paralysis of the abdominal muscles, which allows the abdominal viscera to descend further in the abdominal cavity and hence lowers the resting position of the diaphragm in the sitting position. The excursion of the diaphragm during inspiration is thus reduced. The viscera in the sitting position also offer less recoil to return the diaphragm to its resting position. In the supine position, however, the abdominal viscera exert pressure on the diaphragm at the end of inspiration and a more rostral resting position of the diaphragm results. Diaphragmatic excursion with the next inspiration is thus increased and ventilation is improved. Pulmonary embolism leading to perfusion deficits of the lung parenchyma with consequent ventilation-perfusion mismatching is also an important cause of respiratory embarrassment in persons with stroke or spinal cord injuries.

Discussion of the pathophysiology of emphysema and chronic bronchitis is beyond the scope of this text. Cigarette smoking is the most important etiologic agent in these disorders. Smoking predisposes to chronic bronchitis through inhibition of ciliary activity; at the same time it accentuates mucus secretion in large airways and produces chronic inflammation in small airways. Emphysema likewise is induced through inhibition of α_1-antiprotease activity and accentuation of alveolar leukocyte elastase release by cigarette smoke.

TABLE 20–1
Pathophysiologic Mechanisms in Respiration

Location on Figure 20–1	Anatomic Location	Mechanism
A	Pontomedullary respiratory center	Depression of activity by drugs (such as barbiturates)
		Destruction by infarct, hemorrhage, tumor, for example
B	Upper airway	Mechanical obstruction (such as thyroid tumor)
		Bilateral recurrent laryngeal nerve dysfunction (glottis fails to open with inspiration)
C	High cervical cord	Trauma producing lesions at or above approximately C-3 causes severe weakness of inspiratory and expiratory muscles
		Anterior horn cell disease (such as amyotrophic lateral sclerosis and poliomyelitis)
D	Nerves to respiratory muscles	Inflammatory polyneuropathies (such as Guillain-Barré syndrome)
		Toxic, metabolic, or infectious polyneuropathies (such as mononucleosis or diphtheria-associated conditions)
E	Neuromuscular junction	Myasthenia gravis
		α-Bungarotoxin
F	Respiratory muscles	Myopathy (such as Duchenne muscular dystrophy)
G	Thoracic cage	Crush injuries of chest
		Scoliosis (Cobb angle >90°)
H	Lung and lower airways	Chronic obstructive pulmonary disease (emphysema, asthma, and chronic bronchitis)

TREATMENT

The prevention and treatment of pulmonary complications involve some or all of the following methods: liquefaction and removal of secretions, administration of supplemental oxygen, and mechanical assistance of ventilation.

Pulmonary secretions can be liquefied by the addition of humidity to the inspired gas. Liquefaction is most easily accomplished by bubbling the gas through water. This method, although relatively inefficient, is easily applied to gas being delivered by a face mask or nasal prongs. If the humidifier is heated, the water content of the inspired gas is further increased and prevents drying of secretions within the airways. A more efficient method uses a nebulizer, which, by generating an aerosol, can deliver increased humidity to the distal airways. The intended result is the deposition of the water content of the inspired gas on the airway secretions and, thereby, an increase in their fluidity. Supplemental oxygen is extremely dry and should always be humidified.

Once the secretions have been humidified, their removal can be facilitated by coughing (either spontaneous or assisted), by the maneuvers of postural drainage, by percussion applied by a physical therapist to the chest, and by suctioning of the airway through a tracheal tube.[1]

Both humidification of secretions and their removal can be improved by the additional techniques in incentive spirometry and intermittent positive-pressure breathing. An appropriate incentive spirometer must use inspiration to expand the lungs and must be adjustable to accommodate the small tidal volumes and vital capacities achieved by patients with spinal cord injuries. Support of intermittent positive-pressure breathing, delivered by a mechanical device incorporating a nebulizer, can help with clearance of secretions in three ways: (1) expansion of the airways by positive pressure and the administration of a bronchodilator in the inspired gas, (2) the delivery of humidity to distal airway units, and (3) the expansion of atelectatic lung areas. This treatment is successful only when administered to a cooperative patient by a knowledgeable attendant and with the administration of a bronchodilator.

Supplemental oxygen can be administered either by nasal prongs or by some form of face mask. It should always be humidified, particularly when the airway has been intubated.

In advanced acute respiratory failure, mechanical support of ventilation may be necessary. This requires intubation of the trachea and positive-pressure ventilation. If this level of support of respiratory function will be required for more than approximately 2 weeks, an early tracheostomy is indicated. However, diligent application of the principles of respiratory care may prevent the necessity for this surgical intrusion of the airway. In the presence of an irreversible cause and chronic respiratory failure, a permanent tracheostomy may be necessary, depending on the extent of the pulmonary abnormality. Chronic ventilatory support can be provided by either positive- or negative-pressure ventilation. The "iron lung" is the largest example of a negative-pressure ventilator, and more modern, lighter, and smaller models include the chest cuirass. Positive-pressure ventilation can be provided by any one of the many models available on the market. Positive pressure to the lungs can also be applied by the abdomen and its contents; this principle is utilized in the rocking bed and the pneumatic belt (Pneumobelt), both of which use the rostral movement of the abdominal contents to return the diaphragm to its resting position.

During the acute stages of respiratory failure, adequate monitoring of gas exchange and ventilatory support is essential. In addition to intermittent blood gas analyses, the continuous measurement of arterial oxygen saturation and pulse rate can be very valuable. The pulse oximeter, the latest available monitor, should be used continually during the acute stages and until a satisfactorily stable level of respiratory function has been achieved in the chronically ventilated patient. Patients with acute respiratory failure who require mechanical assistance should be monitored and nursed in a fully equipped intensive care unit, whereas those with chronic respiratory failure and mechanical ventilation may be cared for in a less intense area once respiratory function has stabilized.

Stroke

Prevention of pulmonary complications is essential because frequently respiratory difficulties, such as atelectasis, after acute stroke are transient. However, individuals with brain stem strokes often have difficulties with the handling of pulmonary and oral secretions and with dysphagia. Aggressive clearance of pulmonary secretions, maintenance of adequate hydration to keep pulmonary secretions moist, postural lung segment drainage by chest wall percussion on a regular basis (up to every 4 hours in the presence of severe pulmonary complications), and breathing exercises with incentive spirometry every 2 hours while the patient is awake are indicated in acute stages. If the patient is unable to handle his or her secretions, a tracheostomy should be considered to protect the airway from aspiration of oral secretions and to allow ready access for suctioning of pulmonary secretions. Dysphagia resulting in aspiration of foodstuffs necessitates the use of a nasogastric tube. Placement of a gastric or jejunal feeding tube is usually pursued if the tube feedings are required for more than approximately 4 to 6 weeks because of the risks of nasal, septal, and esophageal erosions with long-term nasogastric feedings.

Spinal Cord Injuries

General treatment principles are outlined in Chapter 14 and in Table 20-2. Assisted coughing (manual compression of the chest wall or abdom-

TABLE 20-2
Prevention of Pulmonary Complications in Spinal Cord Injuries*

Goal	Method
Adequate oxygenation	Oxygen supplementation with humidification to maintain oxygen saturation (SaO_2) > 90%
Prevention of aspiration	Gastric suction acutely to prevent aspiration of gastric contents due to adynamic ileus
Prevention of atelectasis	Side-to-side turning every 2 hours
	Deep breathing, incentive spirometry, and postural drainage with percussion and assisted coughing regularly
	Cessation of smoking
	Isometric strengthening of neck muscles

*Frequent monitoring of pulmonary function and arterial blood gases is needed to detect impending respiratory failure.

inal wall during a coughing attempt by the patient) is helpful to clear retained pulmonary secretions. McMichan et al.[6] demonstrated that aggressive pulmonary toilet prevented death related to respiratory failure in patients with acute quadriplegia who had injury at C-4 to C-8 levels (compared with a mortality rate of approximately 40% before aggressive pulmonary management). Isometric strengthening of neck muscles, which improves strength of accessory muscles of breathing, and breathing exercises, including incentive spirometry, improve inspiratory muscle function but not expiratory muscle function. Frequent monitoring of pulmonary function and arterial blood gases is essential in the acute phases of spinal cord injury, especially after spine stabilization orthoses have been applied, to monitor the adequacy of pulmonary exchange.

Chronically, patients with lesions high on the cervical cord usually require mechanical ventilation through a tracheostomy, both for ventilation and for suctioning of pulmonary secretions. Selected patients with high cord lesions who have physiologically intact phrenic nerves and diaphragms may benefit from implantable phrenic nerve stimulators to improve inspiratory function.[7]

Chronic Obstructive Pulmonary Disease

Important treatment principles include cessation of smoking (if applicable), environmental changes to avoid irritants, pneumococcal and influenza vaccinations, and optimization of pharmacologic management (methylxanthines, β_2-sympathomimetics, anticholinergics, or corticosteroid preparations). In patients who have arterial oxygen tension less than 55 mm Hg while breathing room air and signs of right heart failure, continuous oxygen therapy has been demonstrated to improve exercise tolerance and neuropsychologic function and to reduce symptoms of cor pulmonale. Aerobic exercise programs are task-specific (therefore, walking is recommended). Although they produce no improvement in the results of lung function tests, they do improve exercise tolerance, presumably through enhanced use of peripheral oxygen. Diaphragmatic and pursed-lip breathing exercises and instruction in control of the rate and depth of breathing during exercise may be helpful. Occupational therapists can also teach energy-conservation techniques and can analyze the home and work layouts to simplify daily tasks.

REFERENCES

1. DeLisa JA, ed. Rehabilitation medicine: principles and practice. Philadelphia: JB Lippincott, 1988.
2. Woodburne RT. Essentials of human anatomy. 6th ed. New York: Oxford University Press, 1978.
3. Adams RD, Victor M. Principles of neurology. 3rd ed. New York: McGraw-Hill, 1985.
4. Departments of Neurology and the Department of Physiology and Biophysics,

Mayo Clinic and Mayo Foundation. Clinical Examinations in Neurology. 5th ed. Philadelphia: WB Saunders, 1981.

5. West JB. Pulmonary pathophysiology: the essentials. 2nd ed. Baltimore: Williams & Wilkins, 1982.

6. McMichan JC, Michel L, Westbrook PR. Pulmonary dysfunction following traumatic quadriplegia: recognition, prevention, and treatment. JAMA 1980;243:528–531.

7. McMichan JC, Piepgras DG, Gracey DR, Marsh HM, Sittipong R. Electrophrenic respiration: report of six cases. Mayo Clin Proc 1979;54:662–668.

21

Cardiac Rehabilitation

Ray W. Squires
David G. Hurrell

Cardiovascular disease remains the leading cause of death and disability in the United States. Each year, approximately 1.5 million Americans have a myocardial infarction. Two-thirds of these patients survive, but the incidence of reinfarction and cardiac death is approximately 5% for the entire patient subgroup. More than 300,000 coronary artery bypass graft procedures are performed annually in the United States, and newer revascularization techniques such as percutaneous transluminal coronary angioplasty, atherectomy, and laser angioplasty have continued to be used more frequently during the past few years. Many other patients who do not have infarction receive medical treatment for coronary disease.

During the past 2 decades, cardiac rehabilitation has emerged as an accepted component of patient care after acute myocardial infarction and cardiac operation and for other cardiovascular disorders. It is defined as the process of development and maintenance of a desirable level of physical, social, and psychologic functioning after the onset of cardiovascular illness.[1] Specifically, education, counseling, teaching of nutrition, and exercise training are used in combination in classic cardiac rehabilitation to assist patients in returning to a near-normal life-style as soon as possible after recognition of the disease or in adapting to the limitations imposed by the disease.[2] Goals include risk stratification, limitation of potential adverse psychologic and emotional consequences of the disease, modification of risk factors, reduction of morbidity and mortality, reduction of symptoms, and improvement of function.[3] The need for cardiac rehabilitation is supported by data suggesting that 20% of patients who have had a myocardial infarction have some form of perceived disability after the event. The need to modify cardiovascular risk factors and to use judicious medical and surgical therapy is apparent given the progressive nature of coronary artery disease. More than half of patients who have coronary artery bypass grafting have progressive atherosclerosis that occludes at least one saphenous vein graft within 10 years of the operation.

ADMINISTRATIVE ASPECTS

The components of the rehabilitation program require individualization and are most efficiently provided by using the collective skills and experience of various health professionals (Table 21-1). The primary patient population that may benefit from cardiovascular rehabilitation consists of selected patients with cardiovascular disease, that is, those who have had acute myocardial infarction, angina pectoris, cardiac operation (bypass procedure, balloon angioplasty, laser angioplasty, atherectomy, valve repair or replacement, procedures for congenital abnormalities, cardiac, cardiopulmonary, or pulmonary transplantation), cardiomyopathy, peripheral vascular disease, hypertension, and clinically silent disease demonstrated by angiography. Additional patient subgroups may benefit from exercise training and other rehabilitation services, such as those who have had renal dialysis, renal or renal-pancreatic transplantation, liver transplantation, pulmonary disease, obesity, diabetes mellitus, anxiety and depression, cancer, chronic pain, and drug dependency.

Most patients have the potential to benefit from the educational and counseling aspects of cardiac rehabilitation, such as information regarding the acute event, diet, medications, smoking cessation, stress education and

TABLE 21-1

Members of the Cardiac Rehabilitation Team

Primary physician
Cardiologist
Surgeon
Psychiatrist
Physiatrist
Exercise physiologist
Psychologist
Pharmacist
Social worker
Vocational rehabilitation counselor
Nurse coordinator
Physical therapist
Occupational therapist
Dietitian
Cardiac rehabilitation nurse
Primary nurse
Head nurse
Exercise specialist
Smoking cessation counselor

TABLE 21–2
Absolute Contraindications to Exercise
Training in Cardiac Rehabilitation

Unstable angina pectoris
Dangerous arrhythmias
Overt cardiac failure
Severe left ventricular outflow tract
  obstruction
Dissecting aneurysm
Myocarditis or pericarditis (acute)
Serious systemic disease
Thrombophlebitis
Recent systemic or pulmonary embolus
Severe hypertension
Overt psychoneurotic disturbances
Uncontrolled diabetes mellitus
Severe orthopedic limitations

management, and psychosocial adjustment. The exercise training portion of the program is restricted to patients who do not have any unresolved absolute contraindication to exercise training (Table 21–2).

PSYCHOLOGIC ASPECTS

The usual psychologic responses to an acute cardiac event have been well described.[4] Panic and anxiety may surface during the first 8 hours after myocardial infarction. Precipitating factors include the stress of the illness, unfamiliar surroundings, the threat of death, and discomfort. Depression, probably related to a feeling of loss of physical ability or potential as an individual, may occur within 3 days of infarction or during the early outpatient phase of recovery (homecoming depression). Depression is usually transient and is often characterized by somatization complaints of fatigue or nonspecific discomfort. Denial is common; it may constitute a beneficial response (that is, acceptance of the illness but denial of its seriousness) or may manifest as rejection of the reality of the illness. Beneficial denial is associated with a high potential for rehabilitation and a favorable outcome. Careful education and encouragement are generally all that are required, and particular emphasis is given to the normal psychologic reaction to a cardiac event and to stress education and relaxation training.

PHASES OF CARDIAC REHABILITATION

The cardiac rehabilitation process is arbitrarily divided into four phases (Table 21–3).

TABLE 21–3
Phases of Cardiac Rehabilitation

Phase	Type of Program	Duration
1	Inpatient	Days
2	Outpatient, immediate interval after hospitalization	2–12 weeks
3	Late recovery period	Minimum of 9 months beyond phase 2
4	Maintenance program	Indefinite

Inpatient Rehabilitation

The period of hospitalization is phase 1. Individual patient needs must be addressed, and the family and significant others are included in the rehabilitation process. Program components include controlled low-level exercise, patient and family education, group and individual counseling, and group discussion sessions.

Sexual function should be addressed early in rehabilitation. Typically, the frequency of intercourse is reduced for many months after myocardial infarction and coronary artery bypass grafting, and sexual dysfunction is common.[5] Exercise testing and training are helpful for increasing the confidence of the patient and partner and the patient's sense of well-being. The peak rate of energy expenditure during intercourse is less than 5 METs (equivalent to climbing one to two flights of stairs; one MET is equal to energy expenditure at rest, or 3.5 mL $O_2 \cdot kg^{-1} \cdot min^{-1}$). Most patients are able to return to sexual activity by the third week after the event.

The physical activity program after myocardial infarction follows a step-by-step protocol, and patients typically advance one step each day (Table 21–4). Three stages of activity are identified. Stage 1 begins when the patient is hemodynamically and electrically stable in the intensive care unit. It starts with passive range-of-motion exercises and sitting in an armchair to maintain vasomotor reflexes that prevent orthostatic hypotension. During stage 2 the patient gradually assumes self-care activities and walks (up to 10 minutes three times daily) and performs active range-of-motion exercises supervised by a physical therapist. An upper limit for heart rate response of 20 beats per minute above the rate for standing at rest is used. Limited stair climbing is also performed. Throughout stage 3, the patient dresses in street clothes.

The hemodynamic and electrocardiographic responses to early inpatient low-level exercise are acceptable.[6] Heart rate responses for active range of motion and ambulation are between 5 and 15 beats per minute above resting level (on average). The typical systolic blood pressure response is 4 to 14 mm Hg above resting pressure.

A graded exercise test of low to moderate level performed before dismissal or early after dismissal—either a standard treadmill protocol or nuclear cardiology procedure (radionuclide angiography or thallium perfu-

TABLE 21-4

Mayo Clinic Inpatient Physical Activity Protocol for Cardiac Rehabilitation

Stage	Days of Program			Activity Schedule
	6-Day Plan	9-Day Plan	12-Day Plan	
1	1	1	1	Use bedside commode. Begin physical therapy range-of-motion exercises to each extremity. Sit at side of bed for 5 to 10 minutes
		2	2	Sit in chair for 5 to 15 minutes twice daily. Begin education program at bedside. Continue physical therapy described above
	2	3	3	Sit in chair for up to 30 minutes twice daily. Continue physical therapy described above
2	3	4	5	Move to step-down area. Bathe above waist, shave, and comb hair. Begin self-exercise program supervised by physical therapist. Sit in chair for 60 to 120 minutes twice daily
		5	7	Continue self-exercise program with supervision by physical therapist. Begin ambulation with physical therapist. Sit in chair for 90 to 150 minutes twice daily. Begin attending education classes and discussion groups
		6	8	Take wheelchair shower and use bathroom ad lib. Continue physical therapy as described above
3	4	7	9	Move to general cardiovascular ward. Dress in street clothes if desired. Be up and around room as tolerated. Begin climbing stairs with physical therapist
	5	8	11	Take predismissal graded-exercise test. Continue physical activity as described above. Take standing shower
	6	9	12	Receive final instructions before going home

sion study)—is helpful for risk stratification and prescription of home activities. A home exercise program is provided, and guidelines for graduated general physical activity are reviewed (Table 21-5).

Inpatient cardiac rehabilitation provides important short-term benefits: improvements in orthostatism, impaired physical work capacity, thromboembolism, reduced joint range of motion, and hypoventilation; improved psychologic status during convalescence; a potential for an earlier return to previous activities and work; a potential reduction in the duration of hospitalization; and an increased sense of well-being by the patient.

The recent trend toward shorter periods of hospitalization and more invasive procedures during the hospital stay for patients with a cardiac con-

TABLE 21–5

Guidelines for Graduated Activity After Dismissal From the Hospital After a Myocardial Infarction

Activity	METs	mL $O_2 \cdot kg^{-1} \cdot min^{-1}$	kcal/min (70-kg Person)
Week 1			
Any light activity that can be done while sitting	1½–3	5–11	2–4
Walking, 1–2 mph, on level			
Stationary cycling, minimal resistance			
Light household work			
Dishes or meal preparation (alternate with rest periods)			
Dusting			
Sweeping			
Personal hygiene			
Shaving			
Showering			
Dressing			
Week 2			
Increased social activity	≤4	11–14	4–5
Playing cards at home			
Visiting neighbors			
Car riding			
Walking, 2–3 mph, on level			
Stationary cycling, slight resistance			
Increased household work			
Bed making			
Ironing			
Minor appliance repair			
Bench work			
Supervising farm work			
Week 3			
Driving with another driver present	≤5	14–18	5–6
Household work, vacuuming			
Resumption of sexual intercourse			
Social activity			
Movies			
Church			
Concerts			
Walking, 3–5 mph			
Stationary cycling, slight resistance			
Lifting, 10–15 lb			
Week 4			
Potential return to part-time work	<6	18–21	6–7
Driving alone			
Light gardening			
Pitch and putt golfing			
Social group activities			
Club meetings			
Parties			
Dancing			
Grocery shopping (no heavy lifting)			
Walking, stationary cycling			

dition have resulted in less time for phase 1 activities. A continuation of rehabilitation services during the immediate post-hospitalization period has resulted from these changes.

Outpatient Rehabilitation

Phase 2 rehabilitation begins at hospital dismissal and involves close medical supervision for a period of weeks (Table 21–3). In many respects, phase 2 is the most critical stage of rehabilitation in that patients are usually receptive to prescribed changes in life-style.

Education occurs during consultations with physicians, exercise physiologists, nurses, dietitians, psychologists, smoking cessation counselors, and other team members as needed. Group discussion sessions and educational classes include topics such as medications, stress management, relaxation techniques, cardiovascular pathophysiology, nutrition, physical activity, and risk factor modification and behavior modification techniques. We use a cardiovascular health profile to provide feedback to patients regarding their risk factor status (Fig. 21–1).

A standard phase 2 program consists of three visits per week to the re-

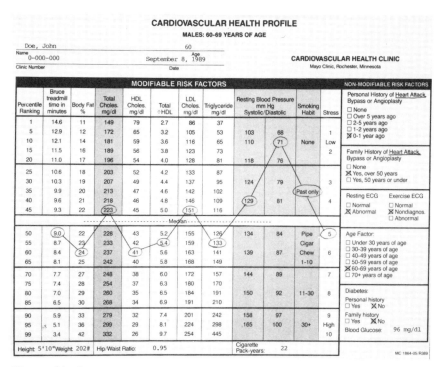

Figure 21–1
Cardiovascular health profile comparing an individual patient's risk factors with established norms.

habilitation center for supervised exercise and education (Fig. 21–2). Additional home exercise sessions are prescribed. Less frequent visits to the center may be scheduled for low-risk patients and for those living outside the immediate area.

The exercise sessions at the medical center are supervised directly by cardiac rehabilitation nurses and exercise specialists, and physicians are available if needed. Continuous single-lead electrocardiographic monitoring and periodic blood pressure measurements are routine. Aerobic activities such as treadmill walking and cycle ergometry form the core of the supervised exercise program at this stage of rehabilitation. Arm ergometry and light weight-training exercise are also used (Fig. 21–3). Upper extremity exercise is an important consideration because there is little carryover in adaptive training responses from one muscle group to another. Warm-up and cool-down activities are always performed. The duration of exercise is progressed gradually to 40 minutes per session with a frequency of five to seven sessions per week (three or fewer at the rehabilitation center). The intensity of exercise is prescribed at a point below which ischemic signs and symptoms are evident; it is based on the heart rate response from the graded exercise test and ratings of 11 to 14 on the Borg perceived exertion scale (Table 21–6). Home exercise during the first weeks of convalescence includes walking, stationary cycling, and gentle calisthenics.

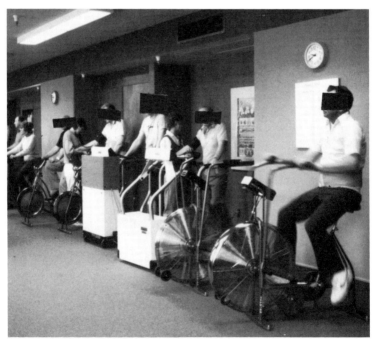

Figure 21–2
Phase 2 cardiac rehabilitation exercise center in operation.

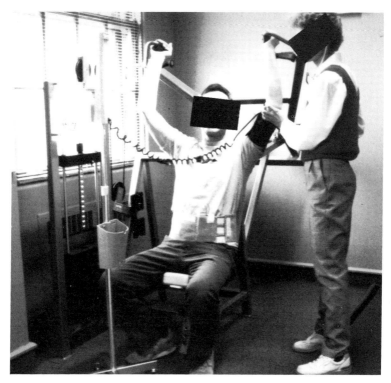

Figure 21-3
Weight training with medical supervision during phase 2 cardiac rehabilitation.

Near the completion of the phase 2 program, a symptom-limited graded exercise test is usually performed. Depending on the clinical situation, a nuclear cardiology test, an exercise echocardiogram, or a standard treadmill test with analysis of expired air is chosen (Fig. 21-4). Results are used to update the exercise prescription and to determine readiness to return to work and other activities. For selected patients, an occupational readiness assessment including strength and endurance testing specific to work tasks is helpful.

Phase 3 of rehabilitation continues for at least 9 months beyond phase 2. The exercise portion of the program either is supervised at the medical center or a community exercise facility or is purely an individual program (at home or at an exercise facility). Participation in patient support groups such as the Coronary Club is encouraged. In our program, patients return to the rehabilitation center for formal evaluations at 3, 6, and 9 months after completion of phase 2. Emphasis is placed on control of risk factors such as blood lipid values, smoking, weight, diet, and exercise. These visits are helpful for maintaining patient compliance with life-style recommendations; in our view, they are critical to the success of the program.

Phase 4 of rehabilitation is the maintenance program used to continue

TABLE 21–6
Borg Perceived Exertion Scale

Scale	Exertion
6	
7	Very, very light
8	
9	Very light
10	
11	Fairly light
12	
13	Somewhat hard
14	
15	Hard
16	
17	Very hard
18	
19	Very, very hard
20	

modification of risk factors; it includes regular physical activity. Evaluations, including graded exercise testing, are recommended on at least a yearly basis.

RISK STRATIFICATION AFTER MYOCARDIAL INFARCTION AND CORONARY ARTERY BYPASS GRAFTING

After myocardial infarction or coronary bypass grafting, patients may be categorized as either low or high risk for reinfarction and sudden death. High-risk patients are identified on the basis of left ventricular dysfunction (left ventricular ejection fraction of 40% or less), congestive heart failure, complex arrhythmia, and ischemia.[7] Exercise testing soon after the clinical event provides information regarding the angina threshold, ischemic electrocardiographic changes, arrhythmia, and exercise capacity, and it forms the basis for the early rehabilitation exercise prescription. Ideally, high-risk patients who are clinically stable should participate in supervised rehabilitation programs.

Many patients with severe left ventricular dysfunction are not referred for cardiac rehabilitation. This decision is based on concerns that such patients may not benefit from exercise training, that the long-term prognosis is dismal, and that exercise training may be potentially dangerous. We recently reviewed the outcome of 20 consecutive patients who had had myocardial infarction and had resting left ventricular ejection fractions of less than 25% (mean, 21%; normal, 55%); these patients participated in our outpatient cardiac rehabilitation program.[8] They had no absolute contraindications to exercise training. No serious complications of exercise

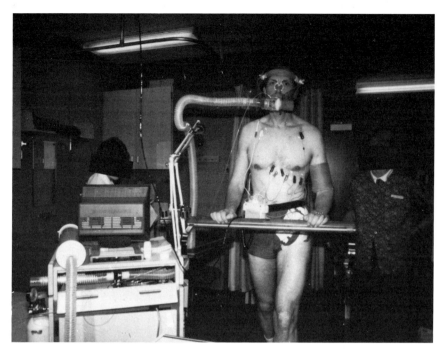

Figure 21-4
Patient performing treadmill graded exercise test with analysis of expired air.

training occurred during the 8-week supervised program, and exercise capacity increased 38%. More than half of these patients returned to gainful employment, and most patients were able to exercise independently after leaving the supervised program. We were encouraged by the relatively low mortality rate of 8% over 3 years of follow-up.

RISKS OF EXERCISE TRAINING

Exercise training in patients with cardiovascular disease is not without risk. Contraindications to exercise (Table 21-2) must be strictly followed. Advanced age and poor left ventricular function are not contraindications. Because patients with cardiac disease may have a limited coronary reserve, the increase in myocardial oxygen demand during exercise may result in ischemia and may precipitate a lethal arrhythmia or myocardial infarction. Cardiac arrest may occur long after the initial clinical event. With proper patient screening and care in prescribing exercise, exercise training may be safely performed by most patients. Reported complication rates are low (one cardiac arrest per 112,000 hours of patient exercise).[9]

Musculoskeletal injuries are common in persons who enter exercise programs. Weight-bearing activities of moderate to high intensity such as jogging, traditional aerobic dance, racket sports, and other court games are more likely to result in injury than other activities. Most patients do not perform these activities but rather opt for walking, stationary cycling, and swimming or other water activities.

EXERCISE PRESCRIPTION

The exercise prescription should be individualized and updated periodically and must include the following: exercise type(s), desired intensity, exercise duration, frequency of exercise sessions, anticipated rate of progression of duration and frequency, specific warm-up and cool-down activities, and warning symptoms.[10] Symptoms requiring termination of exercise sessions and consultation with a physician include new-onset or change in angina pectoris, severe dyspnea, unusual fatigue, light-headedness, syncope, musculoskeletal pain, exceeding the prescribed target heart rate, and new onset of pulse irregularity. Exercise intensity is generally prescribed on the basis of the heart rate response to graded exercise testing and the Borg perceived exertion scale (Table 21–6). Table 21–7 provides general guidelines for exercise prescription.

Adaptations to exercise training are somewhat specific to the muscle groups involved in training. A portion of the exercise session may be devoted to upper extremity activities such as arm ergometry, hand-held weights, rowing, or circuit weight training.

BENEFITS OF CARDIAC REHABILITATION

Exercise training results in impressive benefits for most patients with cardiac disease (Table 21–8). A reduction in the symptoms of angina pec-

TABLE 21–7

Guidelines for Aerobic Exercise Prescription in Cardiac Rehabilitation

Phase	Intensity	Duration (min)	Frequency	Mode
1	RHR +10 to 20 beats/min, RPE 11–13	3–20	2–3 times/day	Slow walk or cycle ergometry
2	RHR +20 beats/min, 50%–70% of HRR, RPE 12–14	10–45	5–7 times/wk	Walk, cycle, arm ergometry, walk-jog
3	50%–70% of HRR, RPE 12–14	20–45	3–6 times/wk	Walk, walk-jog, cycle, swim, games
4	50%–75% of HRR, RPE 12–14	20–45	3–6 times/wk	Same as for phase 3

Abbreviations: HRR, heart rate reserve (for example: HR rest = 60, HR peak [from graded exercise test] = 160, HRR = 160 − 60 = 100; 70% of HRR = 0.7 × 100 + 60 = 130 beats/minute); RHR, resting heart rate; RPE, ratings of perceived exertion.

TABLE 21–8
Benefits From Long-term Outpatient Cardiac
Rehabilitation
_____

Physiologic*
   ↑ $\dot{V} O_2$ max
   ↓ MVO_2 for given work load
   ↑ Muscle strength and endurance
   ↑ Blood fibrinolytic activity
   ↓ Platelet aggregation
   ↓ Catecholamines
Symptomatic
   ↓ Angina pectoris
   ↓ Dyspnea
   ↓ Claudication
   ↓ Fatigue
Anatomic
   ↓ Progression of disease†
  Regression of disease†
Economic
   ↑ Patient productivity†
   ↓ Disability cases†
   ↓ Physician office visits†
   ↓ Medications
Psychologic
   ↓ Anxiety and depression
   ↑ Confidence and self-esteem
   ↑ Knowledge
Epidemiologic
   ↓ Morbidity
   ↓ Mortality
Risk factors
   ↓ Smoking
   ↓ Total cholesterol, low-density lipoprotein
    cholesterol, and triglyceride values
   ↑ High-density lipoprotein cholesterol value
   ↓ Obesity
   ↓ Hypertension
   ↑ Carbohydrate metabolism

*VO_2 max, maximal oxygen uptake; MVO_2, myocardial
  oxygen demand.
†Potential benefits.
_____

toris, exercise-related dyspnea, fatigue, and claudication is an important outcome. The oxygen transport system adapts favorably to exercise training, as indicated by a 10% to 30% or more increase in maximal oxygen uptake. As a result, tasks are performed with less fatigue and dyspnea and reduced perceived exertion, and the productivity and quality of life of the patient may be enhanced considerably.

For a given intensity of exercise, myocardial oxygen requirement, as indicated by a reduction in the product of heart rate and systolic blood pressure, is reduced. Also, evidence indicates that myocardial perfusion is enhanced and that ischemic electrocardiographic changes during exercise testing are lessened. There is no evidence that training improves the coronary collateral circulation. Patients who exercise regularly have an improved psychological profile: less anxiety and depression and more confidence and self-esteem than nonexercising patients.

SECONDARY PREVENTION

The efficacy of risk factor modification in reducing the progression of coronary artery disease and future morbidity and mortality has been established. Progression of disease in the native coronary arteries and in saphenous vein bypass grafts has been associated with continued cigarette smoking, elevated total serum cholesterol values and low values of high-density lipoprotein cholesterol, hypertension, sedentary life-style, and elevated fasting blood glucose concentration.

The Cholesterol-Lowering Atherosclerosis Study demonstrated that the blood lipid profile of patients who had coronary artery bypass grafting could be improved dramatically and that these improvements were associated with less progression of disease and more regression of disease than in control subjects.[11] Cigarette smoking continues to predict cardiac-related death and recurrent infarction after myocardial infarction and coronary artery bypass grafting. Improved survival has been noted in hypertensive patients who have their blood pressure adequately controlled after myocardial infarction or the presence of angina pectoris.

The effects of regular exercise training on the secondary prevention of cardiac disease has been addressed by several investigators. None of the randomized trials have conclusively demonstrated a protective effect of exercise training. Such trials have been plagued by insufficient numbers of patients to achieve adequate statistical power, subject dropouts and crossovers, and short periods of observation. However, pooled data (meta-analysis) have revealed a reduction of 15% to 25% in cardiac mortality in exercising subjects compared with controls.[12]

CARDIOVASCULAR HEALTH ENHANCEMENT

Coronary artery disease is not necessarily an inevitable consequence of a genetic predisposition and the aging process. Multiple environmental risk factors have been elucidated and explain variations in the incidence of the disease around the world. This variation is powerfully illustrated by the observation that migrants, on leaving an area with a low incidence of disease, assume the higher incidence in their new country unless life-style is not altered.

Prevention of coronary disease calls for both a general population strategy for risk factor modification, emphasizing public education, and an

TABLE 21-9
The Relative Risk of the Development of
Coronary Artery Disease for Selected Risk
Factors[13, 14]

Risk Factor	Relative Risk
Smoke ≥ 1 pack/day	2.5
Total cholesterol ≥ 265 mg/dL	2.4
Systolic blood pressure ≥ 150 mm Hg	2.1
Sedentary life-style	1.9

individual patient approach through risk factor profiling. The relative risks of selected risk factors (1 equals average risk) are provided in Table 21-9. An individual program may consist of an evaluation of current cardiovascular status; a profile (Fig. 21-1) of risk factors emphasizing family history, smoking, blood lipid values, blood pressure, body composition (percentage body fat and the waist-to-hip ratio), emotional stress, and aerobic fitness; a counseling session; and referral to appropriate health education programs. We currently provide such services through our laboratory (Cardiovascular Health Clinic). Of paramount importance is the need to assist cigarette smokers to discontinue the habit. Instructions in a dietary and exercise program also receive major emphasis. A diagnostic graded exercise test before initiation of an exercise is indicated for patients older than 40 years or for younger patients with ominous risk factors (family history of coronary disease who are younger than 50 years, diabetes mellitus, familial hypercholesterolemia, end-stage renal disease, inadequately controlled hypertension).

For patients with serious modifiable risk factors, follow-up appointments are advised to measure progress and to motivate patient compliance with recommended life-style changes. It is our belief that efforts to improve cardiovascular health are important and justified, and they warrant more widespread application.

REFERENCES

1. Report of the Task Force on Cardiovascular Rehabilitation: Needs and Opportunities for Rehabilitating the Coronary Heart Disease Patient (DHEW Publication No. [NIH] 75-750). Washington, D.C.: National Heart and Lung Institute, 1974.
2. Squires RW, Gau GT. Cardiac rehabilitation and cardiovascular health enhancement. In: Brandenburg RO, Fuster V, Giuliani ER, McGoon DC, eds. Cardiology: fundamentals and practice. Chicago: Year Book Medical Publishers, 1987:1944-1960.
3. Wenger NK. Rehabilitation of the coronary patient: status 1986. Prog Cardiovasc Dis 1986; 2:181-204.

4. Cassem NH, Hackett TP. Psychological rehabilitation of myocardial infarction patients in the acute phase. Heart Lung 1973;2:382–388.
5. Hellerstein HK, Friedman EH. Sexual activity and the postcoronary patient. Arch Intern Med 1970; 125:987–999.
6. Silvidi GE, Squires RW, Pollock ML, Foster C. Hemodynamic responses and medical problems associated with early exercise and ambulation in coronary artery bypass graft surgery patients. J Cardiac Rehabil 1982; 2:355–362.
7. DeBusk RF, Blomqvist CG, Kouchoukos NT, Luepker RV, Miller HS, Moss AJ, Pollock ML, Reeves TJ, Selvester RH, Stason WB, Wagner GS, Willman VL. Identification and treatment of low-risk patients after acute myocardial infarction and coronary-artery bypass graft surgery. N Engl J Med 1986; 314:161–166.
8. Squires RW, Lavie CJ, Brandt TR, Gau GT, Bailey KR. Cardiac rehabilitation in patients with severe ischemic left ventricular dysfunction. Mayo Clin Proc 1987; 62:997–1002.
9. Van Camp SP, Peterson RA. Cardiovascular complications of outpatient cardiac rehabilitation programs. JAMA 1986; 256:1160–1163.
10. Squires RW, Lavie CJ. New trends in cardiac rehabilitation exercise. Cardio 1988; 5:85–92, 112.
11. Blankenhorn DH, Nessim SA, Johnson RL, Sanmarco ME, Azen SP, Cashin-Hemphill L. Beneficial effects of combined colestipol-niacin therapy on coronary atherosclerosis and coronary venous bypass grafts. JAMA 1987;257:3233–3240.
12. Oldridge NB, Guyatt GH, Fischer ME, Rimm AA. Cardiac rehabilitation after myocardial infarction: combined experience of randomized clinical trials. JAMA 1988; 260:945–950.
13. Powell KE, Thompson PD, Caspersen CJ, Kendrick JS. Physical activity and the incidence of coronary heart disease. Annu Rev Public Health 1987; 8:253–287.
14. The Pooling Project Research Group. Relationship of blood pressure, serum cholesterol, smoking habit, relative weight and ECG abnormalities to incidence of major coronary events: final report of the pooling project. J Chronic Dis 1978; 31:201–306.

PART IX

Rehabilitation in Common Musculoskeletal Disorders

22 | An Approach to the Clinical Evaluation of Physical Impairment

Carl W. Chan
Sherwin Goldman

Injuries resulting from an accident may cause temporary disruption of daily routine or permanent loss of function. In most cases, fortunately, the injured person experiences only minor inconveniences. However, in some cases the accident has serious economic, social, vocational, and avocational ramifications. Whether the disability is short-term or long-term, the injured person will usually be seeking compensation from a third-party insurer.[1] Musculoskeletal disorders are the most frequent type of disabilities that physicians evaluate, and back pain is the most common musculoskeletal cause of disability claims.[1-4] Five percent of American adults have an episode of low back pain each year. Among these, the pain is attributable to an occupational injury in 400,000.[2, 3] Although most of these persons recover, some have chronic, persistent impairments and some become permanently disabled. Currently, more than 11.7 million people are impaired because of low back pain, and more than 5.3 million are disabled because of low back pain.[5] Thus, low back pain causes a substantial socioeconomic impact in terms of medical compensation as well as loss of productivity. The cost of these factors was estimated at $4.5 billion to $16 billion annually.[3, 6] The rate of disability rose alarmingly, at a rate 14 times that of the population growth, between 1977 and 1981. Further analysis of the data shows that a minority of high-cost cases accounted for as much as 85% of the costs.[2, 3]

Because back pain is the leading cause of workers' compensation expenditure as well as the most common musculoskeletal cause of disability claims, the evaluation of back pain is used here as a model for the medical assessment of clinical impairment in the musculoskeletal system.

Before impairment can be determined in a patient with low back pain or a musculoskeletal disorder, the musculoskeletal system must be comprehensively and systematically evaluated. The evaluation should include a clear, chronologic history, a review of systems, a musculoskeletal examination, selected functional tests of the musculoskeletal system, a radiologic examination if necessary, a neurologic examination and consultation if necessary, an orthopedic consultation if necessary, and perhaps a psychologic assessment. Only after this evaluation can a clear diagnosis be made, the need for further treatments be determined, and a plan for comprehensive rehabilitation be developed. In addition, a clinical impairment can be defined only after a comprehensive clinical assessment.

The evaluation of a patient with back pain can be time-consuming and expensive. Many physical and diagnostic tests have been described.[4, 7] The following is a synopsis of our approach.

HISTORY

Important aspects of the history and evaluation of low back pain include careful questioning about the onset of the pain, especially in regard to its cause; the duration of the symptoms; the frequency of the episodes; aggravating or alleviating symptoms; history of prior injuries; previous treatment, including physical therapy and chiropractic or surgical interventions; and treatment results. In particular, physical therapy needs specific delineation, especially in regard to details about heat, diathermy, ultrasound, electrical stimulation, ice and massage, exercises, manipulation, and traction. The result of such treatments should also be described. The history should also include the results of previous diagnostic tests, including electromyography, radiography, neurologic evaluation, neurosurgical evaluation, orthopedic evaluation, and psychiatric evaluation. Specific queries should be directed at the impact of back pain on activities of daily living and on vocational and avocational activities. Information should be obtained about the type of work the patient engages in, the number of work days missed, the date the patient last worked, and current status of employment. Workers' compensation and litigation issues also need to be defined.

Location of pain; symptoms of gait abnormality; patterns of numbness, weakness, and atrophy; bowel, bladder, and sexual dysfunction; and other symptoms that suggest a neurologic component should be specifically addressed. Pain radiation with coughing, sneezing, and the Valsalva maneuver may point to nerve root irritation, but it can also occur in nonradicular acute back pain. Completion of a pain drawing before the examination may provide insight into symptom magnification, nonorganic symptoms, and somatization.[8] The types and amounts of medication being used, including corticosteroids, nonsteroidal anti-inflammatory agents, and narcotic pain medications, should also be determined.[4]

EXAMINATION

The back examination should be systematic. First, the patient should remove enough clothing to allow the physician to observe the back without any camouflage by clothing. The male patient must be in only shorts, and the female patient should have on only a bra and shorts. The patient's posture, movement, and expressions should be observed. The willingness of the patient to move and the pattern of movement should be noted. Clinical observations of posture include determining the presence or absence of scoliosis, kyphosis, and pelvic obliquity. Other factors to be observed are stiffness of movements, total spinal posture, body type, attitude, markings, and gait, including velocity, cadence, and patterns of motion over the lower extremity, pelvis, and trunk.[9] Nonphysiologic components should be differentiated from true antalgia.

Velocity of gait is usually decreased in the presence of back pain, and antalgic gait is characterized by avoidance of pain. With pain on weight bearing on a painful extremity, the stance phase is shortened on the affected side. An antalgic gait of spinal origin is usually characterized by short steps, a symmetric stance phase, and reduced cadence. The hips, knees, and trunk are usually slightly flat and the trunk is held virtually still in an effort to avoid the usual trunk and pelvic rotations that may be provoking the pain.[1] Footdrop, decreased push off, a lock-knee during midstance, or trunk lurches may suggest neurologic impairment or involvement even before the full neurologic examination is conducted. The patient should do a heel-and-toe walk and tandem walking. This portion of the examination may allow for the detection of less severe weakness that may not be detected during the manual muscle test. It may also reveal the presence of an unsuspected extrapyramidal lesion or posterior column lesion. In addition, heel-and-toe walking and tandem walking may also amplify the uncoordinated irregular movements characteristic of astasia-abasia. Step deformity in the lumbar spine indicates the presence of a spondylolisthesis.

Active movements should be performed with the patient standing, and the examiner should specifically look for differences in range of movement and the patient's willingness to do the movement. The range of motion taking place during the active movement is normally the summation of the movements of the whole lumbar spine and not just movement at one level. While the patient is going through the active movements, the examiner should look for limitation of movement and its possible causes, such as pain, spasm, stiffness, or blocking. The greatest motion in the lumbar spine occurs between L-4 and L-5 and between L-5 and S-1 vertebrae.[9-12] The range of motion of the lumbar spine varies considerably among people. The following movements are possible in the lumbar spine: forward flexion and extension, side flexion, and rotation.

For flexion, the maximal range of motion is 40° to 60°. The examiner must ensure that the movement is occurring in the lumbar spine and not in the hips or thoracic spine. Some persons may be able to touch their toes even if no movement occurs in the spine.[1] On forward flexion, the lumbar curve should normally go from its normal lordotic curvature to at least a straight or slightly flexed curve. If this does not occur, there is probably some hypomobility in the lumbar spine. As for the thoracic spine, the examiner may use a tape measure to determine the distance of the increase in the spacing of the spinous processes on forward flexion. With Schober's test, the length between the T-12 spinous process and the S-1 spinous process may be increased up to 8 cm during lumbar flexion. The examiner should know how far forward the patient is able to bend and compare the forward-bending motion while standing with results of the straight-leg raising test, because straight-leg raising, especially bilaterally, is essentially the same movement as forward flexion during standing, except that it occurs from below upward instead of from above downward.

Extension is normally limited to 20° to 35° in the lumbar spine. While performing the movement, the patient places the hands on the small of the back of the hips to stabilize the back. Lateral flexion is approximately 15° to 20° in the lumbar spine; the patient is asked to run a hand down the side of the leg and not to bend forward or backward while performing the movement. Rotation of the lumbar spine is normally 3° to 18° to the left and right and is accomplished by a shearing movement of the lumbar vertebrae on each other.[9]

While the patient is standing, a quick test may be performed. The patient squats down as far as possible, bounces two or three times, and returns to the standing position. This action will quickly test the ankles, knees, and hips for any pathologic condition; if the patient can fully squat and bounce without any signs and symptoms, in all probability these joints are free of an abnormality related to the complaint. The patient is also asked to bounce on one leg and to go up and down on the toes four or five times. While the patient does this, the examiner should watch for a Trendelenburg sign. A positive result is secondary to a weak gluteus medius muscle. If the patient is unable to complete the movement by going up and down on the toes, the examiner might suspect the presence of an S-1 nerve root lesion with weakness involving the ankle plantar flexors.

The examiner should also palpate for the presence of muscle spasms and tenderness. In the presence of low back pain, careful palpation may reveal tenderness in muscle attachment sites at the pelvis and hips, including the regions of the trochanteric bursa and the ischial bursa. Abnormal gait and spinal mechanics, muscle and soft tissue contractures, a lowered pain threshold, and prolonged sitting or sleeping may well contribute to soft tissue fibromyalgia and generalized deconditioning that may be secondary causes of diffuse pain or even major contributors to overall pain.

NEUROLOGIC ASSESSMENT

After the evaluation of gait and spine motion and the assessment of soft tissue tenderness and muscle attachment pain, the neurologic assessment should be conducted. This includes manual muscle testing of the trunk and lower extremities, an assessment of the deep tendon reflexes and pathologic reflexes, and a sensory examination. If muscle weakness or atrophy is present, limb circumference should be determined to document the extent of muscle atrophy.

Straight-leg raising tests should be performed to detect nerve root irritation. The classic positive result of the straight-leg raise is production of radicular pain at 30°. Soft tissue tightness or spasms of the back or gluteal muscles may produce nonradicular back and leg pain. Thus, careful assessment of the patient plays a vital part in the attempt to distinguish true radicular pain from soft tissue pain.

Several variations of the straight-leg raising test can be used to confirm dural or root irritation; these include the crossed straight-leg raising test, the bowstring test, and the Kernig/Brudzinski test. For the crossed straight-leg raising test, when a unilateral straight leg raise is used, 80° to 90° of hip flexion is normal. If one leg ("good" leg) is lifted and the patient complains of pain on the opposite leg, the test is positive. This finding indicates the presence of a space-occupying lesion.[9] The bowstring test is conducted by doing a straight-leg raising test until pain results, at which point the knee is slightly flexed (20°) to reduce the symptoms. Then thumb or finger pressure is applied to the popliteal area to reestablish the painful radicular symptoms. A positive result indicates tension or pressure on the sciatic nerve. The Kernig/Brudzinski test is done with the patient in the supine position with hands cupped behind the head. The patient is asked to flex the head onto the chest. The extended leg is raised actively by flexing the hip until pain is felt. The patient then flexes the knee and the pain disappears. Pain is a positive sign and may indicate meningeal irritation, nerve root involvement, or dural irritation. Of all the results of maneuvers performed during the physical examination, a positive result of the crossed straight-leg raising test has the highest correlation with myelographic findings of a herniated disk (more than 90%).[13]

Inconsistency of results of the sitting and supine straight-leg raising tests may provide insight into psychogenic processes. As part of the clinical assessment of low back pain, the clinical scoring system of nonorganic physical signs reported by Waddell et al.[14] may be used. These are a set of nonorganic physical signs independent of those commonly used to detect organic disease but which correlate with chronic low back complaints and elevation of the hysteria and hypochondriasis scores of the Minnesota Multiphasic Personality Inventory (MMPI) and various other psychological factors. One point is given for the presence of each nonorganic sign; these signs are (1) tenderness, (2) regionalization, (3) simulation, (4) overreaction, and (5) distraction. According to the original article,[14] a score of 3 or more represents significant manifestations of illness behavior and is helpful in distinguishing between organic disease symptoms and symptoms that are psychologically amplified. It is an indicator for further psychological assessment as part of the evaluation and rehabilitation of the patient with low back pain.

OBJECTIVE MEASUREMENTS

In addition to the usual clinical examination, objective measurements of spine and trunk flexibility and strength are used to document physical findings. For example, a gravity inclinometer may be used to measure spinal motion on flexion and extension. The American Medical Association's third edition of *Guides to the Evaluation of Permanent Impairment*[15] requires inclinometer assessment of spinal motion as part of impairment determination (although this requirement may be under review). An electronic digital inclinometer may be used if available. Schober's or modified Schober's test is another simple and repeatable method of objectively measuring spine flexion and can be easily incorporated into the general back examination.

Trunk dynamometers have also been developed that provide information regarding trunk strength and trunk motion in terms of trunk flexion, extension, rotation, and lateral flexion. These machines provide digital and graphic recordings that furnish specific data about power, movement, impulse, torque, and velocity. A graphic display of these data and repeatability are helpful for detecting patterns overall, and they may be useful for defining functional impairment,[1] but only with good patient motivation and effort. The past decade has produced a large volume of literature regarding these dynamic trunk strength machines. However, critical evaluation of this literature shows that scientific evidence still remains inadequate to support the use of these machines in the testing of trunk muscle strength for pre-employment screening, routine clinical assessment, or medicolegal evaluation.[16] In addition to providing information about trunk strength and flexibility, such data may also be helpful for assessing specific weaknesses, and so allow physicians to develop and monitor a comprehensive back rehabilitation program.[17]

RADIOLOGIC AND OTHER TESTS

Plain radiographs of the lumbosacral spine remain one of the cornerstones of radiologic assessment of low back pain. Standard anteroposterior and lateral views as well as oblique views provide useful information. Such testing allows the clinician to determine the presence of degenerative disk disease, spondylitis, compression fractures, metabolic osteopenic disorders, primary or metastatic tumors, congenital anomalies, degenerative spondylosis, spondylolisthesis, kyphosis, and scoliosis.

Most patients with low back pain will not require sophisticated radiologic evaluations beyond these basic views. If a spinal cord abnormality is suspected, a more sophisticated examination, including computed tomography, may be helpful for defining localized processes. Magnetic resonance imaging and computed tomography-enhanced myelography are also being used increasingly for more refined definitions of soft tissue, disks, roots, surrounding ligaments, muscles, and the spinal canal.

The bulging disk is a common finding on computed tomography or magnetic resonance imaging scans of the lumbosacral spine and is of no clinical significance when neurologic structures are not compromised. A careful history and clinical examination are still the cornerstones of diagnosis and management for the patient with low back pain.

Additional laboratory tests such as a complete blood cell count, erythrocyte sedimentation rate, urinalysis, and occasionally rheumatologic studies and psychologic profiles may be necessary for a comprehensive diagnostic workup to identify unusual causes of low back pain.

DIAGNOSIS

The diagnosis is determined after a complete history and physical examination and after appropriate radiologic examinations.

The most common causes of low back pain are usually soft tissue strains, which may progress to chronic fibromyalgia syndrome, degenerative disk disease, and degenerative arthritis. Differential diagnoses that the clinician should bear in mind include spondylolisthesis (usually degenerative); compression fractures; disk space infections; neoplasms, both primary and metastatic; and noninfectious inflammatory disease of the vertebrae and the sacroiliac joint. Other possibilities include sudden visceral conditions such as abdominal neoplasms, pyelonephritis, retrocecal appendicitis, and retroperitoneal abscesses, which may cause symptoms that mimic low back pain. In addition, psychosocial factors may have an influence on pain amplification in the pathogenesis of chronic low back pain syndromes.

WORK TOLERANCE SCREENING AND WORK HARDENING

Physical capabilities and maximal levels at which work can be performed safely can be evaluated through a formalized work tolerance screening. This provides useful information on maximal lifting and carrying capacities, pushing and pulling tolerances, postural biomechanics, and endurance levels. It allows the physician to determine physical limitations and restrictions as well as to assess the need for recommendations of a structured work hardening program to improve a patient's physical endurance and condition, if the patient is unable to work even at a sedentary level.

PERMANENT PARTIAL IMPAIRMENT

The determination that a patient has a permanent partial impairment is based on documented anatomic signs and physical limitations. Some impairment guidelines provide for a rating based on pain. However, the impairment guidelines of the American Medical Association[15] and the Social Security disability guidelines[18] do not allow for the inclusion of pain because it is a subjective component with a wide variation of intensity and leads to physician ratings that tend to be widely variable.

A permanent partial impairment rating is not equivalent to a disability rating. The impairment rating is an assessment of physical limitations based on a patient's physical capacities; it is determined from results of the physical examination and repeatable anatomic signs. Disability is a legal determination of a patient's ability to function; it is based on multiple factors, including physical capacities, psychosocial factors, emotional outlook, and vocational factors. The permanent partial impairment rating is determined after the physician is reasonably sure that the patient has reached maximal medical improvement and that further treatment will not substantially improve the patient's symptoms or function. (Maximal improvement does not necessarily mean full resolution of symptoms.)

IMPAIRMENT REPORT

An impairment evaluation report is prepared after the assessment is completed. A comprehensive impairment evaluation report should address each of the following: (1) chief complaint; (2) history of the present illness with a description of its causal relationship to the traumatic event, if applicable; (3) present symptoms; (4) psychosocial factors; (5) work history; (6) physical examination with documentation of the objective findings; (7) significant laboratory findings, including radiologic reviews and appropriate consultations if requested, especially neurologic, orthopedic, or neurosurgical; (8) clear diagnosis and prognosis; (9) conclusions and recommendations about further medical treatment, current medical status, potential for return to work, restrictions or limitations in work, and whether patient has reached maximal medical improvement; and (10) permanent partial impairment rating (this may be optional).

A particularly helpful approach is to dictate the history, physical findings, laboratory results, consultation information, diagnosis, and conclusions and recommendations, in that order, in the presence of the patient immediately after each particular phase of the consultation. This has proved both timely and efficient. It also allows the patient to verify the accuracy of the history and thus prevents a later claim that misstatements are present in the history.

REFERENCES

1. Merritt JL, Goldman S. Medical assessment of permanent clinical impairment of the musculoskeletal system. In: Gross EL, ed. Injury evaluation: medicolegal principles. Toronto: Butterworths, 1991:51−72.
2. Frymoyer JW, Cats-Baril W. Predictors of low back pain disability. Clin Orthop 1987; 221:89−98.
3. Frymoyer JW, Pope MH, Clements JH, Wilder DG, MacPherson B, Ashikaga T. Risk factors in low-back pain: an epidemiological survey. J Bone Joint Surg [Am] 1983; 65:213−218.
4. Wiesel SW, Feffer HL, Rothman RH. Industrial low back pain: a comprehensive approach. Charlottesville, Virginia: The Michie Company, Law Publishers, 1985.

5. Feller BA. Prevalence of selected impairments, United States, 1977 (Hyattsville, Maryland). Washington DC: U.S. Department of Health and Human Services, Public Health Service, Office of Health Research Statistics, and Technology, National Center for Health Statistics, 1981. (Vital and health statistics. Series 10, data from the National Health Survey; no. 134; DHHS publication no. [PHS] 81–1562.)

6. Snook SH. The costs of back pain in industry. Spine (State of the Art Reviews) 1987; 2(1):1–5.

7. Saunders HD. Evaluation, treatment and prevention of musculoskeletal disorders. Minneapolis, Minnesota: Viking Press, 1985.

8. Ransford AO, Cairns D, Mooney V. The pain drawing as an aid to the psychologic evaluation of patients with low-back pain. Spine 1976; 1:127–134.

9. Magee DJ. Orthopedic physical assessment. Philadelphia: WB Saunders, 1987.

10. Allbrook D. Movements of the lumbar spinal column. J Bone Joint Surg [Br] 1957; 39:339–345.

11. Moll JMH, Wright V. Normal range of spinal mobility: an objective clinical study. Ann Rheum Dis 1971; 30:381–386.

12. Pennal GF, Conn GS, McDonald G, Dale G, Garside H. Motion studies of the lumbar spine: a preliminary report. J Bone Joint Surg [Br] 1972; 54:442–452.

13. Krueger BR. Low back pain and sciatica. In: Spittell JA Jr, ed. Clinical medicine, vol 4, chap 50. Philadelphia: Harper & Row, 1985:1–27.

14. Waddell G, McCulloch JA, Kummel E, Venner RM. Nonorganic physical signs in low-back pain. Spine 1980; 5:117–125.

15. Engelberg AL, ed. Guides to the evaluation of permanent impairment. 3rd ed., revised. Chicago: American Medical Association, 1990.

16. Newton M, Waddell G. Trunk strength testing with iso-machines: Part 1: Review of a decade of scientific evidence. Spine 1993; 18:801–811.

17. Hanson TJ, Merritt JL. Rehabilitation of the patient with lower back pain. In: De Lisa JA, ed. Rehabilitation medicine: principles and practice. Philadelphia: JB Lippincott, 1988:726–748.

18. Disability evaluation under Social Security. U.S. Department of Health and Human Services, Social Security Administration, Baltimore. SSA Publication No. 05–10089, February, 1986.

23

Occupational Rehabilitation Medicine

Richard Paul Bonfiglio

Occupational rehabilitation medicine is an increasingly important area of subspecialization within the field of physical medicine and rehabilitation. The number of potential patients is far larger than that in other areas of rehabilitation medicine. For instance, fewer than 10,000 persons annually suffer spinal cord injuries; in contrast, more than 2 million sustain work-related musculoskeletal injuries each year.[1, 2] Physiatrists and other rehabilitation professionals can often reduce the disability of individuals with pain-related problems to a greater extent than can professionals in other fields of medicine.[3]

Physiatrists are uniquely qualified to reduce disabilities among this patient population through a holistic approach that emphasizes prevention and a team approach to diagnosis and treatment. Frequent rehabilitation goals within this area of medical management include reduction in pain perception, enhancement of functional capabilities, instruction in proper body mechanics and posture, and return to significant gainful employment.[4]

A patient's likelihood of returning to work is directly related to the time off from work because of the disability. The chance of returning to work after 6 months of disability is about 50%. By 1 year, it decreases to about 25%; and by 2 years, almost no patient returns to work without exhaustive rehabilitation measures. In addition, the costs of medical care and disability benefits are great for persons with prolonged disability. Approximately 80% of disability costs result from 10% of claims.[2]

The monetary cost is far exceeded by the impact of work-related disability on the individual and his or her family. Many individuals with long-term work-related disabilities become exceedingly depressed and constrict their activity level. Divorce and other interpersonal disruptions are common.

To practice within the area of occupational rehabilitation medicine, physiatrists must have a sound knowledge regarding the pathophysiology, pathomechanics, diagnosis, and treatment of frequent work-related musculoskeletal injuries and conditions.[5, 6] Additionally, it is important to appreciate the vocational and compensation issues that may have an impact on the patient's motivation, the patient's participation in treatment, and the outcome of the treatment program.[7–9] Practitioners must also be comfortable with the specialized documentation needs and the potential for associated testimony regarding the medical aspects.

ASSESSMENT COMPONENTS

Diagnostic testing must be individualized to the patient's clinical condition. An adequate patient history and examination can provide the basis for accurate diagnosis in most cases. The history should include a description of the patient's pain symptoms, which are generally the most significant. Included must be a description of the nature of the pain and whether it is constant, of variable intensity, or actually intermittent. Inciting and relieving factors should also be delineated. For instance, pain resulting from a radiculopathy is usually aggravated by sitting and improved by standing. Associated lower limb pain, paresthesias, and weakness are common. Associated urinary or fecal incontinence is a poor prognostic factor.

The peripheral nervous and musculoskeletal systems must also be examined. Muscle stretch reflexes are of particular importance because of their objective nature. Because more than 90% of lumbosacral radiculopathies involve S-1 or L-5 nerve roots, the hamstring and gastrocsoleus reflexes must be examined.[10] Evaluation of muscle strength and measurement of muscle bulk to evaluate for atrophy are also important. The sensory examination may be helpful, but it is necessarily somewhat subjective. Patients will often display various pain behaviors or exaggerate their findings during evaluation. Physiatrists must sort out the evidence for true organic abnormality from these other findings.[11]

Patients are generally most worried about having a "pinched nerve" (a radiculopathy). Therefore, evaluation for this condition is essential. Back pain, however, is most often myofascial in nature. The examination must, therefore, include a search for trigger or tender points. Their presence can be secondary to a myofascial pain problem or to an underlying radiculopathy.

Evaluation of lumbosacral mobility is also useful. The presence of muscle tightness and guarding is a sensitive, but nonspecific, indication of back abnormality. Straight leg raising may also help delineate the cause of pain, but unfortunately it is fairly subjective.

Electromyographic evaluation can provide electrophysiologic assessment of the cause of pain.[10] In contrast, radiologic testing—including computed tomography, magnetic resonance imaging, and myelography—demonstrates anatomic abnormalities. It is important to remember that pain is radiolucent and, therefore, radiographic findings must be correlated with clinical findings.[12]

As industry shifts in the United States from being predominantly manufacturing to being service oriented, the incidence of upper limb and neck cumulative trauma disorders is anticipated to increase. Such conditions can be difficult to diagnose and relate to job activities because of their insidious onset and the frequently multifactorial nature of contributing factors. Careful musculoskeletal and peripheral neurologic examinations of the involved limb must be undertaken. Recognizing contributing biomechanical work-related stresses is also important to facilitate assessment and management of the patient. For example, repeated exertions with the wrists flexed or extended can contribute to the development of carpal tunnel syndrome. A work level that is too high or low can contribute to strain of the neck muscles and various musculoskeletal problems of the upper limb.[13]

In addition to medical diagnostic testing, additional evaluations may be helpful, especially for patients with chronic pain problems who cannot return to their former job duties.[14, 15] These studies may include psychologic testing, which can help delineate the individual's response to pain and stress. It may also identify the patient's interpersonal strengths and problems. This knowledge can help determine the best method to motivate the patient to succeed in the rehabilitation program.

Vocational specialists can also help determine the patient's most reasonable return-to-work goals. Vocational testing can include vocational interest inventories, achievement testing, aptitude testing, and assessment of the ability to perform work activities. For patients who are unable to return to their former jobs, transferable skills must be identified.

Occupational and physical therapists also can contribute by performing physical capacity testing or work capacity evaluations to determine a patient's physical capabilities for return to work. This may include standardized testing or specific situational assessments to identify, for example, the patient's sitting and standing tolerances, strength and endurance with lifting and carrying activities, and ability to perform maneuvers such as reaching, kneeling, and climbing. Because material handling, especially lifting with bending and twisting, is correlated with the most frequent onset of lower back pain, evaluation of a patient's lifting technique and maximal weight that can be lifted is of particular significance (Fig. 23–1).

The assessment process should be geared toward identifying the patient's greatest occupational potential. This requires a matching process of the physical limitations based on the medical conditions, the individual's transferable skills, vocational interest and aptitudes, interpersonal skills, and the available job market.[3] The compensation system may have a further impact on this process.

TREATMENT AND ISSUES OF PATIENT MANAGEMENT

Because of the wide variety of possibly contributing medical conditions and the difficulty of delineating a single cause, determination of spe-

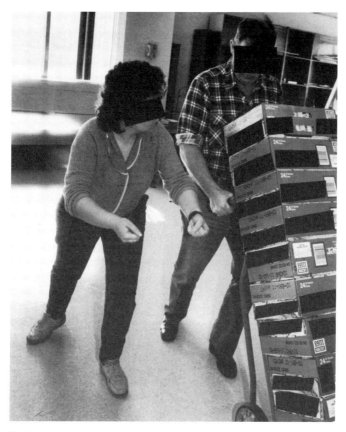

Figure 23–1
Use of situational assessment to delineate a patient's functional capability. (Courtesy of Schwab Rehabilitation Center, Chicago, Illinois.)

cific treatment measures can be difficult. Pain is generally the most significant symptom and greatest complaint. Unfortunately, pain cannot be quantified and is difficult to validate. In fact, pain is a very personal experience. Additionally, many factors can modify the pain experience. These include psychosocial elements such as job satisfaction, premorbid personality, family concerns, and substance abuse.[2]

Medical treatment often includes the prescription of anti-inflammatory medications. Because of the frequent lack of compliance with medication provision, it is valuable to prescribe medications with a simple schedule of administration and relatively few side effects. Tricyclic antidepressants are also often used as a sleep aid because sleep disorders are common among patients with musculoskeletal pain problems. Muscle relaxants and narcotics are generally less helpful for treating work-related musculoskeletal problems.

TEAM APPROACH TO REHABILITATION

Many patients also benefit from a team approach to rehabilitation. The team needs to be cohesive to maximize outcome, especially for patients with limited motivation to return to work.[15-17]

Physical therapy is often helpful for reducing pain perception. Various heating and counterirritant methods are used. However, exercise is the single most important approach for the greatest number of patients. For patients with back pain, the exercise program usually needs to include not only a method to increase the strength and flexibility of lumbosacral paraspinal muscles but also abdominal muscle strengthening and hamstring muscle stretching. Generalized conditioning, especially for patients with chronic pain, is also often very important. Instruction in proper body mechanics and proper posture can also be the key to a successful return to work.

A physical or occupational therapist may also engage the patient in a work hardening program. The patient is first placed in a program to develop endurance for remaining in static positions, including sitting and standing postures, while performing activities. As the individual's tolerance improves, additional work-type activities are added. Depending on the nature of the person's work, these may include lifting, carrying, bending, kneeling, and climbing. Also included may be various activities requiring upper limb function, including reaching overhead and manipulating tools. Foot controls may also be used. The patient's endurance for work activities is slowly increased with supervision. This goal is geared toward maximizing the patient's functional improvement while simultaneously providing it in a safe environment (Fig. 23-2).

Patients also may benefit from instruction in relaxation techniques. This is most often provided by psychologists and may include biofeedback, hypnosis, and progressive muscle relaxation techniques. Patients with mood or thought disorders also benefit from supportive psychotherapy and occasionally from psychotropic medications.

A vocational specialist may develop work-specific activities as part of the work hardening program. The vocational specialist also is instrumental in returning the patient to work, especially when alternative employment must be found.

DISABILITY EVALUATION OF INDUSTRIAL WORKERS

Within some systems of worker's compensation, impairment determinations are of paramount importance. Impairment is defined as "an alteration of an individual's health status that is *assessed by medical means*."[18] Such determinations require careful physical examinations, including, for example, recording of limitations in joint mobility, muscle weakness, and sensory loss. The data must then be "rated" according to a standardized system, such as the American Medical Association's *Guides to the Evalua-*

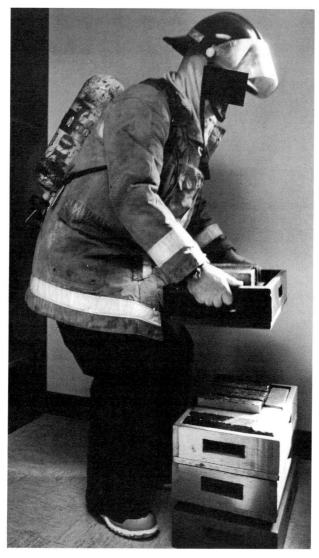

Figure 23–2
Use of a structured rehabilitation setting can help patient to increase endurance safely. (Courtesy of Schwab Rehabilitation Center, Chicago, Illinois.)

tion of Permanent Impairment,[18] for validation. Such impairments are usually translated into a "whole person" impairment rating through the use of a combined values chart. Compensation awards are often based at least in part on such determinations of permanent impairment.

Disability determinations generally require extensive evaluations. A person is considered disabled when there is "an alteration of an individual's capacity to meet personal, social, or occupational demands or statutory or regulatory requirements."[18] This definition takes into account the impact that an individual's medical condition has on residual employability. Such determinations are generally beyond the scope of physician evaluators. The medical evaluation is, however, important for determining the stability of the patient's medical condition. For instance, if the patient has not reached maximal medical recovery, permanent impairment or disability cannot be determined. Projections concerning future medical and vocational outcomes can still be made. In addition, these projections can be bolstered by physical capacity testing that documents the patient's capabilities to perform activities such as static sitting and standing, lifting, and climbing. Such evaluations can be performed by therapists, but they need to take into account the patient's medical condition and limitations.

In addition to the testing of gross physical capabilities, more specific evaluations may be indicated depending on the individual patient's medical problems and vocational options. For example, many tests determine upper extremity dexterity; these include the Purdue Pegboard, Crawford Small Parts, Minnesota Rate of Manipulation, Stromberg Dexterity, and Bennet Hand Tool tests.

In addition to evaluation of the patient's medical and physical capabilities, consideration can also be given to vocational interests, intelligence, aptitude, and achievements. Interest tests are designed to identify broad categories of work with characteristics that an individual would find suitable. Such vocational interests must be matched with the patient's physical and intellectual capabilities. Vocational interest tests include the Wide Range Interest-Opinion Test (WRIOT), the California Occupational Preference Survey (COPS), the Strong-Campbell test, and the Work Values Inventory.

Basic intelligence can be documented with various standardized tests. The Wechsler Adult Intelligence Scale-Revised (WAIS-R) is the most commonly used test of this type; it provides a measure of verbal and performance intelligence quotients. Other tests of intelligence include the Peabody Picture Vocabulary, Stanford-Binet, and the California Test of Mental Maturity. In some cases, memory assessments are useful for providing a memory quotient. In addition, past performance with learning can be determined with achievement testing. Examples include the Wide Range Achievement Test (WRAT), Adult Basic Learning (ABLE), and the Peabody Individual Achievement Test. Aptitude for future training and learning can also be evaluated with various instruments, including the Differential Aptitude Tests (DAT), General Aptitude Test Battery (GATB), and the Oral Directions Test (ODT). These tests are useful in vocational counseling for placement in work settings or training programs. The General Aptitude Test Battery, for instance, has been standardized for more than 450 different occupations, especially in unskilled and semiskilled areas; this testing is useful for individuals with limited transferable skills.

Personality inventories that assess major personality characteristics related to personal and social adjustment help in determining an individual's suitability for adapting to particular work environments. The Minnesota

Multiphasic Personality Inventory (MMPI) has been most widely used for this purpose. Other available personality inventories include Sixteen Personality Factors Questionnaire (16PF) and the Edwards Personal Preference Schedule (EPPS).

After the clinically appropriate tests among those listed above have been interpreted, an individually designed work tolerance program can be provided to serve as a transition to return to work for the individual patient. This may consist of (1) a short-term evaluation with standardized single or multiple work sample stations or (2) an extensive situational assessment combining various work samples designed to simulate a specific occupation. Systems of work sample stations include the Singer Vocational Evaluation System, the Valpar Component Work Sample Series, the Philadelphia Jewish Employment and Vocational Service Work Sample Battery, the Testing, Orientation, and Work Evaluation in Rehabilitation System (TOWER), and the Talent Assessment Program. Specific aptitude tests may also be used for further evaluation of specific aptitudes recognized to be important in particular vocations. Among these tests are the Bennett Mechanical Comprehension Test, the Revised Minnesota Paper Form Board Test, the Minnesota Clerical Test, Computer Operator Aptitude Battery, the Computer Programmer Aptitude Battery, the MacQuarrie Test for Mechanical Ability, the General Clerical Test, and the SRA Tests of Clerical Aptitude.

Actual placement in vocational settings within a rehabilitation program can also allow the patient to work in a supervised setting with a gradual increase in outcome demands.

Thus, injured workers can receive extensive evaluations specifically designed to meet their needs for vocational counseling and job placement or training. Such programs are best provided by interdisciplinary rehabilitation programs.

MEDICAL TESTIMONY

The provision of occupational rehabilitation medicine services often leads to the need for medical testimony. This is usually provided through a deposition at the physician's office (for the physician's convenience). The first step in preparing for such testimony is articulate documentation in the patient's medical record. Perceived inconsistencies or errors in the record diminish the physician's credibility and prolong the testimony process.

The physician must delineate the causal relationship between the individual's work-related injury or disease and his or her ongoing disabling condition. Delineation of the diagnostic considerations and treatments provided is also essential. In addition, prognostication of ongoing medical and rehabilitation needs and vocational outcome is important.

Providers of occupational rehabilitation medicine should recognize that there will often be opposing medical opinion, particularly for a patient with a myofascial pain problem in which there is a paucity of objective findings or a patient with a cumulative trauma disorder without an identified single inciting event. The physiatrist practicing in this area must provide a reasonable and accurate medical perception.

Before testimony is given, it is important to be well prepared by reviewing all available past medical information. Essential issues in the case should be determined, and appropriate answers to possible questions should be considered. Explanations of discrepancies in the record or differences of opinion should be considered. Lack of patient progress with prescribed treatments must be explained.

Comfort with litigation grows with experience. The goal should always be to provide factual information in a precise and credible fashion.

SUMMARY AND CONCLUSIONS

Occupational rehabilitation medicine is emerging as a significant subspecialty within the field of physical medicine and rehabilitation. Physiatrists are uniquely qualified to treat patients with work-related musculoskeletal problems because of the field's use of a holistic approach to treatment that emphasizes prevention, team work, and functional enhancement. Practitioners in this area must have a thorough knowledge of the pathophysiology of common conditions, an understanding of the vocational factors that may have an impact on the condition, and an appreciation of the compensation system and its regulations. Comfort with litigation is also essential.

REFERENCES

1. Andersson GBJ. Epidemiologic aspects on low-back pain in industry. Spine 1981; 6:53–60.
2. Weinstein SM, Herring SA, Shelton JL. The injured worker: assessment and treatment. Phys Med Rehabil: State of the Art Reviews 1990; 4:361–377.
3. Scheer SJ, Wickstrom RJ. Vocational capacity with low back pain impairment. In: Scheer SJ. Medical perspectives in vocational assessment of impaired workers. Gaithersburg: Aspen Publishers, 1991:19–63.
4. Reilly K, Lovejoy B, Williams R, Roth H. Differences between a supervised and independent strength and conditioning program with chronic low back syndromes. J Occup Med 1989; 31:547–550.
5. Bigos SJ, Spengler DM, Martin NA, Zeh J, Fisher L, Nachemson A, Wang MH. Back injuries in industry: a retrospective study. II. Injury factors. Spine 1986; 11:246–251.
6. Bigos SJ, Spengler DM, Martin NA, Zeh J, Fisher L, Nachemson A. Back injuries in industry: a retrospective study. III. Employee-related factors. Spine 1986; 11:252–256.
7. Aronoff GM, McAlary PW, Witkower A, Berdell MS. Pain treatment programs: do they return workers to the workplace? Spine: State of the Art Reviews 1987; 2:123–136.

8. Frymoyer JW, Cats-Baril W: Predictors of low back pain disability. Clin Orthop 1987; 221:89–98.
9. Frymoyer JW, Pope MH, Clements JH, Wilder DG, MacPherson B, Ashikaga T. Risk factors in low-back pain: an epidemiological survey. J Bone Joint Surg [Am] 1983; 65:213–218.
10. Johnson EW, ed. Practical electromyography. 2nd ed. Baltimore: Williams & Wilkins, 1988:229–245.
11. Waddell G, McCulloch JA, Kummel E, Venner RM. Nonorganic physical signs in low-back pain. Spine 1980; 5:117–125.
12. Saal J. Diagnostic studies of industrial low back injuries. Topics in Acute Care Trauma Rehabilitation 1988; 2:31–49.
13. Silverstein BA, Fine LJ, Armstrong TJ. Carpal tunnel syndrome: causes and a preventative strategy. Semin Occup Med 1986; 1:213–221.
14. Herbin ML. Work capacity evaluation for occupational hand injuries. J Hand Surg 1987; 12-A:958–961.
15. Weinstein SM, Shervey JW. Assessment and management of the injured worker with low back pain. Phys Med Rehabil Clin North Am 1991; 2:145–156.
16. Fast A. Low back disorders: conservative management. Arch Phys Med Rehabil 1988; 69:880–891.
17. Saal JA, Saal JS. Nonoperative treatment of herniated lumbar intervertebral disc with radiculopathy: an outcome study. Spine 1989; 14:431–437.
18. Guides to the evaluation of permanent impairment. 4th ed rev. Chicago: American Medical Association, 1993.

24 | Hand Disabilities

Jane L. Reiman

Injury to one or both hands can be serious or devastating to the person who is injured. For someone whose vocation depends on his or her hands, even a small injury can be disabling. Even if it is still possible to perform one's vocation after a hand injury, the effect can be disabling if a favorite hobby has to be abandoned. Most of our activities of daily living such as grooming and hygiene depend on complete use of the hands. The purpose of hand rehabilitation is to restore the most complete function possible to the injured, operated, or diseased hand.

Patients may be referred for hand therapy for various reasons. For example, any number of possible injuries can occur to the hand. Some of the most common are fractures, tendon injuries, crush injuries, amputations, or a combination of these. Hand rehabilitation services may also be needed for patients with arthritis. Many postoperative conditions, such as release of the carpal tunnel in median neuropathy of the wrist, require hand rehabilitation. A patient is most often evaluated in the department of physical medicine and rehabilitation after the hand surgeon has completed the initial operation, treatment, and casting. Even though a patient's hand may be in a cast or dressing, therapy can be initiated.

COMPLICATIONS AND TREATMENT

Certain complications can be prevented or diminished by early evaluation and treatment. Some of the complications are edema, pain, loss of range of motion, loss of strength, adhesions, hypersensitivity, misuse of the extremity, disuse of the extremity, and, occasionally, overuse of the extremity (Table 24-1).

Edema is common after injury or operation. In part, it is due to immobilization of the hand and subsequent loss of the muscle "pump" in moving lymph from the hand. Also, the delicate lymph channels on the dorsum of the hand may be overwhelmed by rapid return of circulation after

TABLE 24-1

Complications of Hand Injury and Some Recommended Therapeutic Measures

Complications	Treatment
Edema	Early active range of motion
	Elevation
	Decongestive massage
	Elastic wrap or glove
Pain	Cold, immediately postoperatively
	Heat methods (avoid swelling)
	Sedative massage
	Transcutaneous electrical nerve stimulation
Loss of range of motion	Control edema
	Range-of-motion exercises
	Joint mobilization techniques
	Splinting
Loss of strength	Progressive resistance exercises, isometric or isotonic
Adhesions	Friction massage
	Ultrasound, usually in water
Hypersensitivity	Desensitization massage
Misuse	
Disuse	Neuromuscular reeducation
Overuse	

release of the tourniquet used during operation. Early active range of motion helps prevent edema and should be started in whichever joints can be moved. Even a small amount of motion can be helpful. Patients are instructed to keep the hand elevated whenever possible when swelling is a problem or a potential problem. They are instructed in decongestive massage, which is a distal-to-proximal massage to push the edema fluid out of the fingers or hand. They also learn to use elastic wrap (Coban) or string to wrap the fingers temporarily to decrease edema. Some patients wear elastic gloves to control swelling. If edema persists, soft tissue fibrosis may develop, which can result in loss of motion of joints and tendons.

Pain is also common after injury or for a short time postoperatively. Various types of hand therapy are used for relief. A whirlpool at moderate temperatures, fluidotherapy, contrast baths, light or deep sedative massage, paraffin baths, ultrasound, and transcutaneous electrical nerve stimulation are some examples. It is important not to increase edema by overuse of heat, especially when the hand is in the dependent position, such as in the whirlpool. If there is a danger of swelling, whirlpool temperatures should be kept lower than the temperature of the limb (that is, lower than 35.5° or 36° C). Severe, persistent pain unrelieved by these treatments requires further investigation and therapy.

Loss of range of motion is another complication of hand trauma or operation. Often, such loss can be prevented by early use of appropriate hand therapy. Several mechanisms contribute to loss of range of motion.

One is edema interfering mechanically with the function of the finger joints. The areas of edema may become fibrosed, causing swelling and stiffness to be persistent or permanent. Another cause for loss of range of motion is capsular and ligamentous tightness after immobilization of joints. Sometimes joints must be immobilized to allow for healing of bones or structures that have been repaired. Any joints that are not immobilized should have range of motion started immediately to help prevent loss. This includes the shoulder and elbow as well as the wrist and finger joints. The shoulder especially has a tendency to become stiff and painful when the patient is unable to use the hand. The purpose of the shoulder is to place the hand where it is needed. If the hand is not used normally, the shoulder will not be used normally, and specific range-of-motion exercises will help the patient use the shoulder and maintain the range of motion.

Although active exercises are most commonly used to maintain and increase range of motion, other forms of maintaining or increasing range of motion are used. Passive range of motion, in which an external force produces the motion, may be used. This does not imply stretching. Such exercises are done within the available range of motion. Active-assisted range of motion involves the patient actively moving the part as far as possible, and an external force completes the movement through the available range without stretching. This external force may be the therapist's hand or the patient's other hand. Gentle prolonged stretch, if desired, must be specified in the therapy prescription. Initially, the patient may tolerate only a few minutes of stretch, but the time ideally is increased gradually to 20 minutes, four times a day. It requires the cooperation of the patient, but the prolonged gentle stretch often achieves the goal of increasing the range of motion.

The addition of ultrasound to the gentle stretching program will enhance the effect of stretch alone. Stretching should be done simultaneously with the application of ultrasound and should be continued for several minutes thereafter while the tissues are cooling. This simultaneous heating and stretching enhances the flexibility of the tissues and makes them more amenable to stretch.

Heat methods other than ultrasound, such as a whirlpool or other superficial heat, during or before treatment may make movement easier.

Joint mobilization techniques, performed by the therapist, may be used to gain full "joint play" or capsular motion. They are not a home treatment, however.

Techniques other than therapeutic exercise can improve range of motion. If scar tissue or skin is tight over an area with loss of range of motion, friction massage will help. Dynamic splints may increase range of motion, and static splints maintain range of motion.

Splints (orthoses) are of many types, but the two basic are static and dynamic. Static splints have no movement built into them (Fig. 24–1), and dynamic splints have movement (Fig. 24–2). Dynamic splints may be made with hinges or external joints and usually have a source of stored energy such as a rubber band or spring that provides movement.

Splints may be used to align, support, resist, assist, and simulate

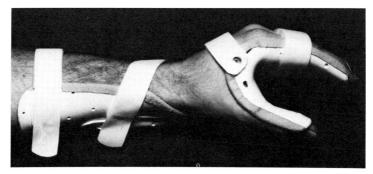

Figure 24–1
Static type of wrist-hand orthosis (splint). This type has no moving parts.

movement. All of these functions are used for hands at various times. Alignment and support are important in the resting splint for the arthritic patient. Static splints may resist abnormal or undesirable movements, such as a splint that prevents the patient from putting tension on a newly repaired tendon. Splints may assist movement dynamically, such as when rubber bands or springs assist movement of a weak muscle, or statically, such as in the wrist cock-up splint that supports the hand with weak or paralyzed wrist extensors. The simulation of function also involves movement built into the splint; also, these splints have a source of stored energy that can be activated by the patient's own muscles or by an external power source.

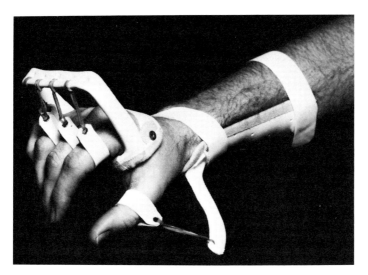

Figure 24–2
Dynamic type of wrist-hand orthosis (splint). The rubber bands assist extension of the metacarpophalangeal joints.

Splints can be made for individual joints, for the entire area of the elbow, hand, and wrist, or for portions of the extremity. Splints can be fabricated from special plastics that soften when heated, or occasionally they are made of metal or of canvas with metal supports; they can also be prefabricated, although a better fit is usually achieved with a custom-made hand splint.

The duration the splint is worn depends on the purpose. Sometimes splints must be worn constantly, such as when sound healing of a tendon or fracture is sought. Dynamic splints, which provide prolonged gentle stretch, are worn for a prescribed time, such as a half hour four times daily.

Failure to control edema, pain, and hypersensitivity and inattention to range of motion may lead to reflex sympathetic dystrophy of the upper extremity. Although this condition may occur spontaneously or after minor trauma or a wrist fracture, it may also occur as a complication of severe trauma or after operation.

Reflex sympathetic dystrophy causes diffuse pain and edema of the hand. The pain may be severe and may involve the entire upper extremity. Initially, there is loss of range of motion due to edema, pain, and unwillingness to move the extremity. Because of instability of the sympathetic nervous system, the hand may be warm or cool, have excessive or decreased sweating, and have blotchy red or blue discoloration. The skin is shiny. Late changes are atrophy of the skin and subcutaneous tissues and severe contractures of joints, including the shoulder and the more distal joints of the extremity. Radiography of the extremity may show patchy loss of bone density.

Physical therapy measures are extremely important in the treatment of this condition; they include antiedema measures and range of motion exercises with care to avoid increasing the pain. Avoiding misuse, disuse, and overuse of the extremity is also extremely important. Transcutaneous electrical nerve stimulation may be helpful for relief of pain. Use of nonnarcotic analgesics or nonsteroidal anti-inflammatory agents for relief of pain is important. Administration of corticosteroids is helpful in severe cases. A series of stellate ganglion blocks in addition to the physical therapy and medications may be of help.

MUSCLE REEDUCATION

The hand therapist will often spend much time on muscle reeducation, regardless of whether tendon transfers have been performed. The classic method of reeducation, as described by Sister Kenny,[1] consists of progression from passive relaxed range of motion to active-assisted and to active range of motion followed by strengthening. The patient must concentrate and be aware of the desired action by feeling the muscle with the other hand and by observing muscle action. Electrical stimulation and electromyographic biofeedback can be used to enhance awareness of the desired action.

During the course of reeducation, the therapist and physician must be aware of and try to prevent misuse, disuse, or overuse of the affected muscles and other muscles of the extremity.

Misuse is using the extremity in the wrong fashion. This includes substitution, cocontraction, and guarding. Substitution is use of the wrong muscles for the desired movement. Cocontraction is contraction of the agonist and the antagonist at the same time while attempting a movement. If one tries to flex the elbow while simultaneously contracting the biceps and the triceps, elbow motion becomes difficult and uncomfortable because of fatigue of the muscles and extra forces on the joint. Misuse of the muscles of the extremity is inefficient and fatiguing. Cocontraction causes trembling and shaking. Guarding is tightening the muscles in a protective fashion.

Disuse is insufficient use of the extremity. Disuse may occur if the patient uses the extremity only for exercises and not for functional activities. Instruction in functional activities is given as soon as the patient is able to do them.

Overuse is using the extremity too much. Too quick a return to normal activities can result in pain and edema. Progression of activities from "light" to "moderate" to "heavy" should be monitored in each patient.

Sensory reeducation is important when the hand has nerve damage. If there is hypersensitivity, desensitization techniques are used. If all or part of the hand is anesthetic, the patient must be instructed in measures to protect the insensate part to avoid injury. As sensation returns, first in very gross rather than fine form, the patient is instructed in activities to practice sensation, thereby making the fullest use of the neurons present and increasing awareness of the sensation that is present. The progression is from identifying textures to differentiating small objects, temperatures, and hard from soft. Small assembly tasks are the final stage.

Although the road to full rehabilitation of hand disabilities may be long, much can be accomplished by the hand physiatrist, the hand therapist (physical or occupational therapist), and other members of the rehabilitation team working with the hand surgeon. Delays in referral to physical medicine and rehabilitation can result in slow or suboptimal rehabilitation; thus, cooperation and communication between the hand surgeon and physiatrist are of extreme importance and are for the benefit of the patient.

REFERENCE

1. Knapp ME. The contribution of Sister Elizabeth Kenny to the treatment of poliomyelitis. Arch Phys Med Rehabil 1955; 36:510–517.

25 | Tension Myalgia

Jeffrey M. Thompson
Mehrsheed Sinaki

The term "tension myalgia" has been used for years. "Tension" suggests a major characteristic—increased muscle tone, whether it is spasm or increased muscle tone related to other factors. One of these factors may be psychologic tension or stress. "Myalgia" refers to the most characteristic finding—muscle pain, including pain in the muscular attachment areas. Through the years, muscle pain disorders have been referred to by a multitude of labels, including muscular rheumatism, fibrositis, fibromyalgia, and myofascial pain syndrome. The most widely used terms for muscle pain syndromes today are "fibromyalgia" (characterized by widespread muscle pain) and "myofascial pain" (characterized by localized muscle pain). The term "tension myalgia" bridges these extremes and includes localized, regional, and generalized subtypes (Table 25−1).[1] Although the precise incidence is unknown, muscle pain syndromes are extremely common. They are the third most common rheumatologic diagnosis; 15% to 20% of outpatients seen by rheumatologists have a muscle pain syndrome.

ETIOLOGY

Most commonly, tension myalgia follows trauma to or overuse of muscles, usually in the shoulder and hip girdle regions. The pain can be perpetuated by poor posture, anxiety or psychologic tension, poor sleep, anatomic variations (short leg), or muscle cocontraction.

SYMPTOMS

The incidence of tension myalgia can only be estimated because no population studies have been done. Most patients are women,[2] and onset

334

TABLE 25–1

Diagnostic Criteria for Tension Myalgia Developed by the Department of Physical Medicine and Rehabilitation at the Mayo Clinic

Generalized tension myalgia
  Diagnostic criteria
    Generalized aches, pains, or stiffness for > 3 mo
    Tenderness in 11 or more of the 18 sites listed in the American College of
      Rheumatology 1990 criteria for fibromyalgia (Table 25–2)
  Associated symptoms and findings (suggestive of, but not necessary for, the
    diagnosis)
    Nonrestorative sleep
    Generalized fatigue
    Modulation of symptoms with activity
    Alleviation of symptoms with heat (or sometimes ice)
    Intensification of symptoms with anxiety or stress
    Type A personality
  Exclusion criteria
    Abnormal values for any of the following factors: antinuclear antibody, erythrocyte
      sedimentation rate, rheumatoid factor, muscle enzymes
    Presence of another disorder that can explain the symptoms—for example, simple
      postexercise muscle soreness, tendinitis, bursitis, or arthritis (although these may
      lead to secondary tension myalgia)
Regional tension myalgia
  Diagnostic criteria
    Generalized aches, pains, or stiffness for > 3 mo
    Tenderness in 3 to 11 of the 18 sites listed in Table 25–2
  Associated symptoms and findings
    Same as those for generalized tension myalgia
  Exclusion criteria
    Same as those for generalized tension myalgia
Acute or localized tension myalgia
  Diagnostic criteria
    Tenderness in fewer than 3 of the 18 sites listed in Table 25–2
    Symptoms present for < 3 mo
  Exclusion criteria
    Same as those for generalized tension myalgia

From Thompson.[1] By permission of Mayo Foundation for Medical Education and Research.

is before age 35 years in more than 70% of patients. Symptoms may include generalized aches and pains, tiredness or fatigue, stiffness, anxiety, depression, disturbed sleep patterns, headaches, irritable bowel symptoms, subjective sensation of joint swelling, and numbness. The most common sites of tender points are the nuchal and upper back muscular attachment areas, lateral epicondyle, pectoralis attachment areas, gluteal attachment areas, gastrocnemius attachment areas, and suboccipital attachment areas.

Cold or humid weather, fatigue (physical or mental), a sedentary state, overactivity, anxiety, and poor sleep aggravate tension myalgia. Relieving factors include warm or dry weather, a hot shower, local heat, massage, modest physical activity, general relaxation, vacation, and restful sleep.

Tension myalgia sometimes may mimic lumbar disk protrusion or cervical radiculopathy.

SUGGESTED CRITERIA FOR DIAGNOSIS

The criteria for the diagnosis of tension myalgia as defined by the Department of Physical Medicine and Rehabilitation at the Mayo Clinic are listed in Table 25–1. The criteria are based on the 1990 criteria for the diagnosis of fibromyalgia (widespread muscle pain) developed by the American College of Rheumatology (Table 25–2)[3] and the criteria for myofascial pain (localized muscle pain) described by Simons.[4] The major finding in tension myalgia is chronic pain at muscle attachments and within muscles which is often made worse by stress (both psychologic and postural) and better with heat. Poor sleep is common; patients often awake unrefreshed after a night's sleep. Results of neurologic and joint examinations are normal, except for often prominent

TABLE 25–2

American College of Rheumatology 1990 Criteria for Classification of Fibromyalgia*

1. History of widespread pain
   Definition: Pain is considered widespread when all the following are present—pain in the left side of the body, pain in the right side of the body, pain above the waist, and pain below the waist. In addition, axial skeletal pain (cervical spine, anterior chest, thoracic spine, or low back) must be present. In this definition, shoulder and buttock pain is considered as pain for each involved side. "Low back" pain is considered lower segment pain
2. Pain in 11 of 18 tender point sites on digital palpation
   Definition: On digital palpation, pain must be present in at least 11 of the following 18 tender point sites:
   Occiput—bilateral, at the suboccipital muscle insertions
   Low cervical—bilateral, at the anterior aspects of the intertransverse spaces at C5–7
   Trapezius—bilateral, at the midpoint of the upper border
   Supraspinatus—bilateral, at origins, above the scapular spine near the medial border
   Second rib—bilateral, at the second costochondral junctions, just lateral to the junctions on upper surfaces
   Lateral epicondyle—bilateral, 2 cm distal to the epicondyles
   Gluteal—bilateral, in upper outer quadrants of buttocks in anterior fold of muscle
   Greater trochanter—bilateral, posterior to the trochanteric prominence
   Knee—bilateral, at the medial fat pad proximal to the joint line.
Digital palpation should be performed with an approximate force of 4 kg.
For a tender point to be considered "positive," the subject must state that the palpation was painful. "Tender" is not to be considered "painful"

*For classification purposes, patients will be said to have fibromyalgia if both criteria are satisfied. Widespread pain must have been present for at least 3 months. The presence of a second clinical disorder does not exclude the diagnosis of fibromyalgia.
From the American College of Rheumatology.[3] By permission.

TABLE 25-3
Partial Differential Diagnosis of Tension
Myalgia

Polymyalgia rheumatica
Hypothyroidism
Bursitis tendinitis
Widespread osteoarthritis
Prodromal phase of a connective tissue
  disease
Polymyositis
Metabolic myopathy
Hyperparathyroidism
Parkinson's disease
Osteopenia, osteomalacia
Primary Sjögren's syndrome
Enthesopathies (for example, tennis elbow)

From Thompson.[1] By permission of Mayo Foundation for Medical Education and Research.

cocontraction with voluntary movement. The differential diagnoses are
listed in Table 25-3.[1]

PATHOPHYSIOLOGY

The pathophysiology of tension myalgia is the subject of much debate
and recently was the subject of an international symposium.[5] Because no
consistent histologic or laboratory abnormalities have been found, the evidence for the prevailing theories is minimal. The most popular hypothesis
involves the development of localized muscle hypoxia (possibly due to
muscle fiber trauma or overuse) leading to sensitization of muscle nocicep-
tors.[5]

TREATMENT

The initial and probably most important step in the treatment of tension myalgia is the establishment of the diagnosis and reassurance and education of the patient. Patients need to know that they have a benign condition that can be treated and that their muscle pain is not "all in their
head," as many have been led to believe.

Elimination of contributing factors (including stress, anatomic variations such as short leg), physical therapy (heat, massage, postural training,
electromyographic biofeedback for specific muscle reeducation), general
aerobic conditioning, and medications (amitriptyline, cyclobenzaprine) to
treat the sleep disturbance, if present, round out the treatment program
(Fig. 25-1).[1]

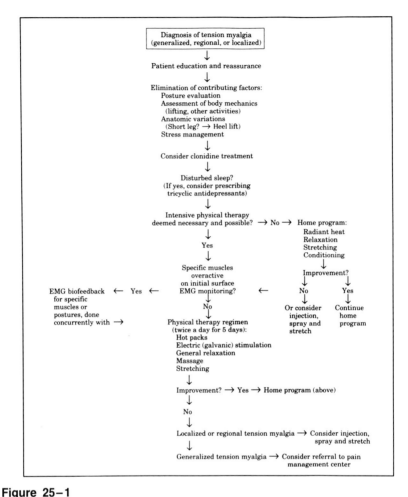

Figure 25–1

Suggested treatment algorithm for tension myalgia, as proposed by the Department of Physical Medicine and Rehabilitation at the Mayo Clinic. See text for complete discussion. EMG, electromyographic. (From Thompson.[1] By permission of Mayo Foundation for Medical Education and Research.)

PELVIC FLOOR TENSION MYALGIA

The syndrome of pelvic floor myalgia is a form of tension myalgia involving the musculature of the pelvic floor and causing pain in these muscles or in their areas of attachment such as the sacrum, coccyx, ischial tuberosity, and pubic rami. The symptoms associated with pelvic floor myalgia are often vague. They are frequently difficult for the patient to describe or localize accurately. Patients usually complain of an aching discomfort in the rectum, pelvis, or lower back. Indeed, many patients are initially treated fruitlessly for low back strain, lumbar disk syndrome, or degenerative joint disease of the lumbar spine. Various terms such as piriformis syndrome,[6] levator ani spasm syndrome, diaphragma pelvis spastica, and coccygodynia (without any traumatic cause) have appeared in the literature, all of them referring more or less to the same entity.

Initial Complaints

A study at the Mayo Clinic[7] demonstrated the major symptoms to be low back pain in 82% of patients, a heavy feeling in the pelvis in 64%, leg pain in 48%, pain with bowel movement in 33%, constipation in 26%, coccyx pain in 19%, dyspareunia in 13%, and urine retention or psychogenic bladder in a few percent.

Aggravating factors are sitting for extended periods, tension, physical activity, standing for a long time, and sexual intercourse.[7]

Alleviating factors are analgesics, muscle relaxants, and sedatives; being in a lying position; relaxing; and a hot tub bath.[7]

Diagnostic Findings

The diagnosis of pelvic floor tension myalgia can easily be missed if the examiner does not consider it in the differential diagnosis. The physical finding that most often leads to the diagnosis is tenderness of one or more pelvic floor muscles on rectal examination. For the examiner to reach the piriformis muscles during rectal examination, the patient should be positioned on the side with the lower limb that is on the top bent at the hip and at the knee. Other reported associated findings are poor posture in about a third of cases, deconditioned abdominal muscles in a third of patients, and generalized muscle tenderness.

Suggested Criteria for Diagnosis

In the absence of a pathologic process in the pelvis, the criteria for diagnosis are tenderness of the pelvic floor muscles on rectal examination, aggravation of pain while in the sitting position, and tenderness of pelvic muscular attachments.

Treatment

The physical therapeutic techniques vary from deep heat (coil diathermy or ultrasound) to hydrotherapy, stretching massage of the pelvic floor muscles via the rectum, relaxation exercises, abdominal and back muscle strengthening exercises, posture instructions, and biofeedback techniques for relaxation. During recent years, significant success has been achieved with superficial heat and relaxation exercises applied with biofeedback techniques[8]; ultrasound therapy and diathermy are used only in selected cases. One or more of these treatments can be used. The duration of the treatment program is usually 5 to 10 days.

Reeducation for Pelvic Floor Muscles[8]

To maintain the skill of keeping pelvic floor muscles relaxed, the patients are instructed to practice the following exercise four times a day: (1) place one's hand over the anal cleft and, to feel the pelvic floor tension, tighten these muscles gently (but do not pinch the buttocks together); (2) tighten the muscles gently and feel the anal cleft being drawn up and in; and (3) in order to relax these muscles, feel the anal cleft bulge against one's hand and keep this relaxed position. Patients should learn how these relaxed muscles feel in order to be able to maintain the relaxed state. When the patient feels confident about keeping the pelvic floor muscles relaxed, indoor and then outdoor activities should be gradually increased. Keeping these muscles relaxed will become easier as the pain and discomfort are diminished.

Treatment Goals

The goals of treatment are (1) to relieve pain by inducing muscle relaxation with deep or superficial heat or exercises with biofeedback measures; (2) to avoid provoking factors; and (3) to teach conscious, frequent relaxation of the pelvic muscles.

Summary

Important points to remember are that (1) this syndrome is little known to some physicians; (2) the diagnosis is obscured by vague complaints in a patient who is often neurotic as a result of pain or a premorbid personality; (3) a diagnostic clue is severe tenderness of the pelvic diaphragm muscles on rectal examination, and the tenderness may be in the posterior or anterior part of the pelvic diaphragm or in the attachment areas of the pelvic floor muscles; and (4) a patient may have a past history of generalized tension myalgia, generalized deconditioning, poor posture, or previous orthopedic or gynecologic operation or pelvic operation.

REFERENCES

1. Thompson JM. Tension myalgia as a diagnosis at the Mayo Clinic and its relationship to fibrositis, fibromyalgia, and myofascial pain syndrome. Mayo Clin Proc 1990; 65:1237–1248.
2. Yunus M, Masi AT, Calabro JJ, Shah IK. Primary fibromyalgia. Am Fam Physician 1982; 25:115–121.
3. The American College of Rheumatology. 1990 criteria for the classification of fibromyalgia: report of the Multicenter Criteria Committee. Arthritis Rheum 1990; 33:160–172.
4. Simons DG. Myofascial pain syndrome due to trigger points. In: Goodgold J, ed. Rehabilitation medicine. St. Louis: CV Mosby Company, 1988:686–723.

5. Fricton JR, Awad EA, eds. Myofascial pain and fibromyalgia. New York: Raven Press, 1990.
6. Thiele GH. Coccygodynia: cause and treatment. Dis Colon Rectum 1963; 6:422–436.
7. Sinaki M, Merritt JL, Stillwell GK. Tension myalgia of the pelvic floor. Mayo Clin Proc 1977; 52:717–722.
8. Department of Physical Medicine and Rehabilitation. Home instructions for relief of pelvic-floor pain. Rochester, Minnesota: Mayo Clinic, 1983.

PART X

Rehabilitation in Soft Tissue Injuries

26

Rehabilitation After Burn Injury

Elizabeth A. Rivers
Steven V. Fisher

Each year, about 1% of the population sustains a burn, and 1 in every 70 burned adults is hospitalized annually. An organized positive approach to rehabilitation can reduce disability and the need for a reconstructive surgical procedure.

CLASSIFICATION OF BURNS

Burn severity is classified according to the patient's age, the agent causing cell damage, the percentage of cutaneous surface injured, the depth of tissue destruction, the body areas injured, and the types of associated injuries or illnesses. Causative agents may include chemicals, thermal means (heat and cold), electricity, and, rarely, radiation. The body surface area is roughly estimated with the "rule of nines" or more accurately calculated with the Lund-Browder chart. Table 26–1 details the classification of depth of injury.

PATHOPHYSIOLOGY

Normal skin is comprised of dermis and epidermis. The epidermal cells begin at the basal layer and flatten and keratinize as they migrate to the skin surface, providing a waterproof bacterial barrier. The dermis consists of a vascular collagen matrix that provides the elasticity and durability of the skin. This tissue does not regenerate. Also included in the dermis are the sweat glands, hair follicles, and sebaceous glands (Fig. 26-1). Burn pathophysiology is complex and therefore the reader is referred to detailed texts.[1-6]

TABLE 26–1
Classification of Depth of Burn Injury

Depth of Injury	Healing Time	Pain	Wound Outcome	Treatment
Superficial epidermis (1st degree)	3–7 days	Painful for 1 to 3 days; ibuprofen or acetaminophen for adequate analgesia	No sequela	Keep clean
Superficial dermis (2nd degree/superficial partial thickness)	5–14 days	Painful for 5 to 14 days; acetaminophen with codeine or oxycodone for adequate analgesia for wound care, exercise, and sleep	Possible pigment changes	Wound care, active exercise, protective garments, sunscreen
Deep reticular dermis (2nd degree/deep partial thickness)	10–30 days for spontaneous healing (if grafted, see below)	Very painful until closure; methadone or oral morphine sulfate for baseline pain control; parenteral morphine or oxazepam and midazolam for dressing changes and stretching exercise	Probable pigment changes; reduced skin durability; severe scarring; sensory changes; apocrine changes; edema in dependent limbs	Wound care; anti-inflammatory agents, analgesics, antipruritics; elevated positioning/orthotics; active exercise; external vascular support; moisturization and lubrication; daily living skills; psychologic therapy;

Subcutaneous tissue (3rd degree/full thickness)	Graft needed/variable healing time	Nonpainful initially because of destruction of nerve endings; pain medication as outlined above	Same as above; additional sweating loss; possible additional sensory loss	Same as above; postoperative positioning/immobilization
Muscle, tendon, bone (4th degree)	Amputation or operation needed/healing time variable	Nonpainful initially because of destruction of nerve endings; chronic pain treatment for neuromas and phantom limb pain	Variable	Same as above; deep tendon massage; adapted equipment; prosthetic fitting if indicated

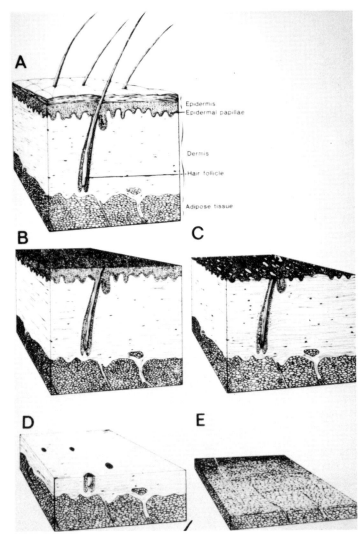

Figure 26–1
Depth of burn. *A,* Normal skin. *B,* Superficial partial-thickness burn, first degree. *C,*
Superficial partial-thickness burn, second degree. *D,* Deep partial-thickness burn. *E,* Full-
thickness burn. (From Fisher SV. Rehabilitation management of burns. In: Basmajian JV,
Kirby RL, eds. Medical rehabilitation. Baltimore: Williams & Wilkins, 1984:305–312. By
permission of the publisher.)

INITIAL REHABILITATION CARE

Emergency medical and surgical management is beyond the scope of this chapter. A burn injury is always of mixed depth and various treatments are needed. In this chapter, the initial phase is considered to begin with the injury and continue until the wound is closed by healing in partial-thickness injury and by autografting in full-thickness injury.

The goals of rehabilitation management during this period are the following: to promote wound closure and prevent infection, to control edema, to maintain joint and skin mobility, to maintain strength and endurance, to facilitate patient and family participation in wound healing and rehabilitation, to improve self-care, and to provide psychologic assistance for pain modification and treatment of posttraumatic stress disorder.

Surgical Management

Surgical consultation is desirable for any wound that will require more than 10 days to heal. Tangential excision and grafting of deep dermal burns preserve dermal collagen and patent capillaries and result in a better cosmetic and functional outcome than occurs with similar wounds permitted to heal spontaneously.

Surgeons may favor excision to fascia and grafting for severe burns because this approach is associated with decreased blood loss and a high percentage of graft survival, but because the contouring fat does not regenerate, cosmetic disfigurement results. Distal lymphedema often occurs in extremity burns with circumferential grafts on fascia. Grafts that permanently adhere to fascia may also limit range of motion. When adequate donor sites for sheet grafts are available, split-thickness sheets may be aligned in cosmetic units along the lines of relaxed skin tension for optimal cosmesis. Difficulty in draining seromas or hematomas is a disadvantage of sheet grafts and therefore the recipient bed must be meticulously dry. Full-thickness sheet grafts are reserved for reconstructive procedures because a full-thickness donor area must be primarily closed or split-thickness grafted. Skin meshing devices allow uniform expansion of the donor skin to cover large recipient areas. The sizes of the cutaneous mesh range from 1:1 to 6:1; the smaller expansion produces more attractive results and more rapid healing. The mesh pattern remains permanently visible, especially with thick-skin grafts. In addition, the wound heals by contraction. The raised collagen scars leave a permanent irregular surface with varied pigmentation. Grafts from areas with similar pigmentation such as scalp to face provide optimal appearance. Final repigmentation in all burn injuries is variable.

If the graft extends across a joint, rehabilitation specialists design orthotics and plan positioning for the immobilization phase of graft healing. The exercise regimen is continued on nonimmobilized body parts.

Biologic dressings can substitute for skin until autografting is undertaken or until partial-thickness burns heal. Range-of-motion exercises resume as soon as the dressing adheres. Cadaver skin homografts and pig-skin xenografts have been widely used to decrease pain and to improve autograft survival. Biobrane, Opsite, Tegapore, and Duoderm are popular temporary dressings.

Local Wound Care

The responsibility for wound care differs from one burn center to another. Wound care, debridement, and subsequent care of the skin affect the final outcome of function and cosmesis. From a rehabilitation standpoint, the outcome is optimal if wound infection is controlled, maximal tissue is preserved, and the wound is closed as soon as possible.

Exercise

Ambulation and active range-of-motion exercises are the most important rehabilitation methods. A wheeled walker with overhead bar (Fig. 26–2) can be used for patients with axillary burns; it promotes increased range of motion with active patient participation. Supervised active range of motion orients the patient to mobility. A progressive ambulation program allows participation of the patient in rehabilitation planning and improves the patient's confidence. Multiple repetitions of range of motion and heavy resistance are painful and unnecessary. However, the healing wound benefits from gentle and slow movement through the full range of active motion at least three times a day; this approach prevents contractures and improves venous return. A therapist provides gentle terminal stretch or prolonged stretch to achieve full motion until the patient is independently able to move fully.

Positioning

Proper alignment of body parts decreases the potential to develop contractures; supervised positioning attempts to assist venous return and minimize contractures (Fig. 26–3). The patient often assumes a flexed, adducted position in withdrawal from pain. An extended position is no more painful, but moving to that position is uncomfortable. A typical anticontracture bed-positioning method consists of neck extension, shoulders abducted to 90° and forward flexed 15°, elbows lacking 15° of extension and supinated, wrists and hands in functional position, hips extended and abducted 10° without external rotation, knees in extension, and ankles at neutral. If ears are burned, they should be protected by avoiding contact with the bed, pillows, or tie tapes. If the mouth is burned, circumoral contracture should be addressed. Any position maintained without active motion becomes a contracture. Wedge pillows, over-bed suspension, deltoid aids, and elevating tables may be used to alternate positions.

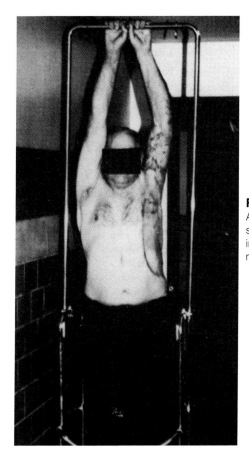

Figure 26-2
A patient using a wheeled walker to stretch axillary contracture while walking. (From Rivers and Fisher.[2] By permission of the publisher.)

Orthotics

Orthotics, a form of positioning, never replaces range-of-motion exercises. However, when antigravity positioning is unsuccessful, an orthosis is fitted. For the comatose or resistive patient, orthotics may protect the healing wound. A resting wrist, hand, finger, and thumb orthosis is often used to immobilize the hand for skin grafting (Fig. 26-4). At this time, finger interphalangeal extension is used rather than the "functional" position. In many instances, orthotics may replace skeletal suspension for postoperative immobilization. A hand continuous passive motion machine may be helpful to decrease swelling. When tendons are exposed, a protective orthosis is fitted to minimize joint movement. Finger extension troughs, secured with a pressure-distributing bandage, protect the proximal interphalangeal joints or dorsal hoods when these structures are exposed. A microstomia correction orthosis may be judiciously used for exercise and for positioning when circumoral burns are present. A foam ankle-foot orthosis

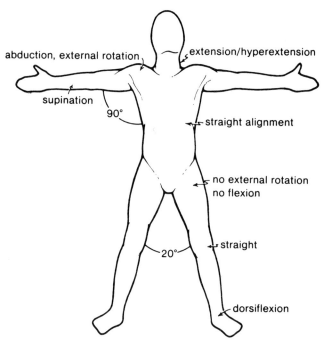

Figure 26–3

A guideline for anticontracture positioning. Patient is lying supine and shown from a ventral view. (From Helm et al.[4] By permission of the American Congress of Rehabilitation Medicine and the American Academy of Physical Medicine and Rehabilitation.)

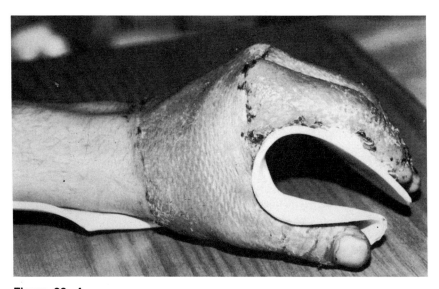

Figure 26–4

Resting orthosis for patients with wrist-hand burn. Ideally, wrist is extended 20°, metacarpophalangeal joints are at 60°, interphalangeal joints are in extension, thumb spacing is wide.

positions the ankle in neutral position more effectively than a foot board. A soft sandal orthosis will decrease pain during walking and helps protect the sole of the burned foot.

Pain Management

Timed, non-pain-contingent administration of drugs and long-acting pain medications maintain relative comfort without painful "valleys" followed by lethargic immobile "peaks." The myth of new narcotic addiction of burn patients needs to be dispelled; for successful rehabilitation, the patient must have relative comfort during the initial phase of therapy. Nearly all medications, including narcotics, are very rapidly metabolized in the seriously burned patient. Therefore, the narcotics given may seem excessive and frighten the novice caregiver.

The rehabilitation team teaches the patient and family behavioral interventions such as hypnosis, visualization, and relaxation procedures to enhance the effects of pain medication. A trauma group, led by a trained professional, decreases stress and improves patient confidence, self-esteem, and comfort. Other interventions to decrease pain include self-controlled exercises such as reciprocal pulleys or the stationary bicycle, cutaneous stimulation, or distraction during exercise.

MATURATION PHASE OF REHABILITATION CARE

The rehabilitation goals during the maturation phase of wound healing include return of normal strength, endurance, dexterity, and coordination; controlling edema; regaining full active range-of-joint motion; fitting total contact, stretching orthotics as needed; minimizing hypertrophic scar formation; achieving independent living skills; knowing compensation techniques for exposure to friction or trauma, ultraviolet light, chemical irritants, and extremes of weather or temperature; awareness of sensory changes, especially in the case of denervation; return to recreation and, as tolerated, full-time school or vocational duties; psychologic adjustment to disability; and initiating discussion of changed body image and related sexuality.

Exercise

Full, active range of motion returns most quickly when minimal inflammatory processes occur (typically when grafts can be applied to dermal remnants) and when the patient continues hourly elevated active motion during waking hours. The secondary benefit of exercise is to speed healing by improving circulation, decreasing edema, and decreasing inflammatory response. The therapist, as coach, provides many choices and written graded programs, which in specific assigned activities can document improvement. Therapists help the patient collaborate with rigorous therapy by breaking projects or exercise into components small enough to ensure success. Active motion and gentle terminal stretch are continued despite open tendons, except for the dorsal hood mechanism over the proximal interphalangeal joint.

The eyelids, mouth, neck, axilla, elbow, wrist, thumb, ankle, and hip are particularly vulnerable to contracture and may require a more intensive exercise program. Each patient can learn to do his or her own terminal stretch with the contralateral hand or with environmental surfaces, for example, stretching the heel cord by pushing off the wall with the heels flat on the floor. The entire length of the scar band must be elongated by combined prolonged stretching of the joints involved. The stretching progresses daily as the patient's tolerance increases. For the severely burned patient, during the first 6 months after healing, rehabilitation is complicated by scar bands that extend over several joints, maximal scar resistance, epithelial and scar sensitivity, and the weakness of the patient. An orthosis that immobilizes one joint at its maximal stretch may be needed. For instance, if a scar extends from the thumb and across the wrist and elbow to the shoulder, a thumb and elbow extension orthosis improves the force angle for prolonged forward flexion or abduction of the shoulder.

Manual resistive exercise, progressive or regressive resistive exercises, Cybex, BTE, bicycle riding, and other therapies done daily help the patient regain strength and endurance. Objectively documented improvement encourages maximal participation of the patient.

Positioning

During rest periods and sleep, the patient benefits from anticontracture positioning. For the motivated patient, the gains in motion during exercise can be maintained with positioning. Antigravity positioning assists venous return, helps prevent blisters, and reduces edema.

Orthotics

Individualized, custom-made orthoses enhance positioning, allow painless maintenance of exercise gains, block undesirable motion, and encourage active motion away from a contracture. Custom-made orthoses assist in minimizing hypertrophic scars by flattening the hypertrophic tissue against the underlying body structures. An example of this type is a clear-plastic face orthosis that has been successful in the preservation of facial contours and management of hypertrophic scarring. Serial dropout casts have the advantage of softening the scar and preventing slippage of the orthosis and removal by the patient. Use of orthoses never replaces exercise. Orthoses should meet specific criteria for each area involved.[6]

Management of Hypertrophic Scar

A hypertrophic scar is a hard, red, collagenous bundle of connective tissue raised above the surface of the burn wound. Myofibroblasts remain active in this hyperemic, dynamically remodeling wound 24 hours a day until some currently unknown factor causes their regression, from 12 to 24 months after wound closure.

One hypothesis is that external vascular support garments decrease nourishment and oxygen supply to the scar, which then matures more rapidly, but this is undocumented. External vascular support is initiated with an elastic bandage wrapped in a figure-of-eight pattern. As skin becomes more durable, soft elastic cloth such as Tubigrip or Isotoner products can be donned without damage. If needed, patients may be treated with more expensive, custom-fitted elastic garments. The burn team must remain alert to delayed growth in children wearing elastic pressure garments for a long period. When scars occur in concave areas, additional inserts must be custom-fitted under the elastic garment.

Pain Management

Neuropathies and sensory abnormalities are common complications in the burn patient. Patients who are severely burned and maintained for long periods on parenteral hyperalimentation also tend to have severe peripheral neuropathy and pain. If the dysesthesias and pain complaints are misinterpreted by the staff as manipulative behavior at about the same time that the use of pain medications is being tapered, cooperation with therapy is undermined. Briefly maintaining the use of narcotics in combination with desensitization techniques will undoubtedly reduce the problem. Most neuropathies resolve slowly. However, in addition to compensation techniques for sensory changes and desensitization, individual counseling and reassurance are helpful.

Itching is a form of pain. As wound healing progresses, alternating oral antihistamine medications every 2 hours may be necessary to prevent scratching. Itchy scales, crusts, and soap residue are avoided by meticulous hygiene with plain water. Hot water is contraindicated because swelling and sweating increase pruritus. Dry tissue is moisturized with an unscented lotion. Massage or tapping is encouraged, and excoriation is discouraged. The use of moisturizing agents is continued even if the rubber in compression garments deteriorates as a result. Use of a vibrator, transcutaneous electrical nerve stimulation unit, or cool pack may relieve itching for several hours. Discomfort from sweating is reduced by air conditioning.

Psychosocial Management

Because more than half of the patients who suffer major burns have severe emotional consequences, psychologic management must be initiated at the outset. The goals of management include helping the patient and family to diminish stress and pain by regaining self-control and greater participation in the rehabilitation process. Favorable outcomes have been shown with counseling that addresses adjustment to disfigurement and management of posttraumatic stress syndrome. Peer groups often provide easily accepted support for return to work. Moreover, these groups share

TABLE 26-2
Vocational Alternatives for Burn Victims, in Order of Escalating Cost

	Job	Employer
Return to work	Same	Same
Return to work	Same (modified)	Same
Return to work	Different	Same
Return to work	Different	Different
Return to work	Different	Different
Return to work*	Different	Self-employment
No return to work*	Financial support from Social Security Disability Income or welfare assistance	

*After extensive, prolonged training or education.

tried and tested tips for easing social embarrassment or interventions for posttraumatic stress symptoms and for adapting the workplace or living quarters if needed.

Vocational Management

The goal is to return the patient to work as soon as possible to the previous job and preferably with the same employer. If needed, a comprehensive individualized vocational rehabilitation plan, including vocational evaluation, work adjustment training, job placement, and sometimes employer development or education, should be formulated shortly after dismissal from the hospital. Table 26-2 lists vocational alternatives in order of escalating cost.

REFERENCES

1. Helm PA, Fisher SV. Rehabilitation of the patient with burns. In: DeLisa JA, ed. Rehabilitation medicine: principles and practice. Philadelphia: JB Lippincott, 1988:821–839.
2. Rivers EA, Fisher SV. Rehabilitation for burn patients. In: Kottke FJ, Lehmann JF, eds. Krusen's handbook of physical medicine and rehabilitation. 4th ed. Philadelphia: WB Saunders, 1990:1070–1101.
3. Covey MH, issue ed. Burn trauma. In: Campbell MK, journal ed. Topics in acute care and trauma rehabilitation. Vol 1 no. 4. Frederick, MD, Aspen, 1987.
4. Helm PA, Kevorkian CG, Lushbaugh M, Pullium G, Head MD, Cromes GF. Burn injury: rehabilitation management in 1982. Arch Phys Med Rehabil 1982; 63:6–16.
5. Johnson CL, O'Shaughnessy EJ, Ostergren G. Burn management. New York: Raven Press, 1981.
6. Fisher SV, Helm PA, eds. Comprehensive rehabilitation of burns. Baltimore: Williams & Wilkins, 1984.

27 | Lymphedema

G. Keith Stillwell

Lymphedema occurs because of obstruction or insufficiency of the lymphatic system.[1] It may be congenital or familial, but in most cases it is acquired. The principal function of the lymphatic system is to return water and proteins from the tissue fluid space to the bloodstream. If the capacity of the system is inadequate for the load of lymph being produced, edema results.

PRODUCTION OF LYMPH

Lymph is derived from tissue fluid, although it is believed to differ from it after being in the lymphatics for a time. The Starling hypothesis dealt with factors believed to affect the transudation of water across the blood capillary membrane. This filtration mechanism is responsible for the production of the major part of the interstitial fluid. The production of water as a by-product of metabolic activity would not be a significant factor in the creation of the lymph load.

Increases in the intracapillary hydrostatic pressure, which result from arteriolar dilatation (for example, with local heating, muscular activity, or high environmental temperatures) or from venous obstruction (for example, congestive heart failure or constricting garments), will lead to the passage of more water from the blood to the tissue fluid. A decrease in the tissue fluid hydrostatic pressure is presumed also to encourage the passage of water out of the capillaries, and an increase will resist this. There is controversy over the measurement of this pressure. It may be close to atmospheric, although the embedded perforated capsule method of Guyton et al.[2] yields a value of -7 mm Hg. The presence of edema does stretch and presumably disrupt the fine structure of the tissues so that they become more compliant, less elastic, and less resistant to repetition of the accumulation of fluid.

The osmotic pressure exerted by the plasma proteins resists the passage of water out of the capillaries. Reduction of it tends to cause edema (for example, in hepatic or renal diseases or starvation). Of more frequent importance is an increase in the osmotic pressure from accumulating proteins in the edema fluid. These proteins hold the water in the tissue space. They are, for the most part, plasma proteins. A small proportion of them may normally return to the bloodstream by the capillaries, but the major portion is returned to the blood by way of the lymphatics.[1] Other macromolecular materials present secondary to trauma or inflammation also exert an oncotic pressure. Removal of the proteins, as well as the water, is important for the treatment of lymphedema.

REMOVAL OF LYMPH

Lymph flow from the extremities seems mainly to be caused by active vasomotion of the lymphatics.[3] The action of their smooth muscle in conjunction with their valves is a strong pumping mechanism by which the tissue spaces are normally kept cleared of mobile or "free" fluid and of the proteins. Subsidiary mechanisms, such as the skeletal "muscle pump," the "thoracic pump" (aspiration of lymph into the thorax, especially during respiratory inspiration), the pulsation of blood vessels adjacent to the lymphatics, and the force of gravity, probably are minor factors normally but become more important when the normal lymphatic mechanism is inoperative.

POSTSURGICAL LYMPHEDEMA

After surgical ablation of axillary or inguinal lymph nodes, there is a considerable incidence of lymphedema. The exact frequency with which it occurs is unknown, although it is expected to be less after a modified radical mastectomy than after the standard Halsted radical mastectomy (after which it occurs in about 30% to 50% of cases). Olszewski[4] demonstrated that dogs had a transitory lymphedema for 4 to 6 weeks after the surgical procedure followed by a latent period lasting months to years before the clinical appearance of chronic edema. During the latent period, that part of the lymphatic system that is obstructed progressively deteriorates. This deterioration includes fibrosis with loss of permeability and lymph-concentrating ability, development of tortuosities and varicosities with incompetence of the valves, and increased compliance of the vessels. Clodius[5] cited the experience in Gottingen where, of 1,155 patients who underwent radical mastectomy, lymphedema subsequently developed in 387. This occurred within the first 10 months postoperatively in 68%, but the onset was delayed more than 3 years postoperatively in 22%.

The deterioration of the impeded lymphatic system proceeds insidiously whether or not the patient has edema. Patients should take reasonable precautions to avoid further damage to their lymphatics from trauma or infections and to avoid overloading the system beyond its limited capacity to remove lymph from the limb, such as by local heating or prolonged active use of the limb, especially in a hot environment.

Other types of lymphedema can be appropriately treated along the same lines as postsurgical lymphedema. With long-standing lymphedema, a hyperplasia of the superficial fascia develops that may prove irreversible. Restoration to normal dimensions will not be possible with nonsurgical treatment. However, the presence of "pitting" indicates movable fluid and offers some hope that the edema can be reduced by physical measures.

The following measures should be of help in the prevention and reduction of edema in the upper extremity after mastectomy:

1. Avoidance of dependent positioning as much as possible
2. Elevation of the arm above the level of the heart during rest as much as possible, but not with the shoulder widely abducted
3. Isometric contraction of the upper extremity muscles with the arm elevated
4. Avoidance of excessive use of the limb, particularly in a warm environment
5. Avoidance of injury to the limb, particularly puncture wounds
6. Decongestive milking massage to decrease edema (infection must be eliminated before this)
7. Use of a pneumatic pumping device
8. Use of elasticized bandaging (to inhibit redevelopment of the swelling between treatments while the edema is being diminished) and of custom-made elastic sleeve to maintain improvement after the condition has stabilized

TREATMENT OF LYMPHEDEMA

Dietary restriction of sodium intake and the use of diuretics are generally of little help in the treatment of chronic lymphedema because removal of the excess protein from the tissue fluid is paramount. Similarly, the routine use of antibiotics is not indicated; however, in patients with evidence of infection in the edematous limb, it is important to control the infection before embarking on vigorous attempts to move the fluid.

Measures to Move the Edema Fluid

When the highly effective normal lymphatic vasomotion pump is rendered inoperative, other methods of moving lymph offer hope of improving the edema. If the fluid cannot be moved through major lymphatic vessels, it can still be moved through the tissues and through the microvascular subdermal lymphatic plexus, which is continuous throughout the body. These methods include most of the time-honored ways to which normal lymph flow was attributed, based on experiments in anesthetized animals. Of course, lymphatics other than those obstructed may drain the limb.

Elevation

Water runs downhill, as does lymph, albeit slowly. The elevated limb need not be vertical. Each period of elevation should be for a half hour or more. Patients are urged to elevate the limb for as much of the night as is compatible with sleep.

Massage

Various pneumatically operated compression devices are available, and all are probably effective. In a study comparing three different devices to the use of no device at all, no significant differences were found, but the patients did have somewhat more improvement with the use of a device.[6] The pneumatic device is usually applied with a pressure of 50 to 70 mm Hg for 45 to 60 minutes at each session.

Manual massage may be helpful for mobilizing pockets of fluid that have been less responsive to the pneumatic device. Questions have been raised about the possibility of damage to the delicate lymphatic terminals, but the significance of this is not established.[7] Massage of an upper extremity usually consumes 10 minutes.

Exercise

Contractions of the skeletal muscles may promote venous and lymphatic flow. When the patient is wearing elastic support, the exercises will also compress the subcutaneous tissues between the muscles and the elastic support. The contractions are performed isometrically or with minimal joint motion, although joint motion is not forbidden. Patients with flaccid paralyses who are unable to perform such exercises have generally not responded as well to the other components of the treatment program.

Measures to Inhibit Accumulation of New Fluid

Because of the increased compliance of the lymphedematous tissue and the skin, there is little natural resistance to recurrence of the swelling. Application of external elastic support is essential if progress is to be made in overcoming the edema. A woven elasticized bandage is preferable for the first few weeks, while the size of the limb is decreasing. Subsequently, the improvement is maintained by the use of an elasticized sleeve or stocking. The bandage should be applied in the morning before arising; it is not worn at night. The bandage must be removed and reapplied about every 2 hours because it does not stay in place indefinitely, particularly around the knee or elbow.

The law of Laplace relates the pressure (P) across the wall of a container, the tension (T) in the wall, and the radius (R) of curvature of the wall, stating that:

$$P = \frac{T}{R}$$

To maintain any given transmural pressure if R is larger, T must be larger too. In the case of the swollen limb, the implication is that it will take less tension in the elastic support (or the skin) to maintain the size of the limb if it can first be made smaller.[8]

RESULTS OF PHYSICAL TREATMENT

Patients with upper extremity lymphedema can generally be treated as outpatients, but it is often preferable that patients with lower extremity lymphedema be hospitalized for more adequate elevation. Treatment, usually applied twice daily, consists of the pneumatic pump, manual massage, and isometric exercise (all used while the limb is elevated) and instruction in the application of the bandage.

After about 4 days of such treatment, a reduction of about 30% of the edema by volume measurement will have been attained in patients with upper extremity lymphedema.[6] The patient then pursues a home program with elevation of the limb for 30 or more minutes every 2 hours, during which time 5 to 10 repetitions of the exercises are done every 5 minutes. At the end of this period of elevation, the bandage is completely removed and then reapplied. After 1 or 2 weeks at home, the interval is lengthened to 3 hours and then 4 hours. The impression is that patients with upper extremity lymphedema obtain a further reduction of about 30% of the edema during 4 to 6 weeks of the home program. They are then fitted with a sleeve.

Because of technical difficulties with measurement of the volume of the lower extremity, there are no comparable data, but the clinical impression is that somewhat less improvement is obtained in the lower extremity. Data on long-term results are spotty, but they suggest that most patients maintain the improvement, a few improve more, and a few have worsening.

CONTINUATION OF EXTERNAL ELASTIC SUPPORT

After the edema has been well controlled for about 3 months, experimenting with removal of the external elastic support is reasonable. By then, the tissue spaces formerly occupied by the edema should have shrunk and the tissues should have regained some of their elasticity. The patient should remove the support 1 hour before going to bed at night. The circumferences of the limb at a few places are measured then and at bedtime. If there is no apparent increase in the size of the limb, the process is repeated an hour earlier each day. In this way, the patient determines how long it is possible to go without the support without having a recurrence of the edema. Most patients with postmastectomy lymph edema can be without support for 4 to 6 hours but cannot abandon the support altogether.

Patients who no longer have an underlying cause for edema usually can be without support.

REFERENCES

1. Földi M. Physiology and pathophysiology of lymph flow. In: Clodius L, ed. Lymphedema. Stuttgart: Georg Thieme Verlag, 1977:1–11.
2. Guyton AC, Granger HJ, Taylor AE. Interstitial fluid pressure. Physiol Rev 1971; 51:527–563.
3. Olszewski WL, Engeset A. Intrinsic contractility of prenodal lymph vessels and lymph flow in human leg. Am J Physiol 1980; 239:H775–783.
4. Olszewski WL. Pathophysiological and clinical observations of obstructive lymphedema of the limbs. In: Clodius L, ed. Lymphedema. Stuttgart: Georg Thieme Verlag, 1977:79–102.
5. Clodius L. Secondary arm lymphedema. In: Clodius L, ed. Lymphedema. Stuttgart: Georg Thieme Verlag, 1977:147–174.
6. Tinkham RG, Stillwell GK. The role of pneumatic pumping devices in the treatment of postmastectomy lymphedema. Arch Phys Med Rehabil 1965; 46:193–197.
7. Casley-Smith JR. The structural basis for the conservative treatment of lymphedema. In: Clodius L, ed. Lymphedema. Stuttgart: Georg Thieme Verlag, 1977:13–25.
8. Stillwell GK. The Law of Laplace: some clinical applications. Mayo Clin Proc 1973; 48:863–869.

28

Athletic Rehabilitation

Edward R. Laskowski

Participation in sporting events of all kinds is reaching record numbers. The "fitness craze" is truly a reality; increasing numbers of all age groups are undertaking activities that will contribute to lifelong aerobic health. A 1984 public health survey suggested that 55% of the population of the United States performs some form of exercise activity at least three times per week. It is estimated that more than 25 million Americans jog or run, and participants in recent marathons have ranged in age from 5 to 84 years. The incredible diversity of sports attracts people from many cultures and people with wide-ranging physical capabilities.

The specialty of physical medicine and rehabilitation is uniquely suited to rehabilitation of the injured athlete. The physiatrist has the skills necessary to evaluate and diagnose acute and subacute injury, refer the patient for surgical intervention if appropriate, and coordinate, plan, and follow the rehabilitation program. Many groups that the physiatrist interacts with on a daily basis may be involved, including physical or occupational therapy and psychology. Successful rehabilitation depends not only on successful diagnosis and initial treatment but also on continued rehabilitation to achieve maximal function of the affected area. Education regarding appropriate sport and disability-specific conditioning, training, and preventive measures is crucial if further injury is to be avoided and new injuries prevented. In addition, the psychological impact of injury on the athlete is an important element of comprehensive rehabilitation.

The field of sports rehabilitation is broad in nature, but there are basic principles, methods, and techniques that apply to a wide variety of situations. This discussion focuses primarily on the musculoskeletal system.

ASSESSMENT OF INJURY

The initial injury can usually be divided into two broad categories: (1) acute and (2) subacute (chronic). The acute injury is often related to a recent breach of integrity of the musculoskeletal system, such as a tibial fracture or an acute disruption of the anterior cruciate ligament. The range of severity can be exceedingly broad, ranging from a mild inversion ankle sprain to an acute injury of the spinal cord that could result in quadriplegia. For this reason, the diagnostic acumen of the evaluator must be concurrently wide ranging. The evaluator must be aware of the signs and symptoms of neurologic compromise. In football, for example, the examining physician must be familiar with return-to-play criteria after head injury with or without loss of consciousness. Equally important is knowledge of the indications for and use of spinal stabilization and transport techniques to prevent spinal cord compromise. Indications for surgical referral also must be appropriate, and guidelines regarding stable and unstable fractures should be followed. It is also essential to consider the age of the patient when evaluating an injury. For example, a high school football player with vague left-sided abdominal pain after a tackle and a history of preceding viral illness should be thoroughly evaluated for mononucleosis. Likewise, older athletes should be evaluated in the context of concurrent medical problems, such as cardiac disease, respiratory compromise, or severe degenerative changes.

The subacute, or chronic, injury can often be thought of as repetitive or "overuse" damage to the muscular system. Examples are the repetitive microtrauma incurred to the forearm extensor muscle mass and tendon group in "tennis elbow" and the stress that the tibia sustains in "shin splints." Treatment of these injuries often does not involve surgical intervention but does involve the principle of "relative rest," in which the injured body part is protected from further trauma and then gradually rehabilitated to normal function while aerobic fitness is maintained. Education plays an important role in the prevention of overuse injuries, and the athlete must understand and use appropriate biomechanics during performance of the activity. Orthotic intervention may be helpful, especially in the lower extremities, where malalignment and foot overpronation can contribute to increased medial tibial stress. Bracing or splints can also be used to rest and protect the damaged body part.

TREATMENT

The initial treatment of an acute sports injury should limit the extent of initial injury as much as possible to aid healing and provide for early institution of rehabilitation measures. The mainstay of early (24 to 48 hours from time of injury) treatment at the Mayo Clinic follows the principles of PRICE (protection, "relative" rest, ice, compression, and elevation). The injured body part should be protected from further trauma by a brace, cast, or limited weight-bearing status. This protection may entail instructing the patient on the appropirate use of crutches or a cane. The injury should be rested initially, with no movement beyond a pain-free range. As mentioned previously, however, general aerobic conditioning should not be neglected, and alternative means of maintaining aerobic fitness should be used. Ice has been shown to be efficacious for both reducing pain and decreasing swelling through local vasoconstriction. Ice packs can safely be applied for 20 minutes out of every hour. If the injury is focal, ice massage to the area may be a particularly effective intervention and one that is easily applied. Compression around the injured area also helps to limit the area of swelling. If compression is initially instituted with Ace wraps, rewrapping should be performed every 4 hours to ensure appropriate compression. Alternative means of compression include elastic fabric, which can be customized to fit the injured body part, and neoprene sleeves. Compression and cold can be applied in combination with an intermittent pneumatic compression pump (Fig. 28-1). Elevation assists venous and lymphatic returns; the injured extremity should be raised higher than heart level to facilitate venous return. In addition to ice, other early measures to reduce pain may include the use of nonsteroidal anti-inflammatory medications (NSAIDs), transcutaneous electrical nerve stimulation, interferential current, and ice-water-slurry whirlpool treatments.

Early treatment of the overuse injury proceeds slightly differently from that of acute musculoskeletal injury. Because significant swelling is usually not a prominent component, there may be no need for compression garments or elevation. Protection and ice, however, remain essential components. The activity that contributed to the microtrauma must be avoided or at least modified to a great degree, especially with respect to frequency. As stated previously, education regarding appropriate biomechanics and kinesiology is essential. Ice may still be an effective method of pain relief, but

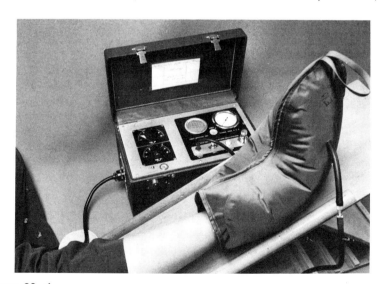

Figure 28-1
Intermittent-pulse pneumatic compression pump (Jobst Institute, Inc., Toledo, Ohio). (From Scott SG. Current concepts in the rehabilitation of the injured athlete. Mayo Clin Proc 1984; 59:83–90. By permission of Mayo Foundation.)

heat may be especially beneficial. Delivery can take the form of radiant heat (heat lamp), moist heat (hot packs), or deeper heat at the bone-tendon interface (ultrasound). Heat provides vasodilatation and pain-relieving properties and can help to reduce muscle tightness. Heat can be used in combination with gentle prolonged stretching to increase range of motion by promoting collagen extensibility[1] (Fig. 28–2). General and muscle-specific relaxation and stretching techniques may be helpful to diminish muscle tightness and enhance whole body relaxation. Massage techniques can also be beneficial adjuncts. Biofeedback is effective for "reeducating" the patient regarding what it feels like to achieve and maintain relaxation in a particular muscle, and it can be helpful in cases of muscle spasm refractory to other treatments. In addition, biofeedback (at times preceded by electrical stimulation) can be effective for enhancing neuromuscular function and activation. For example, the quadriceps (in particular the vestus medialis) can be inhibited up to 60% by even a very small (20 mL) knee effusion.[2] This inhibition can result in a deactivation of the neuromuscular pathway, and the athlete may find it difficult to produce a voluntary quadriceps contraction. Electrical stimulation can help the athlete regain kinesthetic awareness of the particular muscle group, and biofeedback can ver-

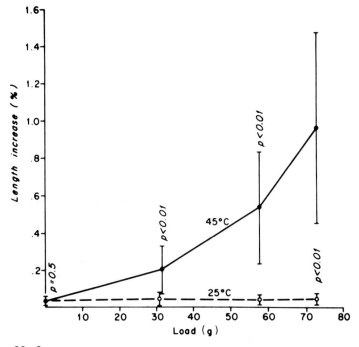

Figure 28–2
Percentage increase in tendon length as function of load in grams at 45° C and at 25° C. (From Lehmann JF, Masock AJ, Warren CG, Koblanski JN. Effect of therapeutic temperatures on tendon extensibility. Arch Phys Med Rehabil 1970; 51:481–487. By permission of the American Congress of Rehabilitation Medicine and the American Academy of Physical Medicine and Rehabilitation.)

ify voluntary activation and be an effective learning tool to enhance selective muscle use.

REHABILITATION

Rehabilitation of an athletic injury should follow in a stepwise progression. The main components are (1) maximization of range of motion, (2) strengthening, and (3) agility, proprioception, and sport-specific exercises. Throughout this progression, maintenance of aerobic conditioning should be emphasized. Fitness exercise can continue through use of the upper extremity (for example, use of an upper extremity ergometer; Fig. 28–3) if the lower extremities are impaired and vice versa. Exercise of the contralateral limb can be continued through the use of devices such as resistance bicycles, which provide for both upper extremity and lower extremity movement for bi- or tri-limb work (Fig. 28–4). "Wet-vest running," which is running in deep water with a buoyant vest to keep the head above water, is an effective method of non-weight-bearing training. The resistance of the water contributes to both lower-limb strengthening and aerobic fitness. Similar benefits can be achieved by walking in shallow water or using a water treadmill. Many athletes forgo aerobic conditioning in favor of focusing on the injured limb; this practice is detrimental, however, because aerobic capacity ($\dot{V}O_2$ max) tends to drop significantly with cessation of exercise, and changes can become evident after only 2 weeks. If training is not continued, the improvements gained tend to be lost rapidly.

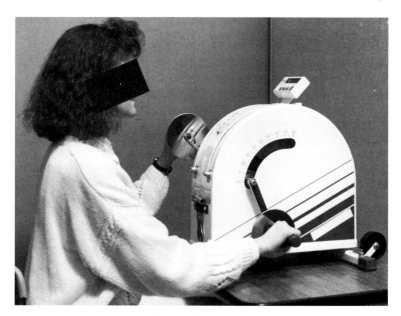

Figure 28–3
Upper arm ergometer.

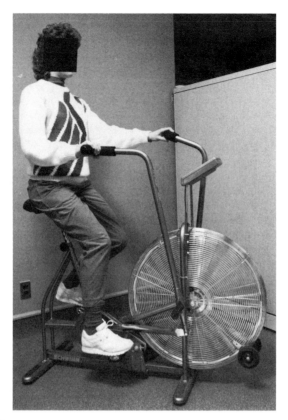

Figure 28–4
Resistance bicycle (Air-Dyne), which enables exercise of both upper and lower extremity muscles.

Aerobic capacity can decrease by 50% after 4 to 12 weeks without training.[3]

Control of pain should be emphasized throughout rehabilitation. This can be accomplished with the previously mentioned modalities and the appropriate, short-term use of medications such as acetaminophen and NSAIDs. Movements should be pain-limited at first, and progression through stages should not occur unless exercises can be performed without pain. Every attempt should be made to eliminate muscle cocontraction and guarding, which interfere with biomechanically correct muscle movements.

RANGE OF MOTION

Early range of motion is essential in rehabilitation of both nonsurgical and surgical athletic injuries. Depending on the injury, range of motion may need to be protected, passive, or limited in the initial stages, but it should progress to full joint range. As stated above, any contribution to limitation of range by pain should be minimized. Joint motion also provides nutrition to articular cartilage and proprioceptive joint and muscle feedback, and it prevents the formation of soft tissue contractures. Gentle terminal stretching may be necessary, especially after superficial heat or ultrasound treatments, to achieve full range. Stretching provides stress to collagen fibers and increases tensile strength by enhancing longitudinal, linear organization during healing.[4] Without stress, fibers tend to arrange in a chaotic fashion. Early postsurgical passive range of motion can be provided by continuous passive motion machines, which are now available for small joints such as the wrist.

STRENGTHENING

After full, pain-free motion is achieved, strengthening can begin. In actuality, the earliest phase (first 2 weeks) of strengthening is enhanced synchronization and recruitment of motor units.[5] Muscle fiber hypertrophy does not occur until after 2 to 4 weeks of strengthening exercises.[6] Nonetheless, the more efficient use of the muscle provided by strengthening exercises will have early functional and performance implications. Various types of strengthening techniques include isometric, isotonic, isokinetic, isodynamic, and plyometric exercise.

Isometric exercise, or muscle contraction while the involved joint is static, can be helpful early in rehabilitation. It entails maximal force exerted against a relatively immovable object, with no appreciable change in muscle length. This technique protects the joint from undue stress and creates less of an inflammatory response within the joint than isotonic exercise. Isometric strength does not transfer, however, to dynamic movements, and the strengthening that takes place is limited to the angle and position in which the exercise is performed. These exercises can prepare the muscle for more formidable strengthening through the lifting of weights or the use of body weight for exercise (squats, push-ups). In addition, isometric exercise can help to limit atrophy during a period of prolonged immobilization.

Isotonic exercise is dynamic in nature, and it occurs when the muscle contraction itself is used to move a load throughout a range of motion. At first, the load may be no more than the weight of the limb. Later, progressive resistance exercises are begun, with progression from light resistance and more repetitions to heavy resistance and fewer repetitions. Isotonic exercise can further be divided into concentric and eccentric contractions. Concentric contractions entail the loading of muscle while shortening, whereas eccentric contractions load the muscle while lengthening. An example of a concentric contraction is a biceps curl, and an eccentric contraction occurs in the quadriceps while running downhill or while letting a weight down slowly. Eccentric contractions are highly efficient and forceful, but they can also cause the greatest amount of post-exercise muscle soreness. Thus, they should be reserved for a later stage in the rehabilitation program after a sufficient foundation of muscle strength has been built.

Isokinetic exercise consists of exercising at a predetermined constant velocity of joint motion. Isokinetic strength is the maximal torque that can be developed at any given velocity of contraction.[7] This type of exercise is valuable in that it can provide objective information regarding peak muscle torque, power, and endurance at reproducible velocities. Side-to-side comparison with an uninjured limb can provide data for research comparisons and in some instances can help to gauge progression through rehabilitation and ability to return to a sport after injury. Ideally, the injured limb should be as close to 100% of the strength of the contralateral limb as possible before return to play is considered. Even if this is achieved, the athlete still must regain agility, coordination, and sport-specific skills before return to competition. Velocities achievable with isokinetic equipment can be higher than those with traditional weight-training equipment but still are much slower than certain sports movements (such as throwing).

Isodynamic exercise usually entails use of a progressive resistance band (i.e., Theraband), which is used to provide gradually increasing resistance when stretched and can be used in multiple planes. This can be used to simulate functional and sport-specific activities such as the throwing motion of a baseball pitcher. This type of functional exercise is increasingly favored over isolated exercise for both upper and lower extremities because it uses the muscles in more of the complex and diagonal/spiral movement planes that a particular sport will require. For the upper extremities in particular, manual resistance strengthening is a variation on isodynamic strengthening and a way of providing carefully gradated resistance in multiple dynamic movement planes. The therapist can adjust the applied resistance according to the patient's pain and range of motion/strength limitations.

Plyometric exercise is a later-stage exercise that emphasizes speed and power. The exercises consist of concentric muscle contractions after a prior stretch of the same muscle groups. In theory, this will help provide neuromuscular facilitation, release neural inhibition, and enable stronger and more forceful muscle contractions. An example of higher-level plyometrics is jumping rapidly on and off different-sized boxes, or jumping back and forth over a low object. These exercises should be performed on an appropriate surface (i.e., grass rather than concrete) with careful supervision and with an adequate foundation of strength in the muscle groups utilized. Nevertheless, they are an important component in developing the speed and explosiveness necessary for many sports, and low-level plyometrics (i.e., skipping, hopscotch variations) can be safely performed by most individuals.

Of increasing interest recently has been the use of "closed kinetic chain" exercises. First conceptualized by Steindler,[8] they can be thought of as exercises in which the distal extremity remains fixed and multiple proximal joints move in a functional manner, with contraction of both agonists and antagonists for stabilization. Examples of such exercise are squats for the lower extremities and push-ups for the upper extremities. These movements entail triarticular motion of either the upper or the lower extremities as opposed to movement around a single joint, which occurs with "open kinetic chain" exercises (that is, isolated leg extension). In many ways, closed kinetic chain exercises are more "function based" and sports specific for the lower extremities than exercises that isolate one specific muscle group. For example, performing squats entails cocontraction and utilization of both quadriceps and hamstrings in a functional manner and in a manner in which they are used in many sports and in life in general (i.e., getting up from a chair). They also provide a great degree of joint and ligament safety if properly performed, and they are one of the prime exercises in rehabilitation of the anterior cruciate ligament.[9] For the upper extremities, open chain exercises are used to a large extent because this is the manner in which the limb is used in most sports (i.e., the throwing motion).

When considering each of the above strengthening exercises, it is important to remember the concepts of muscle balance and the kinetic chain. With respect to muscle balance, agonist and antagonist muscle groups should be exercised equally. As an example many athletes focus on the anterior muscles of the shoulder, such as the pectorals, anterior deltoid, and biceps, but neglect the posterior muscles and scapular stabilizers (trapezius, rhomboids, serratus anterior, and latissimus dorsi). This resulting imbalance can contribute to injury and can contribute to suboptimal performance.

In addition, the biomechanics and kinesiology of a sport and movement must be considered in the context of the entire kinetic chain, and joints and muscle groups both proximal and distal to the area of injury should be evaluated. For example, Whiting et al.[10] showed that elite water polo players throw with one-half the velocity in water as on land. Thus, one can see the importance of the lower extremities and spine in converting ground reaction force to the kinetic energy of a throw. If one looks at only the shoulder, a significant problem with the spine or a lower-extremity flexibility problem may be overlooked. The shoulder may be the "weak link" in a suboptimal biomechanical movement chain, and rehabilitation must address and maximize all elements of the chain.

AGILITY, PROPRIOCEPTION, AND COORDINATION

Once strength has been maximized, or in tandem with strength training, the athlete must work to regain optimal agility and coordination. With many injuries, the muscle, tendon, or ligament and the joint are "detuned" and the proprioceptive feedback that the muscle or joint capsule normally provides is disrupted. Mechanoreceptors, muscle spindles, and Golgi tendon organs may be involved to various degrees. Examples of exercises that help regain this function include "wobble board" exercises, which help to maximize balance and refine coordinating movements of lower extremity muscles. The ankle group muscles "relearn" and are "retrained" to make minute postural adjustments, which are required to stay balanced and upright on the board. Knee proprioception may be better maximized with both standing and supine exercises involving a pediatric ball and "knee-specific" movements. If lower extremity ambulation has been hindered by the injury, therapy will need to focus on higher-order gait activities, including carioca or braid walking, and balance activities specific to the athlete's sport. As an example, a halfback in football may practice timed runs through tires or a rope/maze course.

Many of these exercises should be "sport-specific," that is, they should simulate movements and activities the athlete will perform upon a return to competition. The athlete may have followed a comprehensive and thorough program of exercise to this point, but rehabilitation is incomplete unless exercises specific to both the sport and the athlete's position in the sport can be performed maximally and without pain or loss of function. These exercises, too, must be "reprogrammed," and general exercise alone will not suffice. The ultimate goal is for the athlete to be at both maximal strength and agility to prevent recurrence of injury and maximize performance.

SPORTS FOR THE PHYSICALLY CHALLENGED

Sports for the physically challenged is an area that is experiencing profound growth, both in participation and in adaptive equipment technology. The rehabilitation professional is uniquely suited to serve the needs of the disabled athlete and, thus, should have general knowledge of the many sports and recreation opportunities available to them. National Handicapped Sports, based in Washington, D.C., currently has more than 60 chapters and annually serves nearly 30,000 people who have a wide variety of disabilities. Advances in adaptive sporting equipment and technique have enabled many types of physically disabled individuals to participate in virtually every summer and winter sport, including snow skiing.

The level of competition in physically challenged events has increased to the point that wheelchair road racers routinely finish ahead of able-bodied runners in the Boston Marathon, and disabled ski racers train and compete with their able-bodied counterparts on national teams. Adaptive equipment technology has similarly kept pace, and there are now self-loading "mono-skis" that permit paraplegics to snow ski independently and lightweight wheelchairs that enable persons with quadriplegia up to the C-6 level to complete marathons (Fig. 28–5).

Aerobic conditioning is an important element of exercise for persons whose disabilities preclude them from using their lower extremities. At times in the rehabilitation setting, attention is focused exclusively on functional status in terms of activities of daily living, self-care, and short-distance ambulation. In addition to these crucial areas, therapy should also center on developing a "disability-specific" exercise prescription for aerobic exercise. Numerous studies have shown that aerobic capacity (as measured by $\dot{V}O_2$ max) and cardiovascular status can be improved by using upper arm ergometers and the wheelchair as endurance tools.[11] Also,

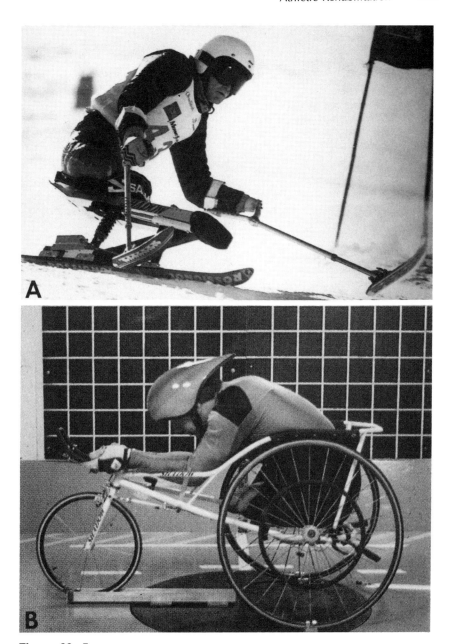

Figure 28–5

A, Mono-ski, new adaptive ski equipment that can be used by patients with paraplegia to experience the same contact with snow as able-bodied skiers. (From Crase N. Winter heat. Sports'n Spokes 1989 May/June; 15:8–14. By permission of Paralyzed Veterans of America. Photograph courtesy of Brooks Dodge.) *B,* Lightweight wheelchair used in road racing and endurance events. (From Magic in Motion, Inc. Four season fun [advertising brochure]. Kent, Washington: Magic in Motion, Inc. By permission.)

wheelchair users often develop rotator cuff problems and carpal tunnel syndrome, and prophylactic programs for each of these emphasizing stretching and balanced muscle strengthening should be provided.

Sports and recreation for the disabled can also provide a means for continued therapy, socialization, and motivation for compliance with exercise. The psychologic impact on self-esteem and outlook cannot be ignored. Also, rehabilitation issues other than performance enhancement and sport-specific issues can be addressed. There is ample opportunity for research regarding the biomechanical aspects of adaptive equipment, technique, and disability-specific training and conditioning methods.

REFERENCES

1. Warren CG, Lehmann JF, Koblanski JN. Heat and stretch procedures: an evaluation using rat tail tendon. Arch Phys Med Rehabil 1976; 57:122–126.
2. Young A, Stokes M, Iles JF. Effects of joint pathology on muscle. Clin Orthop 1987; 219:21–27.
3. Pollock ML, Wilmore JH. Exercise in health and disease: evaluation and prescription for prevention and rehabilitation. 2nd ed. Philadelphia: WB Saunders, 1990:110–114.
4. Gelberman RH, Woo SL-Y, Lothringer K, Akeson WH, Amiel D. Effects of early intermittent passive mobilization on healing canine flexor tendons. J Hand Surg 1982; 7:170–175.
5. Milner-Brown HS, Stein RB, Yemm R. The orderly recruitment of human motor units during voluntary isometric contractions. J Physiol 1973; 230:359–370.
6. Moritani T, deVries HA. Neural factors versus hypertrophy in the time course of muscle strength gain. Am J Phys Med 1979; 58:115–130.
7. de Lateur BJ, Lehmann JF. Strengthening exercise. In: Leek JC, Gershwin ME, Fowler WM Jr, eds. Principles of physical medicine and rehabilitation in the musculoskeletal diseases. Orlando, FL: Grune & Stratton, 1986:25–60.
8. Steindler A. Kinesiology of the human body under normal and pathological conditions. Springfield, IL: Charles C Thomas, 1955.
9. Lutz GE, Stuart MJ, Sim FH. Rehabilitative techniques for athletes after reconstruction of the anterior cruciate ligament. Mayo Clin Proc 1990; 65:1322–1329.
10. Whiting WC, Puffer JC, Finerman GA, Gregor RJ, Maletis GB. Three-dimensional cinematographic analysis of water polo throwing in elite performers. Am J Sports Med 1985; 13:95–98.
11. Franklin BA. Exercise testing, training and arm ergometry. Sports Med 1985; 2:100–119.

PART XI

Pediatric Rehabilitation

29

Cerebral Palsy

Ann H. Schutt

Cerebral palsy is a nonprogressive disorder of brain dysfunction manifested by abnormalities of movement and posture. It is often accompanied by intellectual defects and language and seizure disorders. Aberrant psychosocial behaviors and problems with sensory perception can also occur. This persistent, nonprogressive disorder of qualitative motor abnormalities appears before the age of 3 years. It can affect mobility, self-help, language skills, self-direction, economic self-sufficiency, and capacities for individual living. Two constant features are that cerebral palsy affects children and persists throughout life.

INCIDENCE

The incidence of cerebral palsy is 500 per 100,000 population, and approximately 500,000 persons in the United States are affected.[1] The life expectancy of these patients ranges from 0 to 82 years (mean, 33.9 years). Approximately 60% of children with cerebral palsy have motor disabilities only, 29% have motor and mental disabilities and approximately 2% have other congenital defects such as heart disease and cleft palate.

An intervention that seems to have a positive impact on the outcome of children with cerebral palsy is excellent care in perinatal intensive care units, in which 80% of the children who have brain dysfunctions have mild involvement, 10% moderate, and 10% severe. The incidence of cerebral palsy may be decreasing because of preventive measures such as immunizations for rubella and improved obstetric and perinatal care. Survival of infants born prematurely may increase the incidence.

The morbidity associated with cerebral palsy has decreased because of enrichment programs such as infant stimulation, early infant intervention, mainstreaming in the schools, and the availability of pediatric rehabilitation programs.

ETIOLOGY

When a history is obtained from the parents of a child suspected of having cerebral palsy, some of the salient features are a long labor and a first-born child with a heavy birth weight. In multiparous mothers, a child of heavy birth weight is more likely to have cerebral palsy. The incidence is greater in children whose mothers are older than 35 years or younger than 18 years, and it is more frequent in the white race. Often, the mother has a history of previous miscarriages.

Some of the common correlates are prematurity, anoxia, breech delivery, and toxemia of pregnancy (especially when the mother has convulsions and requires treatment with magnesium). It is not uncommon when fetal distress or birth trauma occurs. Incompatabilities of Rh factor, ABO, or MN can be a cause of cerebral palsy, most commonly of the hyperkinetic type; the occurrence of this type of cerebral palsy decreased from 20% in 1955 to approximately 2% in 1982. Maternal rubella has been largely eliminated by the immunization programs but is known to be a cause of cerebral palsy. Also, precipitous delivery and cesarean sections are common correlates. The study of actual brain specimens in addition to the clinical features allows the pathogenesis of these conditions to be better understood. Noninvasive techniques to study the abnormality, such as brain scanning and nuclear magnetic resonance imaging, can be helpful.

CLASSIFICATION

Pathology

Cerebral palsy can be classified according to the site of abnormality. Extrapyramidal tract lesions in the basal ganglia may result in abnormalities of hyperkinesias and dyskinesias. Lesions in the cerebellar area result primarily in the ataxic and atonic forms of cerebral palsy. Pyramidal tract lesions result in spastic forms of cerebral palsy.

Clinical Symptoms

The clinical classification may be subdivided into spastic forms, hyperkinesias, dyskinesias, ataxia, and mixed forms.[1] The spastic forms are characterized by signs of pyramidal tract involvement, specifically by the presence of hyperactive muscle stretch reflexes. They are also characterized by abnormal increases in tone and a release of postural and labyrinthine reflexes and may involve any combination of the limbs and trunk. Affected patients have a tendency for the development of contractures of muscle.

Hyperkinesias and dyskinesias are characterized by a movement disorder affecting the trunk and extremities. The muscle tone often varies with the age and activity of the patient. Frequently, patients can be very atonic at birth and then develop abnormal movement disorders around age 2½ to

3 years. These movement disorders have been described as athetosis, choreas, ballismus, tremors, dystonias, and occasionally rigidities. These movement disorders are characterized by involuntary and uncontrollable movements that vary in intensity and character. Tremors are pendular or patternlike. The dystonic movement disorders are characterized by postural attitudes, predominantly in the trunk and neck. These involve intermittent muscle spasms and imbalances of muscle tone, primarily in the trunk musculature. Rigidity is manifested by a non-rate-dependent increase in muscle tone; this feature is in contrast to spasticity, which is a rate-dependent increase in tone. Hyperkinesis and dyskinesis often do not present until the age of 2 years.

The ataxic form of cerebral palsy is characterized by a loss of the sense of balance. Most cases are probably due to involvement of the cerebellum. An intention tremor can result in abnormal depth perception, lack of balance, and extreme incoordination, and patients may stagger as they attempt to walk.

The mixed forms of cerebral palsy are a combination of the spastic, ataxic, and extrapyramidal features.

Clinical Presentations

Paraplegia involves the legs only, and most cases are of the spastic variety. *Diplegia* is the most common form of spasticity; it primarily involves the legs, and the arms are affected to a lesser degree. Again, most cases are of the spastic variety. *Tetraplegia* involves all four extremities equally (Fig. 29–1). Cases in which the greatest involvement is in the legs are usually of the spastic type, and those in which the greatest involvement is in the arms are often of the hyperkinetic or dyskinetic type. Of children with cerebral palsy, approximately 54% have paraplegia, diplegia, or tetraplegia.

Hemiplegia involves primarily the arm and leg on one side of the body

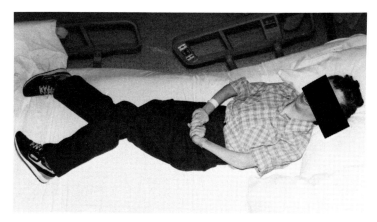

Figure 29–1
Patient with severe spastic tetraplegia.

and is usually of the spastic variety. Muscles controlling the face, tongue, and mouth can be involved. Scoliosis may be an associated problem because of a shorter arm or leg on the side of involvement. *Double hemiplegia* is a term reserved for cases in which all four limbs are involved, primarily the arms, and one side is more involved than the other. Spasticity can also involve the face, tongue, and mouth.

Pseudobulbar-type cerebral palsy involves the muscles of chewing and swallowing and the facial muscles.

Severity of Involvement

The severity of involvement can be classified as mild, moderate, or severe. In mild cases, the children are able to ambulate, use their arms, and speak well. They do not need special care. Children with moderate involvement are handicapped in locomotion, self-help, and communication, but they are not disabled entirely. Such patients may need some special care. Severe involvement results in total incapacitation. Severely affected patients are often bedridden or confined to a wheelchair.

Pathogenesis

Prenatal circumstances associated with abnormal neurologic functions include abnormalities of placental function, abnormalities in brain development, exposure to congenital infections or toxins, chromosome defects, prematurity, congenital defects, anemias of newborns, hypoprothrombinemia, fetal hemorrhages, and polygenic familial syndromes.

The natal factors responsible for cerebral palsy occur from the onset of labor to the birth of a viable fetus. Birth trauma, infections, and respiratory distress syndromes can be the underlying abnormalities. Respiratory distress syndrome with obstruction, bronchial dysplasias, and atelectasis is important. Fetal stress from anoxia can result from placenta previa or abruptio placentae. Anoxia complications can lead to cerebral palsy.

Factors that occur postnatally, defined as from birth to the age of 3 years, include head trauma, infections, and cardiovascular problems. In trauma, contusions to the brain in a battered child or after vigorous shaking have resulted in an increased incidence of cerebral palsy. Anoxia from infection, vascular lesions, hypoxia, and metabolic factors can also be implicated. Occasionally, cerebral palsy has idiopathic causes, such as cases in which the mother has a normal pregnancy and delivery, no abnormalities are noted at birth, and the nonprogressive defect appears before the age of 18 to 24 months.

EXAMINATION

Examination of the patient with cerebral palsy is important but often difficult, and certain features are specific to the disorder. The development, strength, and tone of muscles should be noted. The basic tone should be observed to determine whether spasticity or rigidity prevails and to what degree after exposure to various stimuli such as speech, noise, and excitement. Patterns of movement may be normal in some positions and abnormal in others. Therefore, various positions and attitudes should be checked, including supine, prone, lying on the side, sitting, kneeling, and standing.

Tonic reflex activity should be noted and described as symmetric tonic neck reflex, asymmetric tonic neck reflex, or labyrinthine neck reflex; these are useful reflexes for determining functional goals. How the child uses his or her hands and whether they cross the midline or are properly positioned should be noted. Basic automatic reactions such as head posture, balance, and protective movements should be monitored during developmental stages, and gaps in all levels of development should be noted. Contractures and deformities should be noted early in order to provide treatment. The motor patterns responsible for contractures and deformities should be determined.

DIAGNOSIS

One of the diagnostic procedures that can be helpful is computed tomography of cerebral hemorrhage or calcification and other structural abnormalities that can be visualized. Further investigations such as radionuclide brain scanning, magnetic resonance imaging, and electroencephalography are also useful diagnostic tools.

ASSOCIATED MEDICAL PROBLEMS

An associated medical problem is gastroesophageal reflux. This can occur in approximately 50% of severely handicapped, brain-injured children. A potential complication of this problem is failure to thrive and aspiration pneumonia. Seizure disorders are more common in spastic types than dyskinetic types, and from a third to a half of children with cerebral palsy will have a seizure or recurrent seizures.[1] Mental retardation does not necessarily accompany the motor handicaps of cerebral palsy.[2] It is most common in children with bilateral and widespread cerebral injury, and it is less common in children with extrapyramidal forms of cerebral palsy and spastic diplegia.

When appropriate, psychologic testing and communication evaluation should be completed. Pseudoretardation may be apparent when the handicaps are so severe that they interfere with both communication and self-help skills. Dysarthrias can occur in approximately three-fourths of patients with cerebral palsy. The sensory defects in hemiplegic persons can be more disabling than the motor weakness. Associated dental abnormalities are bruxism (grinding of the teeth), enamel defects, jaw deformities, and drooling. Emotional problems are common, and about 80% of adults with cerebral palsy are unemployed because of these emotional problems.[1]

AIMS OF TREATMENT

Functional self-care is the first aim of treatment. Ambulation is often desired by the parents. In terms of the handicapping condition, ambulation can be accomplished by wheelchair (Fig. 29–2 and 29–3) or with aids such as walkers, canes, crutches, or bracing. Communication is extremely important in patients with cerebral palsy, and augmentative communication is often necessary by computer, word boards (Fig. 29–4), or sign language. Without communication, affected children are locked into their own world. Vocational or avocational skills should be addressed. In school-age children and teenagers, it is particularly important to strive for a near-normal appearance. Recreational capabilities should not be overlooked. Emotional stability is important. In the area of exercise, it is important to work for substitution of weak muscles, stabilization of joints, alignment of the trunk and extremity, and posture. Prevention of contractures is most important in an exercise program. Relief of weight-bearing surfaces such as the sacrum, ischial tuberosities, or the curvature of the spine is important. The exercise program should have functional goals. Also, positioning for function is extremely important.

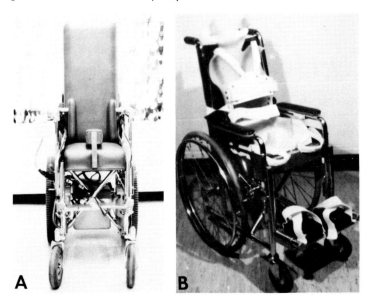

Figure 29–2
A, Electric wheelchair with adapted seat insert. *B,* Wheelchair with molded sitting orthosis.

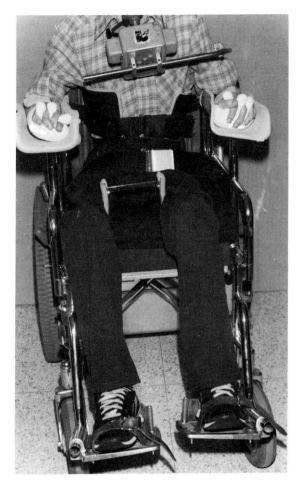

Figure 29–3
Chin-operated electric wheelchair with hand splints, adductor bar, lateral trunk supports, and wedge seat.

THE MEDICAL TEAM

The interdisciplinary team approach is needed for the care of children with cerebral palsy. Fragmentation of care should be avoided but can happen because of the need for many disciplines. The team includes physiatrists, orthopedists, neurologists, pediatricians, neurosurgeons, dentists, psychiatrists, physical therapists, occupational therapists, speech therapists, teachers, nurses, psychologists, parents, and vocational counselors. Interrelationships and full cooperation are essential in a multidisciplined team approach to treatment.

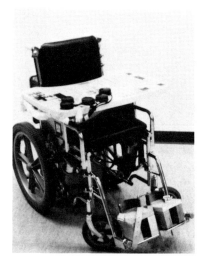

Figure 29–4
Specially adapted electric wheelchair with word board on tray table.

TREATMENT

Treatment in early infancy is used to stimulate normal motor activity and prevent deformities. Abnormal muscle activities must be suppressed or inhibited. Facilitation of postural adjustment reactions is important in early treatment, as are positioning and handling techniques during daily activities, and one should consider correction of disturbances of reciprocal inhibition.[2]

The basic approach is to teach motor skills that affected children cannot acquire spontaneously.[3] This treatment must include social experiences, sensory motor stimulation, and provision of activities of daily living.[4] Early treatment goals are to accomplish rolling, raising the head, scooting, sitting, feeding, and creeping and to develop an ongoing home treatment program. The Bobath method of treatment is aimed at reducing spastic patterns. Activities in the lower extremity that should be avoided are stimulation of extensors and extension, inversion of the foot, retraction of the pelvis, and external rotation of the thigh. Activities in the upper extremity that should be avoided are retractions of the shoulder, depression of the shoulder girdle, adduction, and internal rotation of the shoulder. Also, prolonged flexion of the elbow, wrist, and fingers should be avoided if at all possible. Pronation and ulnar deviation of the wrist and adduction of the thumb and fingers should be prevented.

Motor skills are best done manually with muscle reeducation. Muscle reeducation is necessary through successful voluntary efforts, and repetition is important. Repetition of proper volitional motor patterns is extremely important. Developmental sequencing must occur. Simplicity of environments, regardless of chronologic age, avoids distractions. The therapy setting should be quiet.

Principles of behavior modification and reinforcement of positive behaviors are important. In physical therapy, the general treatment routine is stretching, range of motion, relaxation, muscle reeducation, coordination, conditioning, dominance, and repetition. Occupational therapy addresses eye-hand coordination, skills in activities of daily living, two-handed activities, sensory reeducation and development, and proprioceptive motor development.

ORTHOSES

The philosophy of the Mayo Clinic is to use orthoses as little as possible and only when necessary. Many types of shoes, used with or without bracing, are available. Wedges can be attached to the shoes; these can be medial, lateral, heel, or sole wedges. Longitudinal arch pads can also be used. Metatarsal bars can be applied. The many varieties of short leg braces can be most helpful. Often, a solid plastic (polypropylene) ankle-foot orthosis is helpful (see Figs. 9–9 and 9–10), in which inhibition of extensor spasm is built into the foot areas. The knee-ankle-foot orthoses consist of calf and thigh bands, molded lacers, and fastening-tape (Velcro) closures. Orthoses for specific cases may need to be fabricated. Many knee and ankle mechanisms approach normal anatomy.

Prone standers or standing tables can be used for standing. Scoliosis can sometimes be managed with polypropylene (Fig. 29–2 *B*) or Orthoplast jackets.[5] The Milwaukee brace is helpful in children with progressive scoliosis or kyphosis. Before surgical stabilization, the sitting orthosis is often helpful. Serial casting for tight heel cords and hamstrings is occasionally advocated. With casting, precautions should be taken to prevent ulcers from pressure areas. Casting is time consuming. Inhibiting casting for severe spasticity of the gastrocnemius-soleus muscles is often done early.

Proper positioning of the lower extremity can be accomplished with night orthoses for prevention and stretching of contractures at the hips, knees, and ankles. Dislocated hips can be managed with orthoses to maintain the hips widely abducted. In the upper extremity, dorsal cock-up and volar cock-up splints can be helpful for wrist positioning. Orthoses to hold the thumb in opposition and abduction can counteract adducted, flexed thumbs. Night-resting orthoses are used to maintain proper wrist and hand positioning (see Fig. 24–1). Dorsal dynamic orthoses are alternatives.

DRUGS

Atropine or propantheline bromide can be used for excessive drooling. Frequently, anticonvulsant drugs are necessary. Spasticity can be pharmacologically managed with diazepam, dantrolene, or baclofen.[1] For increased concentration in school, dextroamphetamine sulfate or methylphenidate has often been proposed. Chlorpheniramine maleate is used for nasal congestion. Dextroamphetamine sulfate has also been proposed for psychologic disturbances.

OPERATIVE PROCEDURES

Orthopedic surgical procedures for patients with cerebral palsy are often tenolysis and tendon lengthenings. Occasionally, bone reconstructions such as osteotomies or rotational or derotational osteotomies are done for dislocated hips.[1] Fusion of wrists, fingers, or ankles may be needed. Tendon transfers promote ankle dorsiflexion and wrist extension.[6]

The neurosurgical procedure advocated for children with cerebral palsy is often destruction of the dentate nucleus and a stereotactic operation.[1] Hemispherectomies have been done for intractable seizures. Intraoperative electromyography-monitored posterior rhizotomies can be done to decrease spasticity. Neurectomies such as obturator neurectomy, tibial neurectomy for spasticity, and Jacobson's plexus neurectomy for drooling are helpful. Nerve or motor point blocks can be used for similar objectives.

PSYCHOSOCIAL AND VOCATIONAL ISSUES

Some of the persistent difficulties in treatment of children with cerebral palsy are psychosocial, intellectual, and educational issues. Sexuality, independence, and employment also need to be addressed.

PARENTS AND THERAPY

Parental instruction in and understanding of the physical and occupational therapy programs are essential. The parents must understand the program and its objectives. They must be aware of the limitations imposed on their child by specific types and degrees of handicaps. Educational programs for the parents and parental groups for mutual support are helpful. The parents must understand that the fundamentals of movement have to be learned by the child before complicated motor activities can be accomplished. Parental understanding and help are important factors in treatment. Psychologists, social workers, and educators can help the parents in these groups understand a child with cerebral palsy and their reactions to this child. Everyone treating a child with cerebral palsy must work toward common aims and have an understanding of the physical and occupational therapy and educational and psychosocial needs of the child with cerebral palsy. These needs are ongoing, changing, and progressive.

REFERENCES

1. Molnar GE, ed. Pediatric rehabilitation. Baltimore: Williams & Wilkins, 1985:420–467.
2. Finnie NR. Handling the young cerebral palsy child at home. 2nd ed. London: Heinemann Medical Books, 1974.
3. Köng E. Very early treatment of cerebral palsy. Dev Med Child Neurol 1966; 8:198–202.
4. Mead S. The treatment of cerebral palsy: presidential address 1967. Dev Med Child Neurol 1968; 10:423–426.
5. Alexander MA. Orthotics, adapted seating, and assistive devices. In: Molnar GE, ed. Pediatric rehabilitation. Baltimore: Williams & Wilkins, 1985:158–175.
6. Bleck EE. Orthopaedic management of cerebral palsy. Philadelphia: WB Saunders, 1979.

30

Myopathies

Stephen F. Noll

The neuromuscular diseases account for a myriad of diagnoses that are not infrequently encountered by physicians in rehabilitation medicine. An important subset of the neuromuscular diseases is primary muscle disease, which of itself includes a vast array of disorders (Table 30–1). Although each of these disorders has its peculiarities, certain characteristics are common to their presentation, and certain principles are common to their management.

A common fallacy associated with neuromuscular disorders, including muscle disease, is that if they are not curable, neither are they treatable. Although rehabilitation does not alter the pathophysiologic course of these diseases, it certainly, and often significantly, alters their functional impact.

PRESENTATION

Whatever other characteristics may be present, the hallmark of primary muscle disease is muscle weakness. But rather than complain of general fatigue, patients with true muscle weakness often volunteer specific difficulties, and the difficulties vary depending on where weakness is most apparent.[1] For example, patients commonly complain of the inability to place objects on a high shelf, to hammer overhead, or to comb their hair. These particular complaints indicate proximal more than distal upper extremity weakness. Patients with hand weakness, however, complain of difficulty opening jars or buttoning shirts. Alternatively, weakness in the proximal lower extremities results in complaints of difficulty getting out of chairs or off the toilet or perhaps with ascending and descending stairs. Yet, if patients have weakness of the distal lower extremities, they complain of tripping and stumbling, especially when walking on uneven surfaces.

Just as the complaint of weakness is important to the diagnosis of muscle disease, so too is the demonstration of weakness. Formal manual mus-

TABLE 30–1

A Brief Classification of Myopathies*

Categories	Examples
Dystrophies	Duchenne
	Facioscapulohumeral
	Limb-girdle
	Myotonic
Congenital myopathies	Central core disease
	Nemaline (rod) myopathy
	Centronuclear myopathy
	Sarcotubular myopathy
Metabolic myopathies	Glycogen storage diseases (for example, acid maltase deficiency)
	Lipid storage myopathy (for example, carnitine deficiency)
Endocrine myopathies	Hyperthyroidism or hypothyroidism
	Hyperparathyroidism
	Corticosteroid-induced
Toxic myopathies	Alcohol-induced
	Chloroquine
Inflammatory myopathies	Polymyositis
	Dermatomyositis

*This table is not meant to be an all-inclusive list of myopathies.

cle testing is the accepted method to determine muscle weakness. Equally as helpful, however, is functional or task-oriented muscle testing. Table 30–2 itemizes several functional tasks or tests and the major muscle or muscles with which they are associated.

Gait analysis is another functional evaluation that may give clues to muscle weakness. Several typical gait alterations occur with weakness. For

TABLE 30–2

Functional Tasks Used to Determine
Muscle Weakness

Functional Task	Key Muscles Tested*	Strength
Toe walk	Gastrocnemius, soleus	+
Heel walk	Tibialis anterior	+
Deep knee bend	Quadriceps	+
Gower's maneuver	Gluteus maximus, quadriceps	−
Froment's sign	Adductor pollicis	−
Arms overhead	Supraspinatus, deltoid	+

*Several other muscles must often work synergistically to accomplish such tasks.

example, weakness of the gluteus medius results in a waddling appearance referred to as a Trendelenburg gait. Likewise, with weakness of the gluteus maximus, gait is characterized by a sudden forward lurch and marked lumbar lordosis that provide for stability at the hip. If the quadriceps are weak, genu recurvatum will be prominent during the stance phase of walking to provide stability at the knee. Finally, weakness of the tibialis anterior results in a "steppage" gait, so called because, in order to clear the foot during the swing phase of walking, patients must actually lift the leg high as if to step up.

The presentation and finding of muscle weakness, of course, are not specific to any one type of muscle disease. Other signs and symptoms may narrow the possibilities. For example, in a hypotonic infant with enlarged heart, liver, and spleen, Pompe's disease is suspected. A peculiar facies and percussion myotonia suggest myotonic dystrophy. In addition, the distribution of weakness and course of illness may help distinguish one disease from another, such as Duchenne's dystrophy from facioscapulohumeral dystrophy. But for a definitive diagnosis, clinical suspicions must be documented with laboratory and histologic data.

Furthermore, the presentation and finding of muscle weakness are not specific to muscle disease alone. Any disease process that affects the motor unit can result in weakness; therefore, other signs and symptoms may be helpful insomuch as they support a diagnosis other than muscle disease. For example, sensory loss is suggestive of a neuropathy. Fasciculations favor a diagnosis of motor neuron disease. Atrophy and hypoactive reflexes, especially if found early in the course of the illness, are more indicative of a neuropathic process.

Because the clinical findings only suggest a diagnosis, laboratory data are important for confirmation. The creatinine phosphokinase value is an essential, although nonspecific, factor in the diagnosis of muscle disease. When increased, it suggests muscle destruction secondary to active muscle disease. The creatinine phosphokinase value, however, is not always increased in active disease, and when it is, the degree of elevation does not necessarily correlate with the degree of clinical impairment. In Duchenne's muscular dystrophy, for example, the highest values of creatinine phosphokinase are recorded early in infancy and early childhood when, clinically, the disease is least evident.[2]

Electromyography is another important study in the evaluation of the patient with suspected primary muscle disease. Electromyography consists of two types of studies: nerve conduction studies and needle examination. An abnormality in conduction studies is often indicative of neuropathic disease, although the amplitude of a compound muscle action potential is sometimes low in muscle disease because of the decreased number of muscle fibers. The needle examination samples various muscles at rest and with effort. In muscle disease, the action potentials on needle examination often show a distinctive pattern: low amplitude, short duration, and polyphasia. Although the electromyogram cannot always determine a specific diagnosis, it is valuable in at least two respects when primary muscle disease is a consideration. First, it can differentiate myopathic from neuropathic disease, which at times is clinically confusing. Second, it can disclose characteristics of a myopathic process. For example, fibrillation potentials are more abundant in an inflammatory myopathy; a "dive-bomber" sound of high-frequency potentials suggests myotonia.

Despite the clinical, laboratory, and electromyographic data, a specific diagnosis can often be made only by muscle biopsy. Multiple histochemical staining techniques allow classification of a specimen into the various types of muscle disease. The recent discovery of dystrophin, a large-molecular-weight protein, is helpful for differentiating types of neuromuscular disease (Duchenne's dystrophy from Becker's dystrophy) and determining the severity of disease.[3]

CONSIDERATIONS FOR REHABILITATION

As stated above, primary muscle disease includes multiple types of disorders. However, rehabilitation is not as specific to a diagnosis as it is to functional disability. With any muscle disease, it is important to ask certain questions that pertain to decision making in rehabilitation, irrespective of the diagnosis.

Is it reversible or irreversible? Most primary muscle diseases are irreversible, but not all. Steroid myopathy or polymyositis may be amenable to treatment—steroid myopathy to withdrawal of steroids, and polymyositis to their introduction. The answer to this question has a bearing on what is to be done. For example, if an ankle-foot orthosis is needed, prescribing an off-the-shelf orthosis may be most practical when the condition is temporary, and a more expensive and durable custom-fitted orthosis may be a better choice if the process is permanent.

Is it stable or progressive (and if progressive, at what rate)? The course of a disease has a significant influence on decision making. In classic Duchenne's muscular dystrophy, for example, loss of ambulation can be predicted to occur approximately 6 to 12 months after the loss of ability to climb stairs.[4] Consequently, the need for a wheelchair can be easily anticipated. In contrast, the need for a wheelchair is more delayed in Becker's variant of muscular dystrophy, which is much slower to evolve.

Is it genetic or acquired? The impact of a primary muscle disease is related not only to the person with the disease but also to other family members and to their environment. As part of the rehabilitation effort, incorporating a genetic counselor, psychologist, and social service worker into the team approach is often imperative.

REHABILITATION EFFORTS

The goal of rehabilitation in muscle diseases is the same as that for any other disease: to maximize independent functional capacity. This process may involve attempts to restore lost function (for example, with an orthosis) or to prevent further loss of function (for example, with regular therapeutic exercise). Several rehabilitation measures are available to improve function.[5]

Physical Modalities

Physical methods are sometimes useful for the management of primary muscle disease. Hot or cold applications, whether packs or a radiant heat lamp, may effectively relieve the pain sometimes associated with inflammatory myopathies. Use of a Hubbard tank is often helpful for facilitating range-of-motion exercises in the case of severe muscle weakness and for providing comfort for the myalgias that may be associated with muscle disease. Treatment with ultrasound is particularly effective when used in conjunction with prolonged stretching exercises for joint contractures that often plague patients with chronic myopathies. Finally, biofeedback can enhance muscle reeducation efforts in a recovering but weakened muscle.

Therapeutic Exercise

In any muscle disease, contracture formation is a major concern. Weakness often prevents full active range of motion, and resting postures tend to become fixed. Although all muscles can tighten, at most risk for this complication are those that cross more than one joint, such as the hamstrings, the gastrocnemius, and the tensor fasciae latae. Thus, a common pattern for contractures in the lower extremities is hip flexion and abduction, knee flexion, and plantar flexion. Likewise, because of a predisposition for contracture formation, special attention should be given to the shoulder adductors, elbow flexors, pronators, and metacarpophalangeal extensors in the upper extremities.[6] Regardless of the stage of disease, range of motion of all joints related to weakened muscles is important, as is gentle, prolonged stretching of key muscles such as those mentioned above.

The applicability of strengthening exercises in myopathies remains controversial. The fear associated with exercising to the point of muscle fatigue has been that the exercise will actually produce overwork weakness rather than promote strength. In a small, controlled study of a group of boys with Duchenne's muscular dystrophy, submaximal isokinetic exercise resulted in no overwork weakness and a statistically nonsignificant increase in strength.[7] More extensive study is needed in several of the myopathies to clarify this matter. Nonetheless, exercise training seems to be beneficial provided that the degree of weakness is minimal, the rate of disease progression is slow, the intensity of the exercise program is mild, and the exercise program takes into consideration the patient's overall physical activity level.[8] Currently, a practical approach to therapeutic exercise seems to be (1) strengthening early in the course of the disease rather than late and (2) strengthening at submaximal exercise levels.[9] Corollaries to this approach might also be to strengthen muscles that are only minimally affected rather than those that are severely affected and to strengthen primarily the muscles of functional importance such as the hip extensors and quadriceps.

Specific training in functional skills, such as transfers from bed to a chair, onto the toilet, or into a car, is often the most important component of an "exercise" program for patients severely impaired with primary muscle disease. Aids may be necessary to augment these skills, such as a sliding board, an overhead trapeze, or ultimately even a Hoyer lift.

Mobility Training

Independent mobility is an important goal. Although this goal is usually thought of in terms of ambulation, wheelchair mobility may be best functionally. Both assisted ambulation and wheelchair mobility have their advantages. Walking, for example, has an advantage in overcoming some architectural barriers; however, wheelchair propulsion usually is more energy efficient.

Assistive Devices. Ambulation can be maintained, in part, by means of assistive devices, such as a cane, quadripod cane, hemiwalker, crutches, or walker. These devices provide various amounts of stability. Their use, however, implies fair to good strength in the so-called crutch muscles of the upper extremities, some of which include shoulder depressors, shoulder abductors and adductors, and triceps. For patients with diffuse or proximal muscle weakness of the upper extremities, such as occurs in Duchenne's muscular dystrophy or facioscapulohumeral dystrophy, crutch or cane-assisted ambulation may not be feasible.

Bracing. Another means of assisting ambulation is with orthotic devices. Bracing serves several functions that assist gait. A brace may protect a joint. A jointed knee brace, for example, may prevent progression of genu recurvatum and provide knee stability in a patient with significant quadriceps weakness. A brace also positions the joint and may prevent contracture formation. A person with marked weakness of the tibialis anterior muscle can be placed in a molded polypropylene ankle-foot orthosis that will hold the foot and ankle in near neutral position. In doing so, the orthosis stabilizes the joint, prevents tripping and falling from footdrop, and prevents equinus-positioned contractures at the ankle. Finally, an orthotic device may, in fact, augment function. For example, the reciprocating hip-knee-ankle-foot orthoses provide assisted hip flexion and extension by means of passive movement of a cable.[10] Likewise, the elastic qualities of materials used in a posterior leaf-spring ankle-foot orthosis may provide dynamic ankle dorsiflexion.

Orthoses may also have merit unrelated to mobility itself. Standing and walking are thought to decrease disuse osteoporosis, retard the development of scoliosis in some cases, and provide a psychologic lift to the patient.

Unfortunately, orthoses are not without disadvantages. The use of an ankle-foot orthosis in Duchenne's muscular dystrophy, for example, may in fact, collapse the patient. Passive stability of stance[11] is dependent on maintaining the center of gravity weight line posterior to the hip and anterior to the knee. This task is, in part, accomplished by toe walking. Therefore, if the foot and ankle are braced independent of other joints, this compensatory posture is broken and the patient may collapse. Another disadvantage is the energy requirement for braced ambulation. Braces significantly increase the energy expenditure of walking.[12] The rate of ambulation is often decreased to compensate for this increased workload. Because of the increased workload and the decreased efficiency, in some instances bracing may not always be worth the effort required. Nonetheless, with proper selection of patients, knee-ankle-foot orthoses may prolong ambulation for as long as 2 to 4 years in children with Duchenne's muscular dystrophy.[13]

Wheelchairs. Although there is often a hesitancy to use it, a wheelchair is a reasonable alternative to ambulation for mobility and may offer the most efficient means of mobility. The energy cost of propelling a wheelchair is approximately the same as that of normal ambulation. Furthermore, a wheelchair need not be the sole means of mobility. For example, a patient with facioscapulohumeral dystrophy may walk well on smooth surfaces for short distances (a household ambulator) but may benefit from the use of a wheelchair for mobility around the community and for sports activities.

Because of their expense, electric wheelchairs are often viewed as luxury items. In fact, however, they should be prescribed as would any other medical device to provide for lost function, just as one would prescribe a catheter for urinary drainage or a cast for stability of a fracture. The electric wheelchair provides for lost independent mobility.

The wheelchair provides more than mobility.[14] Through proper positioning, it has the potential to retard scoliosis and contracture formation, especially in young persons. Therefore, it is important to prescribe a wheelchair with certain specifications, as shown in Figure 30–1: (1) a firm seat, with or without a cushion, to discourage pelvic obliquity; (2) removable and adjustable desktop armrests to prevent "slumping" (a lap tray is also often helpful for positioning); (3) a lumbar support and firm backrest to position the spine in extension in an attempt to stabilize facets and discourage scoliosis; and (4) swing-away, detachable footrests to prevent equinus posturing at the ankles. Lateral pads, or even a custom-molded seating orthosis, may be additional needs.

Activities of Daily Living

Because of weakness, whether proximal or distal, the ability to accomplish basic self-care activities may be significantly impaired by primary muscle disease. With specific training in techniques, energy conservation,

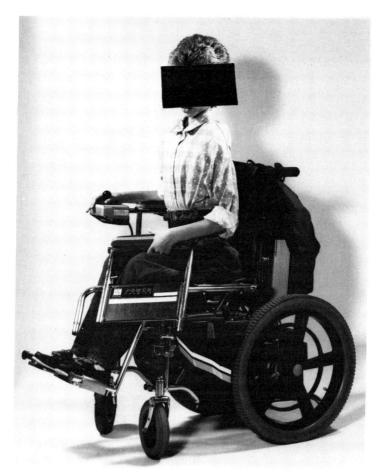

Figure 30–1
Prescribed electric wheelchair for an adolescent with facioscapulohumeral dystrophy.

and the use of adaptive aids (Table 30–3 and Figure 30–2), the safe performance of activities of daily living is often possible.

In addition to assistive devices, static or dynamic splints can be fabricated to prevent contractures and to promote or improve function. For example, a wrist cock-up splint in a patient with distal myopathy may improve grasp by means of stabilizing the wrist and providing a tenodesis effect.

Other Concerns

Prevention of contractures, maintenance of muscle strength, mobility, and independence in self-care are the usual and traditional goals in the re-

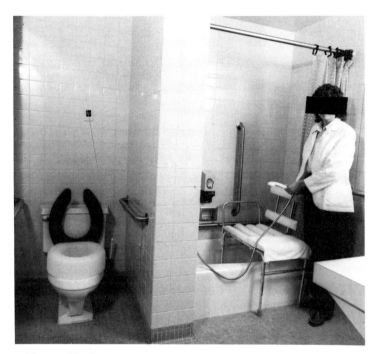

Figure 30–2
Adapted bathroom and hygiene aids for patients with muscle disease.

habilitation of patients with primary muscle disease. Other problems arise, however, that require rehabilitation efforts, and, although there can be many, two of these problems deserve special comment.

Dysphagia is a disorder that plagues patients with certain primary muscle diseases, such as myotonic dystrophy. Swallowing difficulties may be significant and result in malnutrition or aspiration pneumonia. Proper positioning, modification of food consistencies, and compensatory and facilitation techniques for swallowing may, in fact, resolve this problem. If not, home enteral feeding programs are feasible. Dysarthria often accompanies dysphagia. It, too, at times, is amenable to treatment (for example, with a palatal lift).

Respiratory failure is the most feared complication of primary muscle disease. Options now exist for patients with advanced disease and impending respiratory failure.[15] For example, life may be prolonged in Duchenne's muscular dystrophy by using an iron lung or a chest cuirass at night for temporary respiratory support. Tracheostomy with portable ventilatory support is also an option for some patients. Such treatments have both advantages and disadvantages for patients and their families. Therefore, decisions regarding respiratory support must be reached far in advance of the "crisis" of respiratory failure.

TABLE 30–3
Examples of Assistive Devices for
Activities of Daily Living

Dressing aids
    Fastening-tape (Velcro) closures
    Buttonhook
    Sock loops
Eating aids
    Universal cuff
    Built-up grips
    Balanced forearm orthosis
Hygiene aids
    Bath bench
    Grab bars
    Toilet seat riser
    Long-handled sponge and brush

SUMMARY

Management of primary muscle disease from a rehabilitation stand-point varies considerably with the particular disease entity, its course, and its extent. In some cases, rehabilitation may involve only the prescription of an exercise program to prevent contractures. In other cases, it may demand a comprehensive program involving a full complement of services, including medical or surgical consultations, rehabilitation nursing, physical, occupational, and recreational therapy, speech therapy, orthotics, genetic counseling, educational and vocational counseling, and psychologic and social service work evaluations. Regardless of the extent of involvement, treatment must be directed not only at the disease process itself but also at the restoration and preservation of a patient's functional capacity for as long as possible.

REFERENCES

1. Brooke MH. A clinician's view of neuromuscular diseases. 2nd ed. Baltimore: Williams & Wilkins, 1986:1–35.
2. Munsat TL. Review of neuromuscular diseases. Phys Med Rehabil 1988; 2 no. 4:467–479.
3. Hoffman EP, Fischbeck KH, Brown RH, Johnson M, Medori R, Loike JD, Harris JB, Waterston R, Brooke M, Specht L, Kupsky W, Chamberlain J, Caskey CT, Shapiro F, Kunkel LM. Characterization of dystrophin in muscle-biopsy specimens from patients with Duchenne's or Becker's muscular dystrophy. N Engl J Med 1988; 318:1363–1368.
4. Vignos PJ Jr. Rehabilitation in progressive muscular dystrophy. In: Licht S, ed. Rehabilitation and medicine. Baltimore: Waverly Press, 1968:584–642.

5. Fowler WM Jr. Rehabilitation management of muscular dystrophy and related disorders: II. Comprehensive care. Arch Phys Med Rehabil 1982; 63:322–328.

6. Johnson EW, Alexander MA. Management of motor unit diseases. In: Kottke FJ, Stillwell GK, Lehmann JF, eds. Krusen's handbook of physical medicine and rehabilitation. 3rd ed. Philadelphia: WB Saunders, 1982:679–690.

7. de Lateur BJ, Giaconi RM. Effect of maximal strength of submaximal exercise in Duchenne muscular dystrophy. Am J Phys Med 1979; 58:26–36.

8. Fowler WM Jr. Management of musculoskeletal complications in neuromuscular diseases: weakness and the role of exercise. Phys Med Rehabil 1988; 2 no. 4:489–507.

9. Fowler WM Jr, Taylor M. Rehabilitation management of muscular dystrophy and related disorders: I. The role of exercise. Arch Phys Med Rehabil 1982; 63:319–321.

10. Douglas R, Larson PF, D'Ambrosia R, McCall RE. The LSU reciprocation-gait orthosis. Orthopaedics 1983; 6:834–839.

11. Johnson EW. Pathokinesiology of Duchenne muscular dystrophy: implications for management. Arch Phys Med Rehabil 1977; 58:4–7.

12. Fischer SV, Gullickson G Jr. Energy cost of ambulation in health and disability: a literature review. Arch Phys Med Rehabil 1978; 59:124–133.

13. Vignos PJ Jr. Management of musculoskeletal complications in neuromuscular diseases: limb contractures and the role of stretching, braces and surgery. Phys Med Rehabil 1988; 2 no. 4:509–536.

14. Alexander MA. Orthotics, adapted seating, and assistive devices. In: Molnar GE, ed. Pediatric rehabilitation. Baltimore: Williams & Wilkins, 1985:158–175.

15. Alexander MA, Johnson EW, Petty J, Stauch D. Mechanical ventilation of patients with late stage Duchenne muscular dystrophy: management in the home. Arch Phys Med Rehabil 1979; 60:289–292.

31

Orthopedic Management of the Disabled Child

Dennis J. Matthews
Lynne M. Stempien

GENERAL CONSIDERATIONS

Treatment of disabled children poses some unique considerations. Congenital neuromuscular or skeletal dysfunction and acquired disabilities are superimposed on a growing, changing organism. These disabilities can influence the child's ultimate functional outcome and also treatment decisions.

From birth to adulthood, dramatic somatic changes take place at different times in maturation. During the first year of life, height increases 50% to 55% and weight increases 180% to 200%. During the preschool years, the limbs elongate relative to the trunk. During adolescence, the distal extremities elongate first, but later the trunk length increases greater than that of the limbs.[1] There are also seasonal variations; the warm summer months bring a faster velocity of growth.[2]

There are changes in the anatomic relationship of some structures with normal skeletal maturation. At birth, the spinal cord lies with neural segments adjacent to the bony vertebral segments. With greater longitudinal growth of the vertebral column, the spinal cord ends at L-12, and the lumbosacral roots subsequently become obliquely oriented to their respective foramina as they leave the cauda equina. The brain is 15% of total body weight at birth and reaches the adult proportion of 5% by age 5 years.

As the immature nervous system develops, a series of "primitive reflexes" are extinguished. These reflexes, such as asymmetric tonic neck reflex, cause movement in predictable patterns. With congenital or acquired neurologic insult, these reflexes persist or are unmasked. This will influence the balance of muscle pull across specific joints and will influence expectations for certain contractures and functional outcome. Also, several abnormal motor control patterns that occur with injury to the immature brain influence the types of musculoskeletal deformity that can occur. For example, the spastic diplegic "scissoring" of cerebral palsy, with lower extremity adduction, internal rotation, knee extension, and plantar flexion, leads to limitation of abduction and dorsiflexion.[3]

SPECIFIC CONSIDERATIONS

The Spine

The spine provides trunk stability, the basis for head and limb function. Spinal deformity can occur in several planes: kyphosis (increased posterior apex curve in the anteroposterior plane), lordosis (increased anterior apex curve in the anteroposterior plane), or scoliosis (increased curvature in the sagittal plane). Because of the complex intervertebral relationships, an increase in curvature is often accompanied by some degree of vertebral rotation. These changes in vertebral alignment alter the position of many other structures and can serve as a clue for detection. Unilateral shoulder elevation, a "rib hump" posteriorly on forward bending, pectus excavatum, unequal breast development, and pelvic obliquity may result.[4]

Spinal deformity may be congenital or acquired. Among the myriad of congenital causes are many systemic, bony, and connective tissue diseases. The presence of simultaneous abnormalities, particularly of the skin, nails, eyes, ears, and joints, may suggest inherited skeletal disorders or bone dysplasias such as osteogenesis imperfecta. Acquired spinal deformity is very common in conditions associated with childhood neuromuscular weakness, such as spinal cord injury and myelomeningocele. Acquired neuromuscular spinal deformity generally progresses more rapidly than the congenital conditions. Peripheral vertebral growth may be affected by mechanical factors on the spine, such as paraspinal tone.[4] Ambulatory or sitting ability and the symmetry of paravertebral muscle function may contribute to subsequent spinal deformity.

The most serious complication of spinal deformity is the decrease in pulmonary function subsequent to the accompanying changes in the shape of the chest, compliance, and respiratory muscle function. Spinal curvature tends to progress throughout childhood and can continue to progress even after skeletal maturity. Once scoliosis has reached 60°, vital capacity progressively declines.[4] The subsequent respiratory compromise is estimated to double mortality in adults with spinal deformity, and mortality is 4 times expected in persons with thoracic spinal deformity.

Spinal deformity also affects functional ability by influencing sitting and standing posture. Accompanying pelvic obliquity changes the pressure distribution on the skin and increases the risk for pressure sores.

The Hip

The hip is a major weight-bearing joint and an important portion of the pelvis. Its components, the acetabulum and femoral head, influence the bony development of each other. Any change in the relationship of these components before completion of bony ossification during puberty can significantly alter the structure of the joint. Such alteration may occur with congenital dislocation of the hip as an intrinsic deformity. Congenital dislocation of the hip is also associated with other deformities such as torticollis (15% to 20% of cases) and metatarsus adductus (5% to 10% of cases).[4]

Neuromuscular disabilities that cause weakness, a change in muscle tone, or posturing can affect the femoral head-acetabulum relationship. When these components are not maintained in proximity, the result is dysplastic components, a more shallow acetabulum, and flattening of the femoral head. These changes disrupt the normal ball-and-socket mechanics and make hip subluxation and dislocation more likely. Hip deformity can cause pain, loss of range of motion, and pelvic obliquity with a consequent impact on seating position, hygiene, mobility, posture, ambulation potential, and comfort. Yearly clinical examination for decreased abduction, asymmetric thigh folds, femoral inequality on hip flexion in the supine position, and signs of hip instability in combination with radiologic examination is needed for "hips at risk" until the disabled child reaches skeletal maturity.

The Knee

A major concern in knee mechanics of the disabled child is range of motion, particularly at the hamstring muscles. Limitations in range are frequent with spastic conditions such as cerebral palsy or spinal cord injury, and they are increased by predominant sitting in wheelchair-dependent children. Hamstring limitation causes posterior pelvic tilt, with subsequent "sacral sitting," which complicates sitting and standing postures. Use of supported standing (for example, in a prone or supine stander in small children) can assist in maintaining range of motion of the hamstrings while providing alternative positioning for developmental stimulation.

Foot and Ankle

A myriad of congenital foot deformities such as clubfoot, arthrogryposis, and vertical talus (rocker bottom) require surgical intervention or orthotics to provide a weight-bearing surface. Neuromuscular impairment can impose unbalanced forces across the hindfoot and forefoot to cause acquired deformity such as equinovarus, equinovalgus, or cavovarus pattern. In some cases, bracing can assist in balancing these forces and can also affect knee biomechanics by influencing ankle position in weight bearing.

Upper Extremity

In addition to the congenital limb malformations, the major cause of upper extremity disability is loss of functional range of motion. Reaching and fine motor abilities are required for the child to develop independence in activities of daily living and aid in development of cognitive skills by enabling manipulation of the environment.

CEREBRAL PALSY

Management of cerebral palsy requires an understanding of the interaction of biologic and environmental factors with normal development. By integrating a basic knowledge of the child's anatomic-physiologic abnormalities with a clear concept of the interaction between structure and experience, team management seeks to encourage development of the handicapped child to a maximal level of motor, intellectual, and social function.[5]

Cerebral palsy is the most common permanent physical disability of childhood. It is not a single disease but includes a collection of diverse syndromes with diverse causes, pathologic features, and clinical manifestations. Cerebral palsy is a categorical term that designates motor disorders resulting from static, nonprogressive lesions of the immature central nervous system. Associated with these motor deficits may be sensory or learning deficits. Because the anatomic structures involved may include the cerebral cortex, basal ganglia, midbrain, pons, and cerebellum, the term "cerebral palsy" is not scientifically correct but is a descriptive term.[3, 6]

Orthopedic surgical procedures are an important adjunct to management of the child with cerebral palsy. The purpose of and expectation for operation must be clear to all involved with care of the child.[7] The timing of the operation in conjunction with the functional status is important. Goal-oriented management requires that the child's problem be analyzed consistent with the priorities and need for independent living.

Upper Extremity

Surgical management of the spastic upper extremity requires an understanding of dynamic muscle imbalance, tendons and ligamentous contractures, and bony abnormalities. Analysis of the patient must include documentation of adequate hand sensation, including light touch, two-point discrimination, and proprioception. The patient also should have sufficient intellectual function and emotional stability to comprehend the goals of the operation and to cooperate in the restoration of hand function postoperatively. Goals are to improve the function and appearance of the hand.

Thumb deformities are common in cerebral palsy. Most frequent is a thumb-in-palm deformity due to spasticity of the adductor pollicis and flexor pollicis longus muscles. Management includes tendon lengthening, release of contracted muscles, Z-plasty of the web space, and arthrodesis of metacarpophalangeal joints (especially on unstable thumbs with extensive capsular stretch).

A spastic wrist flexion deformity is often due to a combination of both wrist and finger flexor spasticity. Various techniques to lengthen the finger flexor tendons along with distal advancement of the flexor tendon origins from the medial epicondyle have been described. It is important to avoid overlengthening of the finger flexor tendons to ensure normal tension when the hand is relaxed and the wrist is in the neutral position. If the wrist extensors are weak or absent, a transfer of the flexor carpi ulnaris to the extensor carpi radialis brevis is frequently performed to provide some extension. Tendon lengthenings and transfers require 4 weeks of immobilization with dressings and splints. This is usually followed by 6 to 8 weeks of intermittent splinting during the day and all-night splinting with the wrist in the neutral position and the fingers extended; the splints can be removed for guided functional activities and restoration of motion.[3, 8]

Pronation spasticity and early contracture are common. Posterior subluxation of the radial head frequently occurs early and often accounts for a fixed deformity that limits elbow extension. Pronator teres tenotomy has improved active supination.

Surgical approaches to elbow flexion deformity are important to evaluate in light of physical function. Generally, if the elbow lacks only 30° to 40° of range of motion, therapy is directed toward maintenance of motion with splinting and exercise. When there is greater limitation, various surgical techniques can be used, including medial lengthening of the biceps tendon and brachialis aponeurosis. If contractures have been persistent for a significant time, a capsulotomy and Z-plasty skin lengthening may be needed. Postoperative splinting should include enough extension to prevent excessive stretch of the nerve and vessels. Intermittent, supervised flexion-extension exercises can be started within a week.

Orthopedic surgical techniques are rarely applied to the shoulder. Occasionally, a spastic pectoralis major and subscapularis may preclude neutral or slightly externally rotated position of the shoulders and interferes with function.

Lower Extremity

Operative procedures for the lower extremity, especially in the spastic types of cerebral palsy, address the adducted, internally rotated lower extremity with the equinovarus foot. Various early, nonoperative management techniques, including orthotics, casting, and phenol motor point blocks,[9–11] may assist in maintaining and increasing range of motion. Operation is generally indicated for triceps surae contracture. The various surgical techniques include neurectomy of the gastrocnemius, gastrocnemius lengthening, gastrocnemius origin recession, tendo-Achilles lengthening, and Achilles tendon translocation. All are designed to reduce the increased stretch reflex and lengthen the muscle. Whether part of the Achilles tendon is exposed and lengthened or cut in the proper places by the percutaneous technique, the principle is the same. Postoperative management includes plaster immobilization for 3 to 6 weeks, followed by a weight-bearing program and consideration of the use of orthotics.

Deformity of the foot in cerebral palsy is due to spastic muscle imbalance.[3, 8, 12] Where the force of the invertor muscles of the spastic foot exceeds that of the spastic evertors, varus deformity results. Generally, two muscles are involved in the varus deformity: the posterior tibialis and the anterior tibialis. Surgical correction of this deformity involves a lengthening or transfer of the posterior tibialis tendon. Fixed hindfoot varus may also require a wedge osteotomy of the calcaneus.

Pes valgus deformities occur less commonly in children. The foot has an eversion and equinus inclination of the calcaneus and abduction of the midfoot, which result in a prominence of the head of the talus medially. Generally, this deformity is flexible until adolescence. Obvious and severe pes valgus can be corrected only with operation. Correction by extra-articular subtalar arthrodesis (Grice technique) is indicated by incipient development of hallux valgus. The objective is to prevent eversion of the hindfoot by permanently eliminating subtalar motion. This is generally performed on children younger than 13 years to preserve tarsal bone growth. Long-term results have been satisfactory; corrections have been good in about 50% of cases. Triple arthrodesis is the standard operation for severe pes valgus in adolescents and adults. This is a fusion of the talus, calcaneus, navicular, and cuboid bones that requires 6 to 8 weeks of reduced weight-bearing immobilization.

Metatarsus adductus in the child with cerebral palsy appears to be secondary to a spastic abductor hallucis muscle. Early, the deformity is dynamic and later evolves into a fixed skeletal adduction and subsequently a bunion. The different surgical approaches include abductor hallucis release, capsulotomies, and osteotomies of the first metatarsal.

Torsional Deformity: Tibia and Fibula, Internal or External

Excessive external tibial-fibular torsion is more common than internal torsion in cerebral palsy. This may represent a compensation for femoral torsion and surgical lengthening of the medial hamstring muscles. Internal tibial-fibular torsion is of the congenital type and is superimposed on spastic diplegia. Spontaneous correction is rare. There is no evidence that orthotics correct the torsional deformity in either direction. Indications for surgical correction include subjective disability due to severe in-toeing or significant interference with active ambulation. The choice is either proximal or distal rotation osteotomy.

Knee

Knee flexion deformities may be due to spastic and contracted hamstring muscles or secondarily due to weakened triceps surae muscles. They are often accompanied by a hip flexion deformity. This is a result of the persistent knee-flexed posture secondary to contractures of the posterior capsule of the joint and includes shortening of the sciatic nerve. Flexion contracture releases are indicated when the knee flexion posture is more than 40°. This condition reduces energy efficiency in ambulation and decreases stride length. Surgical techniques include hamstring tenotomy, transfers, or lengthening. Because of the risk of knee hyperextension due to excessive hamstring weakness, maintenance of the semimembranous integrity decreases possible recurvatum of the joint.

Frequently, the crouched-gait pattern in children with spasticity produces significant lengthening and pain of the patellar tendon. This is better addressed by control of the crouched gait rather than patellar surgical procedures.

Hip

Hip adduction deformity originates from spasticity of the adductor muscles.[3, 12] In the ambulatory patient, operation to relieve adduction spasticity is indicated when each hip is limited to abduction of 20° or less with the hip extended or when there is scissoring. When there is doubt about the need for operation, intramuscular neurolysis[9–11] may help evaluate the effect of passive range of motion. Fixed adductor contractures generally require a release of the adductor longus and gracilis, occasionally paired with a neurectomy of the anterior branch of the obturator nerve. Other surgical approaches include an adductor origin transfer to the ilium.

Three weeks of postoperative immobilization with long leg casts connected by an abduction splint to keep each hip in 30° to 40° of abduction is generally sufficient. The casts can be removed at this time for activities to regain strength and range of motion and early gait training.

Hip flexion deformities are secondary to sartorius, rectus femoris, adductors, or iliopsoas contracture. In general, if the hip flexion deformity is more than 15° to 20°, surgical correction is indicated.[3, 8, 12] Surgical lengthening of the iliopsoas is frequently done because this is the major flexor of the hip. The iliopsoas also has a function in walking and, for this reason, it is desirable to preserve its strength and function. In a nonambulatory patient, tenotomy is satisfactory. Various Z lengthening methods, along with iliopsoas recession, have been described.

Hip Internal Rotation Deformities

The internal rotator muscles of the hip are the gluteus medius and minimus, semitendinosus, and adductors.[3, 13] The hip internal rotation deformity from contracture of these muscles is further compounded by excessive femoral anteversion. Most infants have angles of femoral anteversion of 10° to 60°. During skeletal maturation, this angle decreases to the adult value of 19°. This spontaneous decrease in most children is biomechanically aided by normal muscle balance and weight bearing. Spastic, nonambulatory children tend to maintain a higher degree of femoral anteversion. Procedures to correct hip internal rotation include posterior transposition of the origin of the adductors, adductor myotomy, and gluteus medius and minimus tendon transfer.[3, 8, 12]

Hip subluxation occurs in children with cerebral palsy when muscle imbalances cause acetabular and femoral dysplasia.[3, 4, 8, 12–14] Reducing spasticity and contracture of the muscles, especially the adductors, before the age of 5 years results in success in most patients. When abduction is less than 40°, adductor myotomy with or without anterior branch neurectomy may arrest or prevent further lateral subluxation. This is done to prevent progressive subluxation and allow remodeling of the acetabulum. Generally, after age 5 years or if there is significant loss of femoral head coverage with acetabular and femoral dysplasia, tenotomy needs to be paired with femoral varus derotational osteotomy and occasionally pelvic osteotomy. Derotational femoral osteotomy has produced definite and permanent results. The osteotomy is either subtrochanteric or supracondylar. This requires internal fixation and the use of a long leg plaster or hip spica cast to maintain position. This procedure corrects the excessive femoral anteversion and coxa valga. It also reestablishes the femoral head-acetabular relationships and allows remodeling of the acetabulum to occur.

The acetabular dysplasia is not likely to self-correct in older children. Various pelvic osteotomies with acetabular cup procedures are used to correct this problem. These procedures require internal fixation and 6 to 8 weeks of immobilization or modified ambulatory activity to decrease weight bearing. Later in life, subsequent hip deformity can occur with significant deformation of the femur and cartilage degeneration. If the hip has become painful in the adult, four salvage procedures have been proposed, including 1) subtrochanteric femoral osteotomy, 2) femoral head and neck resection, 3) hip arthrodesis, and 4) total hip replacement.[3, 4, 12]

Scoliosis

The prevalence of structural scoliosis in cerebral palsy differs between ambulatory and nonambulatory individuals. The mechanism that triggers the onset of spinal curvature in cerebral palsy has not been specifically defined. Theories include central nervous system imbalance, asymmetric muscle pull, and postural mechanisms. Numerous studies of scoliosis progression in both idiopathic and paralytic types have been published.[3, 8, 15] Spinal growth ceases for all practical purposes when the iliac apophyses are fully ossified and fusion with the body of the ilium occurs. If the curvature is less than 50° when skeletal maturation occurs, then progression due to growth usually does not occur in ambulatory patients with cerebral palsy who have a spinal curvature that does not involve the sacrum or pelvis.

Orthoses of various types appear to be effective. Electrical stimulation of the spinal muscles has had intermediate results. Surgical treatment is indicated when scoliosis is progressive despite adequate orthotic use or a severe degree of curvature is reached. Generally, if the curve measures more than 40°, orthoses are not likely to be effective. If curves approach 90° to

100°, respiratory function is severely compromised and operations become much more hazardous. Surgical decisions are based on the total functional involvement of the patient. The surgical principles in paralytic scoliosis include 1) spinal fusion is essential, 2) the site of arthrodesis for the spine should be as far lateral as the transverse process, and 3) the facet joints should be excised. Generally, both an anterior and a posterior spinal fusion produce the best results. When pelvic obliquity is present, the fusion should extend from the sacrum to the uppermost thoracic vertebra. The pelvic obliquity should be corrected as much as possible. The correction should always aim for compensation of the spine deformity with the occiput remaining directly over the sacrum. Note that correction should not be forced beyond the limits of passive mobility of the spine. Most approaches now include some sort of segmental spinal instrumentation for rotational control in combination with an anterior discectomy and fusion. Postoperative management may include no sitting for 5 to 6 days postoperatively. Orthotics may or may not be necessary depending on the type of fixation and the functional mobility level of the child.

MUSCULAR DISORDERS

Orthopedic management of neuromuscular dystrophies is based on an understanding of the pathokinesiology of neuromuscular diseases, which is essential to the proper timing of physical therapy, bracing, and operation.[2, 6, 16] Treatment of the muscular dystrophy is not limited to palliation but should include appropriately timed surgical intervention to change muscle balance, reduce deformity and contracture development, and preserve maximal physical capacity.

Many orthopedic surgical procedures have proved successful in reestablishing balance and maintaining mobility in selected patients.[2, 6, 8, 16, 17] The timing of these procedures is of prime importance. It is generally agreed that operative techniques should permit early postoperative mobilization and a minimum of resting and immobilization. Some children are poor anesthetic risks, particularly because of inadequate pulmonary reserve, the depressant effects of barbiturates on compromised pulmonary mechanics, cardiotoxic properties of anesthetic agents on a compromised myocardium, and possible malignant hyperthermia.

Principal functional loss is noted in the musculature of the limb girdles. The most severe contractures occur in muscles that span two joints or in those that exercise a postural function. Three muscle groups that limit ambulation are hip flexors, tensor fascia lata, and triceps surae. Several authors have reported a maintenance of ambulation in boys who have undergone a program of early tenotomy and myotomy. Various percutaneous and open operative techniques have been described. Early postoperative ambulation and mobilization are essential. Frequently, proper bracing is required to maintain independent ambulation for up to 5 years after operation.

Paralytic scoliosis is one of the most serious complications of muscular dystrophy. Spinal curvature appears to occur with increasing age and advancing disability. Its presence depends on the type of dystrophy. Generally, its progress is related to the severity of the disease. The paraspinal weakness is symmetric, and scoliosis is unusual in the well-balanced boy with Duchenne muscular dystrophy who is still ambulatory. As weakness of the back extensor and hip extension muscles increases, the classic posture is lumbar lordosis without scoliosis. Once weakness progresses to prevent ambulation, a scoliosis develops in almost all patients with Duchenne muscular dystrophy. These curves are generally rapidly progressive, and their major convexity is usually toward the dominant hand. Because an erect spine is necessary for proper sitting balance, various orthotics have been developed. Generally, children tolerate a thoracolumbar sacral orthosis or a sitting support orthosis until the curve reaches more than 40°. Once the curve is more than 40°, a relatively rapid progression continues that cannot be managed orthotically.

Surgical stabilization of the spine has been used in various neuromuscular disorders.[2, 6, 8, 16] Various segmental instrumentation and fusion techniques are used. The procedure is extensive and accompanied by significant blood loss. Complications are primarily pulmonary. There is a move to perform earlier spinal stabilization to minimize the pulmonary and cardiac complications.

Children with spinal muscular atrophy have a spectrum from slowly to rapidly progressive motor neuron disease. Generally, infants with Werdnig-Hoffmann disease (spinal muscular atrophy, type I) require little orthopedic surgical intervention because their life expectancy is significantly reduced. In Kugelberg-Welander disease (spinal muscular atrophy, type III), the emphasis is on early spinal stabilization using segmental technique, lower extremity tendon releases, and lightweight bracing to prolong weight bearing.

Patients with hereditary sensorimotor neuropathies have significant weakness of distal muscles. Classic foot deformities (champagne-bottle calves with high arches) are evident in Charcot-Marie-Tooth disease. They frequently require plantar fascia release, various tendon transfer techniques, and occasionally triple arthrodesis to prevent progressive foot deformities. Hammertoe and clawtoe surgical procedures, along with bunionectomies, are frequent in end-stage Charcot-Marie-Tooth disease for persistent painful foot deformities. Orthotics have some limited success because of the concurrent sensory abnormalities present in some of these disorders.

SPINAL DEFECTS

Myelodysplasia is the most frequent spinal disorder and one of the leading causes of disability in children. The cause of neural tube defects is unknown, but inheritance patterns indicate a multifactorial interaction of environment and genetic influences. Motor and sensory dysfunction is dependent on the degree and amount of neural tissue involved in the myelodysplasia. Hydrocephalus is present in about 90% of children affected with myelodysplasia and generally requires ventriculoperitoneal shunting. Accurate assessment of sensory and motor function is the basis for anticipating musculoskeletal paralytic deformity and formulating long-term and short-term objectives.

The principal goal of orthopedic operations is to ensure satisfactory joint alignment for sitting and stance posture.[2, 8, 15, 18] Vertebral and costal anomalies frequently accompany the spinal defect and contribute to further weakening of the stability of the vertebral column. By interfering with stable balance, stance, and sitting, severe scoliosis can compromise ambulation, pulmonary function, self-care, and wheelchair stability. Progressive curves require early application of an orthosis and frequently surgical stabilization. Scoliosis and kyphosis are primarily controlled with segmental instrumentation with fusion. Severe thoracolumbar kyphos deformities may require kyphectomy and subsequent surgical fusion and stabilization.

Major concerns involve the maintenance of symmetric hips with adequate mobility of the hip and knee joints. Later, soft tissue contractures develop as a result of muscle imbalance. Treatment initially involves passive range of motion and stretching exercises. If adequate range cannot be obtained, surgical intervention should be considered. Children with low thoracic lesions frequently have bilateral hip dislocation. They frequently have hip flexion, abduction, and external rotation deformities. Extensive surgical procedures are frequently required to relocate the hips, and they have limited long-term benefits to maintain desired position.[19] Contractures are frequently accompanied by poor acetabular cup development and may require significant surgical intervention, including varus derotational osteotomies and pelvic and acetabular procedures. Some authors believe that bilaterally dislocated hips in this level of dysfunction should not be surgically corrected.

With upper lumbar defects, the child frequently has hip flexion and adduction with dislocation of the hip. Iliopsoas as a primary hip flexor potentiates dislocation. Iliopsoas transfer has had inconsistent results. The patient frequently requires anterior soft tissue releases, femoral osteotomies, and muscle transfer to maintain hip position. The lowest recurrence rate is with an abdominal external oblique transfer to the greater trochanter in association with adductor recession to the ischial tuberosity and intertrochanteric varus osteotomy.

In the lumbar defect, there is a slow progression of hip flexion and an increase in lumbar lordosis. Late hip dislocation can be prevented by appropriately timed soft tissue release of the hip flexors. Children frequently have calcaneovalgus foot deformity, depending on the involved musculature. The foot deformities are frequently correctable by muscle transfer to balance the foot. Frequently, bony procedures may be required, including relocation of subluxation and triple arthrodesis.

The most common foot deformity, the clubfoot, is an inversion and adduction of the forefoot, inversion of the heel, and equinus (talipes equinovarus).[8, 12] Treatment should be started early. Most commonly, casting is used with changes every 2 to 3 weeks. Sequential casting first corrects the forefoot and the hindfoot. If the deformity is too rigid for correction within 4 to 5 months, surgical releases of the medial soft tissue and tendo-Achilles lengthening are needed.[6] If the hindfoot is not fully corrected, a triple arthrodesis may be needed at skeletal maturity.

Sacral deformities include minimal significant motor involvement. There may be some difficulties with a cavus foot or vertical talus causing a poor weight-bearing surface. Fixed vertical talus requires a talectomy. Cavus foot may require soft tissue releases.

ARTHROGRYPOSIS

Arthrogryposis multiplex congenita (multiple congenital contractures) is characterized by upper and lower extremity joint contractures and muscle weakness. This is frequently associated with causes of neuromuscular weakness such as central nervous system defects. A vigorous program of daily range of motion and stretching of the joints in addition to serial casting will improve joint range early in life. Most children require surgical myotomy and tenotomy for functional upper and lower extremities.

LEG-LENGTH DISCREPANCY

Leg-length discrepancy results from undergrowth or overgrowth, hip dislocations, pelvic obliquity, and contractures. Undergrowth frequently results from bony abnormalities, including dysplasias and traumas, or from neuromuscular abnormalities, such as cerebral palsy and poliomyelitis. Discrepancy from overgrowth follows fractures, septic arthritis, hemangioma, and neurofibromatosis. Serial scanography or computed tomography measures leg length more precisely than clinical measurements. This length can be plotted along with bone age according to the Greulich and Pyle tables.[4, 8] These tables predict remaining growth and can help with the appropriate timing of an epiphysiodesis of the longer extremity. Timed appropriately, treatment can compensate for discrepancies of 3 to 18 cm. Various leg-lengthening procedures have been developed, most recently the Ilizarov technique. This requires external skeletal fixation and can be used to lengthen long bones in the arm, forearm, thigh, and leg. Major complications include nonunion, infection, nerve injury, and hematoma.

REFERENCES

1. Falkner F, Tanner JM, eds. Human growth: a comprehensive treatise. 2nd ed. New York: Plenum Press, 1986.
2. Gans BM. Rehabilitation of the pediatric patient. In: DeLisa JA, ed. Rehabili-

tation medicine: principles and practice. Philadelphia: JB Lippincott, 1988:391–409.

3. Bleck EE. Orthopaedic management in cerebral palsy. Philadelphia: JB Lippincott, 1987.
4. Carroll NC. Assessment and management of the lower extremity in myelodysplasia. Orthop Clin North Am 1987; 18 no. 4:709–724.
5. Molnar GE, Gordon SU. Cerebral palsy: predictive value of selected clinical signs for early prognostication of motor function. Arch Phys Med Rehabil 1976; 57:153–158.
6. Molnar GE. Pediatric rehabilitation. Baltimore: Williams & Wilkins, 1985.
7. Bleck EE. Locomotor prognosis in cerebral palsy. Dev Med Child Neurol 1975; 17:18–25.
8. Staheli LT, guest editor. Common orthopedic problems. Pediatric Clinics of North America. Vol 33 no. 6. Philadelphia: WB Saunders, 1986:1269–1580.
9. Carpenter EB, Seitz DG. Intramuscular alcohol as an aid in management of spastic cerebral palsy. Dev Med Child Neurol 1980; 22:497–501.
10. Halpern D, Meelhuysen FE. Phenol motor point block in the management of muscular hypertonia. Arch Phys Med Rehabil 1966; 47:659–664.
11. Spira R. Management of spasticity in cerebral palsied children by peripheral nerve block with phenol. Dev Med Child Neurol 1971; 13:164–173.
12. Hensinger RN. Congenital dislocation of the hip: treatment in infancy to walking age. Orthop Clin North Am 1987; 18 no. 4:597–616.
13. Chung SMK. Hip disorders in infants and children. Philadelphia: Lea & Febiger, 1981.
14. Katz JF, Siffert RS, eds. Management of hip disorders in children. Philadelphia: JB Lippincott, 1983.
15. Horan F, Beighton P. Orthopaedic problems in inherited skeletal disorders. New York: Springer-Verlag, 1982.
16. Sutherland DH. Gait disorders in childhood and adolescence. Baltimore: Williams & Wilkins, 1984.
17. Siegel IM. Management of muskuloskeletal complications in neuromuscular disease: enhancing mobility and the role of bracing and surgery. Phys Med Rehabil: State of the Art Reviews 1988; 2 no. 4:553–575.
18. Shurtleff DB, ed. Myelodysplasias and exstrophies: significance, prevention, and treatment. Orlando: Grune & Stratton, 1986.
19. Crandall RC, Birkebak RC, Winter RB. The role of hip location and dislocation in the functional status of the myelodysplastic patient: a review of 100 patients. Orthopedics 1989; 12:675–684.

PART XII

Psychosocial Aspects of Disability

32

Psychologic Aspects of Disability

James F. Malec

This chapter briefly reviews the psychologic aspects of rehabilitation. Specific psychologic problem areas are discussed, followed by a brief summary of standardized assessment and treatment techniques.

PSYCHOLOGIC SEQUELAE

Psychosis

Persistent psychosis (disorganized thinking and behavior typically accompanied by hallucinations or delusions) is rare after the onset of disability. Persistent psychosis, if present, is most likely associated with severe premorbid personality disorder (for example, schizophrenia or schizotypal or borderline personality) or with brain injury. Even among brain-injured patients, psychotic episodes occur in only a small minority and are usually short-lived.

Transient, acute psychotic episodes may also occur among patients whose disability or treatment imposes long periods of sensory deprivation. Some patients with burns or spinal cord injuries must lie in a fixed position with little change in visual or auditory stimulation on a specially designed mattress that reduces tactile irritation (for example, a water bed, mud bed, or bead bed). These patients may experience a loss of reality contact in reaction to such sensory deprivation, as may patients who are deprived of sensation because of impaired peripheral vision, hearing, or touch.

Depression

Criteria for a major depressive episode and for dysthymia (neurotic depression), as defined by the American Psychiatric Association's *Diagnostic and Statistical Manual of Mental Disorders* (DSM-III-R), third edition-Revised,[1] are outlined in Table 32–1. Depression is more common than psy-

TABLE 32–1
Diagnostic Criteria (DSM-III-R) for Major Depressive Episode, Dysthymic Disorder, and Adjustment Disorder

Diagnostic Criteria for Major Depressive Episode
   A. At least five of the following symptoms have been present during the same two-week period and represent a change from previous functioning; at least one of the symptoms is either (1) depressed mood, or (2) loss of interest or pleasure. (Do not include symptoms that are clearly due to a physical condition, mood-incongruent delusions or hallucinations, incoherence, or marked loosening of associations.)
      (1) depressed mood (or can be irritable mood in children and adolescents) most of the day, nearly every day, as indicated either by subjective account or observation by others
      (2) markedly diminished interest or pleasure in all, or almost all, activities most of the day, nearly every day (as indicated either by subjective account or observation by others of apathy most of the time)
      (3) significant weight loss or weight gain when not dieting (e.g., more than 5% of body weight in a month), or decrease or increase in appetite nearly every day (in children, consider failure to make expected weight gains)
      (4) insomnia or hypersomnia nearly every day
      (5) psychomotor agitation or retardation nearly every day (observable by others, not merely subjective feelings of restlessness or being slowed down)
      (6) fatigue or loss of energy nearly every day
      (7) feelings of worthlessness or excessive or inappropriate guilt (which may be delusional) nearly every day (not merely self-reproach or guilt about being sick)
      (8) diminished ability to think or concentrate, or indecisiveness, nearly every day (either by subjective account or as observed by others)
      (9) recurrent thoughts of death (not just fear of dying), recurrent suicidal ideation without a specific plan, or a suicide attempt or a specific plan for committing suicide
   B. (1) It cannot be established that an organic factor initiated and maintained the disturbance
      (2) The disturbance is not a normal reaction to the death of a loved one (Uncomplicated Bereavement)
   Note: Morbid preoccupation with worthlessness, suicidal ideation, marked functional impairment or psychomotor retardation, or prolonged duration suggests bereavement complicated by Major Depression.
   C. At no time during the disturbance have there been delusions or hallucinations for as long as two weeks in the absence of prominent mood symptoms (i.e., before the mood symptoms developed or after they have remitted).
   D. Not superimposed on Schizophrenia, Schizophreniform Disorder, Delusional Disorder, or Psychotic Disorder NOS.
Diagnostic Criteria for Dysthymic Disorder
   A. Depressed mood (or can be irritable mood in children and adolescents) for most of the day, more days than not, as indicated either by subjective account or observation by others, for at least two years (one year for children and adolescents)

B.   Presence, while depressed, of at least two of the following:
   (1)   poor appetite or overeating
   (2)   insomnia or hypersomnia
   (3)   low energy or fatigue
   (4)   low self-esteem
   (5)   poor concentration or difficulty making decisions
   (6)   feelings of hopelessness
C.   During a two-year period (one-year for children and adolescents) of the disturbance, never without the symptoms in A for more than two months at a time.
D.   No evidence of an unequivocal Major Depressive Episode during the first two years (one year for children and adolescents) of the disturbance.
   Note: There may have been a previous Major Depressive Episode, provided there was a full remission (no significant signs or symptoms for six months) before development of the Dysthymia. In addition, after these two years (one year in children or adolescents) of Dysthymia, there may be superimposed episodes of Major Depression, in which case both diagnoses are given.
E.   Has never had a Manic Episode or an unequivocal Hypomanic Episode.
F.   Not superimposed on a chronic psychotic disorder, such as Schizophrenia or Delusional Disorder.
G.   It cannot be established that an organic factor initiated and maintained the disturbance, e.g., prolonged administration of an antihypertensive medication.

Diagnostic Criteria for Adjustment Disorder
A.   A reaction to an identifiable psychosocial stressor (or multiple stressors) that occurs within three months of onset of the stressor(s).
B.   The maladaptive nature of the reaction is indicated by either of the following:
   (1)   impairment in occupational (including school) functioning or in usual social activities or relationships with others
   (2)   symptoms that are in excess of a normal and expectable reaction to the stressor(s)
C.   The disturbance is not merely one instance of a pattern of overreaction to stress or an exacerbation of one of the mental disorders previously described.
D.   The maladaptive reaction has persisted for no longer than six months.
E.   The disturbance does not meet the criteria for any specific mental disorder and does not represent Uncomplicated Bereavement.

From American Psychiatric Association.[1] By permission.

chosis after the onset of disability, but it occurs in only a minority of cases. Fullerton et al.[2] found that 10% of patients with spinal cord injuries suffered a major depressive episode and 20% had a minor depression or a mixed affective disorder. Patterson and Foliart[3] reported that 18% to 25% of patients with multiple sclerosis experienced depression. Robinson et al.[4] reported that 26% of patients with stroke experienced major depression and 20%, minor depression during the acute period; they also noted that the prevalence of depression increased at 6 months after stroke. Malec et al.[5] found a similar incidence of major depression (30%) among patients with stroke during acute rehabilitation, and they identified three other common types of affective response to stroke: (1) emotional stability, (2) distress (that is, minor depression, adjustment disorder, or grief) without vegetative depressive symptoms, and (3) sleep or appetite disturbance without reported distress. Estimates of the incidence of major and minor depression after traumatic brain injury are not available. Clinical experience suggests that limited self-awareness and self-control pose more frequent problems than depression for patients with traumatic brain injury during acute rehabilitation and that depression becomes more prevalent after the acute phase.

Estimates of suicide after spinal cord injury range from 0.3% to 1.5%.[6] Although *active* suicide attempts or completions are easily identified, disabled or chronically ill persons may also invite *passive* suicide through noncompliance with medical recommendations. The incidence of passive suicide is difficult to estimate, but it may be one to two times that of active suicide.[6]

It is important to recognize that the incidence of depression after disability varies with social and environmental factors affecting the patient. For instance, the Mayo Clinic experience is that depression is not nearly as frequent after the acute phase in patients with stroke from rural areas and small towns who return to stable family and social networks as in the urban population studied by Robinson et al.[4]

Patients with certain central nervous system lesions causing pseudobulbar palsy may show a type of emotional uncontrol termed *pathologic laughing or crying* in the absence of significant depression. This disorder sometimes occurs in patients with stroke or multiple sclerosis. The patient may respond with laughter or tears without any subjective sense of strong emotion. In severe cases, even the production of speech may trigger a pathologic laughing or crying response. The neurologic mechanism responsible is poorly understood, but it is believed to be associated with anterior cerebral lesions possibly involving the basal ganglia.

Anxiety

Fears of specific things or situations (phobias) are uncommon after a disabling event, but they may occur, particularly in reaction to a traumatic experience. A person severely injured in a car accident, for instance, may experience debilitating anxiety when trying to enter a car. A patient who has fallen several times may begin to experience interfering anxiety during ambulation training.

Some patients become so anxious to do well in rehabilitation therapy that a high level of emotional arousal interferes with learning and performance. Performance anxiety may also result from fear of failure in specific performance situations.

Adjustment Reaction

A broad generalization is that about a third of patients experience depression or other severe psychologic disorder after the onset of disability, a third adjust to disability without any emotional or behavioral disturbance requiring professional attention, and a third experience mild adjustment problems. These mild affective disorders often fit the DSM-III-R category of adjustment disorder (Table 32–1). An adjustment disorder may be characterized primarily by depressive mood, anxiety, or inappropriate behavior.

Many adjustment problems and stressors affect the disabled patient. People often find self-worth and a means for dealing with stress in their activities. Disability may limit work, hobbies, and social and recreational activities and thus result in diminished self-esteem, boredom, or frustration. At the same time, the patient is prevented from engaging in activities that may have formerly provided a distraction from or a method of addressing such stress. Patients may need considerable time and support to discover new, rewarding activities.

Communication problems, sexual problems, and other disabilities that interfere with interpersonal relationships and intimacy can result in particularly severe stress. Disability and disfigurement can also produce self-consciousness and concerns about body image, more so for persons whose self-worth was based on physical beauty, strength, or skill.

Grief Reactions

Other mild affective or behavioral problems after becoming disabled do not clearly fit the DSM-III-R scheme. Some patients, for instance, seem to experience genuine grief for a lost body part, physical function, or activity. The grief does not seem inappropriate in degree and usually resolves if the patient is allowed a period of grieving.

A grief reaction is not a universal phenomenon after the onset of disability. At one point in the study of the psychology of rehabilitation, it was vogue to believe that, after becoming disabled, all persons went through a period of grief or through predictable stages of adjustment. Contemporary research, however, has failed to identify any predictable course or series of stages of emotional adjustment to disability.[6] Brasted and Callahan[7] reviewed stage theories of grief and presented an alternative behavioral model. The behavioral model describes grief as a process of extinction of response to the lost object. Extinction is a behavioral term that refers to the decrease and ultimate cessation of responses that no longer result in reinforcement (reward). Extinction is usually accompanied by emotional behavior. In the behavioral model, an initial, possibly universal, reaction of shock to the loss is assumed. After the initial shock, subsequent emotional reactions resulting from an extinction process (such as denial, depression, or anger) will vary greatly among individuals, depending on factors such as personality, experience with loss, and value of the lost object.

Denial

After brain injury, some patients are unable to recognize their illness (anosognosia) or to recognize an impaired body part (autotopagnosia). Such extreme denial rarely occurs on a purely psychologic basis, that is, as a defense against negative feelings associated with illness or disability.

When extreme denial does occur without brain injury, it raises a strong suspicion of premorbid personality disturbance.

Alternatively, many patients tend to minimize the permanence or consequences of their disabilities. Most contemporary clinicians believe this form of mild "denial" can be an effective means for emotional coping, particularly during the acute period after the onset of disability, and becomes problematic only if it interferes with participation in the rehabilitation process. At a time when medical and rehabilitation staff are often themselves uncertain about the ultimate degree of recovery that can be expected, the patient who does not have the background knowledge to appreciate the subtleties of medical prognosis often hopes for the best. Just as it may be appropriate for medical staff to advise patients of the possibility of a less-than-hoped-for outcome at this time, patients may appropriately be more optimistic. Their optimism allows them to find the energy to manage negative feelings, to learn more about their conditions, and to participate fully in the rehabilitation process.

Cognitive Impairment

In addition to nonrecognition of disability, brain-injured patients may show an array of impaired cognitive abilities that interfere with social functioning, such as poor concentration, language disturbance, visuoperceptual disturbance, confusion, poor judgment, impulsiveness, and limited self-awareness and social awareness, including sexual inappropriateness. Cognitive impairment may interfere with coping abilities and may be associated with episodes of significant distress.

Substance Abuse

Among drivers requiring emergency hospital treatment after a nonfatal automobile accident, 25% to 35% are intoxicated (that is, they have a blood alcohol level of 0.10% or more).[8] In a prospective study, Rimel[9] reported that ethanol was present in the bloodstream of 72% of 1,330 patients with central nervous system trauma and that 55% of these patients had a blood alcohol level of more than 0.10%. This relatively high percentage indicates the need for evaluation for substance abuse disorders among this patient group.

For the evaluation of substance abuse disorders, a distinction can be made between patients who are substance dependent or have a pattern of abuse and those who are not chemically dependent but were intoxicated at the time of an injury. Substance-dependent or substance-abusing patients typically show a pattern of regular, problematic use that interferes with occupational or social functioning. They often have a family history of substance dependency. Such patients are appropriately treated in traditional programs that emphasize total abstinence.

Nonalcoholics are not physically or psychologically dependent on alcohol. Their use of ethanol does not significantly interfere with work or social adjustment. In fact, an episode of irresponsible use leading to injury in these persons is often associated with a work or social function. The non-alcoholics who are intoxicated at the time of injury often resist traditional treatment because—with some justification—they do not see themselves as "alcoholic" or "hooked" and are unwilling to commit themselves to life-long sobriety. A behavioral treatment program emphasizing moderation and responsible use may be most appropriate for these patients. It must be emphasized, however, that differentiating the chemically dependent or substance-abusing patient who denies and minimizes the extent of use from the nonalcoholic with a history of intoxication is very difficult.

Personality

The DSM-III-R makes a valuable distinction between acute psychologic disorders (Axis I) such as depression or psychosis and more long-standing personality disorders (Axis II) evidenced in maladaptive coping and interpersonal styles. A thorough discussion of personality theory is beyond the scope of this chapter. However, an assessment by a psychologist or psychiatrist of personality style and of possible premorbid maladaptive personality tendencies can be invaluable for planning a rehabilitation program that maximally elicits the patient's cooperation and reduces interpersonal friction between patient and staff.

The possibility of a relationship between specific personality traits and specific disabilities is controversial. Shontz[10] presented the argument that personality traits are not associated with specific disabling illnesses or events. Rohe and Athelstan[11] and Malec[12] presented evidence that identifiable personality traits predispose patients to severe traumatic injury and must be considered in rehabilitation planning.

The person who is most likely to sustain a severe traumatic injury, such as a spinal cord injury, is likely to be an activity-oriented, risk-taking person who learns best by doing rather than through study and introspection. This type of person, whose traits resemble Eysenck's[13] description of extroversion, typically prefers occupations in which tangible effects are produced by physical labor. Because of their risk-taking behavior, persons with this sort of personality may rebel against the cautious, conservative restrictions of inpatient rehabilitation but eventually are more likely to adjust successfully to disability than persons who are less willing to try new things.[14] Frictions may develop between the more extroverted patient and staff, who often value introspection, conceptual thinking, caution, and careful planning. Such frictions can be avoided if rehabilitation planning is activity oriented and incorporates some planned "risks" that allow patients to test themselves. Often employed as a mechanic, plumber, welder, or carpenter, for example, patients with extroverted personality often find great difficulty in shifting vocational interests to less physically demanding occupations such as accounting or computer programming. Vocational counseling thus requires creativity in discovering occupations in which the more extroverted patient's limited physical abilities can still be used to produce a tangible (and marketable) product or service.

Family Reactions

Close family members may also experience significant affective or adjustment disorders after the onset of disability in a loved one. Spouses often find they must exchange responsibilities; for instance, a wife may become the primary wage earner and her disabled husband assume the role of homemaker and primary caregiver for the children. Such role reversals may result in loss of self-esteem, guilt, sexual problems, and affective distress for one or both partners.

Family members often find that a loved one who has sustained brain damage shows subtle—or not so subtle—changes in personality. Unlike when a loved one is lost in death, however, society offers no avenue for the family's grief. On the contrary, the family is expected to be overjoyed that the loved one has not died and to maintain love and responsibility for that person despite personality changes. Lezak[15] offered an excellent discussion of problems facing families after brain injury of a family member.

ASSESSMENT

As a supplement to the clinical interview, practitioners in clinical psychology and neuropsychology have developed methods for standardized assessment of various factors of psychologic functioning, including mood, acute psychopathology, personality, intelligence and cognitive functioning, interpersonal relationships, and vocational interests and aptitudes. Standardized assessment means that such procedures are conducted in a standard, invariable manner. Typically, results are then interpreted with reference to a normative group, usually a sample of persons whose age and sex are similar to those of the patient and who exhibit normal functioning. Selection, administration, and interpretation of standardized assessment instruments are technical enterprises for which qualified clinical psychologists have specialized training.

TREATMENT

Antidepressant medication is often of benefit to patients who meet criteria for a biologically based depression. Pathologic laughing or crying may be reduced with antidepressant medication given at doses lower than those typically recommended for treating depression, probably because of the dopamine agonistic, not the antidepressant, properties of the medication.[16] Levodopa has also been reported to decrease pathologic laughing or crying.[17]

Beck et al.[18] described an alternative treatment approach in which depressed patients are guided to rethink ideas that maintain depression, such as overgeneralized assumptions (for example, "no one cares about me" or "I can't do anything right") or selectively negative perceptions (for example, "I'm not making any progress in ambulation training" when the patient is making good progress in all other areas). Contemporary psychologic treatment involves increasingly sophisticated procedures and thus is best offered by or in consultation with a qualified psychiatrist or clinical psychologist. The most effective treatment for depression is often a combination of antidepressant medication and Beck's cognitive-behavioral approach. Medication reduces dysphoria and improves energy level during the initial stages, and therapy teaches improved self-control and the interpersonal skills needed to maintain adjustment.

Cognitive-behavioral therapy can also help people learn to make decisions, reassess life-styles, think constructively, and plan activities in order to resolve an adjustment disorder. Yet another approach that has been found to reduce dysphoria is systematically increasing pleasant and valued activities.[19] Active involvement in a comprehensive rehabilitation program offers many patients the opportunity to participate in various activities that they enjoy and value.

Resolution of grief requires a somewhat different approach involving the acknowledgment and experience of feelings related to loss in association with psychologic support.

Changing maladaptive personality traits may be accomplished in long-term psychodynamic psychotherapy, but it is usually an unrealistic goal for the relatively short period of inpatient physical rehabilitation. During inpatient rehabilitation, patients are typically focused not on psychologic but on physical change. Behavioral programs (in which desired behaviors are consistently rewarded and undesirable behaviors are not rewarded), behavioral contracts, or simple limit setting offers rehabilitation staff the avenues for restricting the expression of maladaptive personality tendencies and for increasing compliance with medical and rehabilitation treatment. To obtain cooperation from patients with less flexible and adaptable personalities, the rehabilitation staff must also adapt. In consultation with the staff psychologist, the rehabilitation team may attempt to elicit the patient's participation by accommodating their expectations and their own style of interpersonal interaction to those of the patient.

REFERENCES

1. American Psychiatric Association. Diagnostic and statistical manual of mental disorders. 3rd ed. revised. Washington DC: American Psychiatric Association, 1987.
2. Fullerton DT, Harvey RF, Klein MH, Howell T. Psychiatric disorders in patients with spinal cord injuries. Arch Gen Psychiatry 1981; 38:1369–1371.
3. Patterson MB, Foliart R. Multiple sclerosis: understanding the psychologic implications. Gen Hosp Psychiatry 1985; 7:234–238.
4. Robinson RG, Lipsey JR, Price TR. Diagnosis and clinical management of post-stroke depression. Psychosomatics 1985; 26:769–778.
5. Malec JF, Richardson JW, Sinaki M, O'Brien MW. Types of affective response to stroke. Arch Phys Med Rehabil 1990; 71:279–284.

6. Trieschmann RB. Spinal cord injuries: psychological, social, and vocational rehabilitation. 2nd ed. New York: Demos Publications, 1988.
7. Brasted WS, Callahan EJ. A behavioral analysis of the grief process. Behav Ther 1984; 15:529–543.
8. Lowenfels AB, Miller TT. Alcohol and trauma. Ann Emerg Med 1984; 13:1056–1060.
9. Rimel RW. A prospective study of patients with central nervous system trauma. J Neurosurg Nurs 1981; 13:132–141.
10. Shontz FC. Physical disability and personality: theory and recent research. In: Marinelli RP, Dell Orto AE, eds. The psychological and social impact of physical disability. New York: Springer-Verlag, 1977:105–129.
11. Rohe DE, Athelstan GT. Vocational interests of persons with spinal cord injury. J Counsel Psychol 1982; 29:283–291.
12. Malec J. Personality factors associated with severe traumatic disability. Rehabil Psychol 1985; 30:165–172.
13. Eysenck HJ. Dimensions of personality. London: Routledge & Paul, 1947.
14. Athelstan GT, Crewe NM. Psychological adjustment to spinal cord injury as related to manner of onset of disability. Rehabil Counsel Bull 1979; 22:311–319.
15. Lezak MD. Living with the characterologically altered brain injured patient. J Clin Psychiatry 1978; 39:592–598.
16. Schiffer RB, Herndon RM, Rudick RA. Treatment of pathologic laughing and weeping with amitriptyline. N Engl J Med 1985; 312:1480–1482.
17. Udaka F, Yamao S, Nagata H, Nakamura S, Kameyama M. Pathologic laughing and crying treated with levodopa. Arch Neurol 1984; 41:1095–1096.
18. Beck AT, Rush AJ, Shaw BF, Emery G. Cognitive therapy of depression. New York: Guilford Press, 1979.
19. Lewinsohn PM, Hoberman HM. Depression. In: Bellack AS, Hersen M, Kazdin AE, eds. International handbook of behavior modification and therapy. New York: Plenum Press, 1982:397–431.

33

Sexuality and Disability

Daniel E. Rohe

Concern about the sexual functioning of persons with disabilities began in earnest in the late 1960s in the United States. This concern was an outgrowth of various social forces operating at the time, such as the human rights movement, alternative life-styles, and increased societal willingness to examine sexual attitudes. During the early 1970s, an experiential learning program entitled Sexual Attitude Restructuring (SAR) was devised through the Glide Urban Center, an agency of the United Methodist Church, and implemented to help professionals examine their sexual beliefs and values. These programs helped raise consciousness about the topic of sexuality, and soon SAR workshops were devised for persons with physical disabilities.

The rehabilitation literature blossomed with articles expounding the importance of sexuality issues, commonly encountered sexuality concerns, and how to provide counseling.[1-3] The heightened interest in this area led to publication of the journal *Sexuality and Disability*.[4] Interest became so intense that rehabilitation professionals actually overestimated the importance of sexual function for recently disabled persons.[5] Addressing the sexuality concerns of disabled patients has now become a well-established and accepted part of comprehensive rehabilitation services.

The goal of this chapter is to provide a succinct overview of how sexuality is affected by the presence of a physical disability. The sexual response cycle and common sexual dysfunctions in nonphysically disabled persons are summarized, and the conceptual distinctions among sex drive, sex acts, and sexuality are delineated. Disabilities are classified according to their effect on sexual function, and associated interfering medical conditions are explained. For purposes of illustration, the sexuality concerns of persons with spinal cord injury, a disability affecting multiple areas of sexual functioning, are discussed. The topic of sexual counseling is also addressed.

SEXUAL RESPONSE CYCLE AND COMMON DYSFUNCTIONS

Understanding sexuality in physically disabled patients presumes a working knowledge of the sexual response cycle and common sexual difficulties encountered in nonphysically disabled persons. The work of Masters and Johnson demonstrated that male and female responses are similar and can be divided into four phases: excitement, plateau, orgasm, and resolution. The excitement phase occurs when psychologic or physical stimuli result in increased muscle tension, blood pressure, and heart rate. It is accompanied by penile erection or vaginal lubrication. During the plateau phase, maximal vasocongestion of the sexual organs occurs with additional increases in heart rate and blood pressure. Orgasm involves rhythmic contractions of the penis in men and the vagina in women and the perineal muscles in both sexes. The resolution phase involves return to the body's normal resting state.

Common male sexual difficulties include premature ejaculation, impotence, and retarded ejaculation. Common female sexual difficulties include preorgasmia, secondary orgasmia, dyspareunia, sexual aversion, and vaginismus. Various publications[6-8] have detailed descriptions of the sexual dysfunctions. Not infrequently, professionals fail to understand that persons with physical disabilities are subject to the same sexual dysfunctions as nondisabled persons. The treatment approaches are frequently similar, if not identical.

SEX DRIVE, SEX ACTS, AND SEXUALITY

A proper understanding of human sexuality requires careful differentiation among sex drive, sex acts, and sexuality.[9] Sex drive is a primary drive similar to others such as hunger, thirst, and avoidance of pain. These drives are innate and involve complex interrelationships among bodily receptors, hormone levels, and autonomic and central nervous system functions. Because the sex drive does not have immediate consequences for survival, other drives usually take precedence. For example, if a person is experiencing pain, the probability of the sex drive being expressed is greatly diminished. In a physically disabled person, difficulties with anxiety, pain, malaise, or fatigue may interfere with the sex drive.

Sex acts are behaviors that result in pleasurable sensations through contact with one's own or another person's body. Contact is most frequently made with the erogenous zones or genitals, which are maximally responsive to such stimulation. Yet, it is important to understand that many other areas of the body may provide pleasurable sensations. This fact is especially important for physically disabled persons, who may have reduced or absent sensation in certain areas of the body. The various human behaviors that result in pleasurable sensations are exceedingly diverse.[10] Sexual intercourse is but one of an infinite number of sex acts.

Sexuality can be defined as the expression of one's sex drive, through learned sex acts, within the context of the sexual identity of the person. Sexuality is more than sexual organs or sexual behaviors. Berkman et al.[11] described sexuality as a dynamic process grounded in developmental learning experiences and having three components. These components are the individual's self-concept, relationships with others, and specific repertoire of sexual behaviors. Sexuality is frequently confused with intimacy because physical closeness is often equated with psychologic closeness. Intimacy is a special state of mutual understanding, trust, and acceptance. Intimacy may or may not involve the satisfaction of a sex drive through sex behaviors. Although physical disability may interfere with sex drive and sex behaviors, the ongoing basic human need and capacity for intimacy remain.[3]

SEXUAL DYSFUNCTION IN DISABLED PERSONS

Sexual dysfunction in disabled persons can be categorized according to four causes. First, those constantly under the stress of pain, fatigue, or malaise may have decreased sexual activity due to a reduction in sex drive. A second cause of sexual dysfunction is limited learning opportunities involving sexual behaviors or the lack of social skills necessary for initiation and maintenance of relationships. Third, sexual dysfunction may arise because of bodily changes that directly interfere with the ability to either receive sexual pleasure or engage in previously learned sex acts. Examples include spinal cord injury, stroke, arthritis, and multiple sclerosis. Fourth, major changes in self-image, self-esteem, and body image may result in sexual dysfunction. These changes are especially likely with the sudden onset of disability.

For all of the above-mentioned conditions, the ultimate goal of the helping professional is to increase comfort with changes in sexual function and encourage a willingness to experiment with alternative methods of expressing one's sexuality. Persons with the fewest inhibiting attitudes and greatest willingness to use alternative methods have the most potential to achieve a satisfactory sexual life-style.

TYPES OF DISABILITY ACCORDING TO THEIR IMPACT ON SEXUAL FUNCTION

Cole and Cole[12] suggested that severe disabilities can be grouped into four types with respect to their impact on sexual function. Type I disabilities are nonprogressive and occur at birth or before puberty. Examples include congenital loss of sight or hearing, spina bifida, and mental retardation. Persons with these disabilities often fail to encounter the social learning opportunities associated with adolescent sexual development. This occurs for various reasons, including overprotective parents and societal ambivalence about sexuality training for developmentally disabled persons. The naive belief, associated with this group to an even greater degree than for nondisabled persons, is that sexuality education will be interpreted as an endorsement and thus increase the frequency of sexual behavior.

Type II disabilities also begin before puberty but are progressive. Examples include cystic fibrosis, muscular dystrophy, diabetes mellitus, and juvenile rheumatoid arthritis. Persons with these disabilities find it difficult to establish a stable body image and constantly face the uncertainty of further physical deterioration. As in the case of persons with type I disabilities, these persons frequently miss important socializing opportunities of a psychosexual nature.

Type III disabilities occur after adolescence and are nonprogressive. These stable, late-onset disabilities include spinal cord injury (discussed below), amputation, and burns. Affected persons have gone through the socializing experiences connected with adolescence and often have engaged in various sexual behaviors. They have developed the interpersonal skills required to initiate and maintain intimate social relationships, particularly of a sexual nature. After injury, their task is to adapt already developed skills in order to maximize the likelihood of a fulfilling sexual lifestyle.

Type IV disabilities include progressive degenerative diseases and are usually found in older adults.[13] These disabilities include arthritis, multiple sclerosis,[14] heart disease, stroke, cancer, and chronic renal disease. Affected patients usually have a long history of intimate relationships. They face the problem of coping with either a discrete event or slow deterioration that may impair their intellectual and physical ability to communicate sexually. Others face negligible impairments but may harbor fear of further losses should they engage in strenuous physical activity.[15] These fears coupled with the necessity of frequent medical interventions often result in marked changes in sexual behavior.

SEXUAL CONCERNS OF PERSONS WITH SPINAL CORD INJURY

Spinal cord injury is a disability with widespread impact in all areas of sexual functioning. Currently, more than 400,000 persons in the United States have a spinal cord injury. About four-fifths of these persons are male, and most are in their early twenties at the time of injury. Hohmann[16] provided data suggesting that male patients with spinal cord injury may have some reduction in sex drive, possibly due to disruption of the autonomic nervous system. Many of his subjects reported reduced sexual interest and fewer sexual feelings. The author concluded that the quality of the relationship with the partner becomes a critical issue in maintaining sexual activity after injury.

The sexual behaviors of male and female patients with spinal cord injury are often significantly altered by the disability.[17-20] Male patients have two types of potential erections after injury: psychogenic and reflexogenic. Psychogenic erections result primarily from mental stimulation and occur in approximately 30% of male patients with lower motor neuron lesions; they are absent in those with complete upper motor neuron lesions. Reflexogenic erections result when an external stimulus is applied to the genitals or pelvic area. These erections occur in 90% of male patients with upper motor neuron lesions. Rates of ejaculation have improved dramatically in recent years with use of techniques such as vibromassage[21] and electroejaculation. Those unable to achieve a usable erection have the option of obtaining a penile prosthesis; these have proved useful, and their reliability has steadily improved.[22, 23] Newer techniques for achieving erections include intracavernous injections of vasoactive substances and vacuum tumescence constriction therapy.

Male patients with a complete spinal cord injury frequently become infertile because of reduced sperm motility and viability. Fertility rates have improved in recent years because of advances in semen collection, but they still remain below those of males without cord injury.[21]

Women with spinal cord injury remain fertile; menstruation usually resumes 2 to 3 months after injury. Both sexes report the loss of orgasm as experienced before injury. Some describe the presence of a "phantom orgasm"; this consists of a buildup of muscle tension accompanied by pleasurable sensations in body areas that are still innervated followed by a feeling of relaxation. Sexual behaviors of persons with spinal cord injury are usually altered because of limitations in body movements. If the partner who incurs the injury was previously the most active, significant changes in roles may be needed. Sexual positions may have to be changed and new methods of stimulating the partner used.[17]

The effect of spinal cord injury on a person's sexuality and the resulting social and economic changes place tremendous stress on any already established relationship. Studies examining marriage among persons with spinal cord injury are confounded by several factors, including the amount of time since the onset of disability. Early studies of male veterans suggested that divorce rates were not significantly different from those of nondisabled persons.[24, 25] A recent study of a civilian sample, however, showed that persons with spinal cord injury have fewer marriages and more divorces than the general population.[26] Divorce was more likely if the person with spinal cord injury was young, female, black, childless, previously divorced, or more dependent in self-care activities. Data from another nonveteran sample suggested that persons who married after injury were happier and more satisfied than those married before injury.[27]

SEXUAL COUNSELING: PLISSIT MODEL

All physicians, physiatrists in particular, are in a central position to detect and provide help to patients with sexually related concerns. Persons who have sexually related difficulties typically turn to either their physician or their pastor. Until the relatively recent introduction of sexual medicine courses into the curriculum of medical schools, few physicians had any specific training to deal with these concerns.

Effective instruction with sexual concerns requires that physicians have a thorough understanding of their own sexual values, a knowledge of sexual function and dysfunction, and the interpersonal skills to establish rapport and obtain a sexual history. Wiens and Brazman[28] stated that taking a sexual history produces a therapeutic effect by giving the patient permission to be sexual, filling knowledge gaps, and providing reality-based feedback. Estimates are that as many as half of all sexual concerns can be ameliorated through the provision of information alone. Physicians are often ambivalent when asking about sexuality concerns. Annon and Robinson[6] described a simple yet useful model to help guide interventions for sexual concerns primarily related to response difficulties connected with orgasm, arousal, or desire. The system is the PLISSIT model or, more accurately, the P-LI-SS-IT model. The letters refer to three levels of brief therapy—permission, *l*imited *i*nformation, and *s*pecific *s*uggestions—and a fourth level of *i*ntensive *t*herapy.

The first and most basic level of intervention is permission. Often, disabled individuals seek a knowledgeable person in a position of authority to listen to their sexual concerns, reassure them that they are not unique or unusual, and, in most instances, provide permission to continue doing what they have been doing. This level of intervention may provide reassurance and affirm the individual as a sexual being. Permission is most appropriate when directed toward a patient's thoughts, fantasies, feelings, and sexual acts. Permission should be limited to activities that do not carry the risk of being dangerous or illegal.

Limited information entails provision of specific information relevant to a sexual concern. This level of intervention seeks to remove sexual myths that may be the basis of much anxiety and fear. Such myths might include issues such as genital size, masturbation, sexual frequency, and sexual performance. Disabled persons might need information about alternative methods of giving and receiving sexual pleasure, changes in sexual response secondary to disease or medications, and fertility. The focus of this intervention is on information directly relevant to the client's concerns.

The final level of brief therapy involves providing specific suggestions. The first step in this process is to obtain a limited history about the sexual problem. This history would include items such as a description of the problem, information about problem onset and course, the client's concept of cause and maintenance of the problem, past treatment outcome, and current expectations and goals of treatment. Once this history is obtained, specific interventions are provided that have proved helpful and usually reliable for ameliorating a particular problem. Descriptions of these interventions are available in standard texts of sexual therapy. These interventions are usually simple, have a behavioral focus, and emphasize the necessity to engage in practice sessions alone or with a partner at home.

Intensive therapy is usually initiated for sexual problems other than those related to sexual response, such as sexual identity problems. Because few persons require intensive therapy, physicians are less likely to encounter them. This level of intervention involves obtaining a comprehensive developmental history of the patient or partner or both. The goal is to define a person's sexual identity, behaviors, and fantasies thoroughly. Therapeutic intervention in such cases is usually lengthy, involves multiple areas of sexual functioning, and is usually done by a therapist having extensive training and appropriate credentials.

In summary, the PLISSIT model provides a method for conceptualizing appropriate levels of intervention for the physician. Given the likelihood that persons will expect their physician to be knowledgeable about sexual function, the physician must have appropriate self-knowledge and factual knowledge to guide the patient appropriately. All physicians working with physically disabled patients can achieve the skills needed for the first two levels of therapy—permission and limited information. Some may have further training and develop the skills needed to intervene at the third level—specific suggestions. Problems requiring intensive therapy require referral to appropriate sources.

REFERENCES

1. Eisenberg MG, Rustad LC. Sex education and counseling program on a spinal cord injury service. Arch Phys Med Rehabil 1976; 57:135–140.
2. Robinault IP. Sex, society, and the disabled: a developmental inquiry into roles, reactions, and responsibilities. Hagerstown, Maryland: Harper & Row, 1978.
3. Romano MD, Lassiter RE. Sexual counseling with the spinal-cord injured. Arch Phys Med Rehabil 1972; 53:568–572.
4. Daniels SM, Nowinski J. Sexuality and disability. Vol 1, Spring. New York: Human Sciences Press, 1978.
5. Hanson RW, Franklin MR. Sexual loss in relation to other functional losses for spinal cord injured males. Arch Phys Med Rehabil 1976; 57:291–293.
6. Annon JS, Robinson CH. Treatment of common male and female sexual concerns. In: Ferguson JM, Taylor CB, eds. The comprehensive handbook of behavioral medicine. Vol 1. New York: SP Medical & Scientific Books, 1980:273–296.
7. Lief HI, ed. Sexual problems in medical practice. Monroe, WI: American Medical Association, 1981.
8. Leiblum SR, Pervin LA, eds. Principles and practice of sex therapy. New York: Guilford Press, 1980.
9. Griffith ER, Trieschmann RB, Hohmann GW, Cole TM, Tobis JS, Cummings V. Sexual dysfunctions associated with physical disabilities. Arch Phys Med Rehabil 1975; 56:8–13.
10. Ford CS, Beach FA. Patterns of sexual behavior. New York: Harper & Brothers, 1951.
11. Berkman AH, Weissman R, Frielich MH. Sexual adjustment of spinal cord injured veterans living in the community. Arch Phys Med Rehabil 1978; 59:29–33.
12. Cole TM, Cole SS. Sexual adjustment to chronic disease and disability. In: Stolov WC, Clowers MR, eds. Handbook of severe disability. Washington

DC: United States Department of Education, Government Printing Office, 1981:279–288.

13. Schover LR, Jensen SB. Sexuality and chronic illness: a comprehensive approach. New York: Guilford Press, 1988.

14. Barrett M. Sexuality and multiple sclerosis. New York: National Multiple Sclerosis Society, 1982.

15. Tardif GS. Sexual activity after a myocardial infarction. Arch Phys Med Rehabil 1989; 70:763–766.

16. Hohmann GW. Some effects of spinal cord lesions on experienced emotional feelings. Psychophysiology 1966; 3:143–156.

17. Mooney TO, Cole TM, Chilgren RA. Sexual options for paraplegics and quadraplegics. Boston: Little, Brown & Company, 1975.

18. Narum GD, Rodolfa ER. Sex therapy for the spinal cord injured client: suggestions for professionals. Prof Psychol Res Pract 1984; 15:775–784.

19. Trieschmann RB. Spinal cord injuries: psychological, social, and vocational rehabilitation. 2nd ed. New York: Demos Publications, 1988.

20. Willmuth ME. Sexuality after spinal cord injury: a critical review. Clin Psych 1987; 7:389–412.

21. Yarkony GM. Enhancement of sexual function and fertility in spinal cord-injured males. Am J Phys Med Rehabil 1990; 69:81–87.

22. Beutler LE, Scott FB, Karacan I, Baer PE, Rogers RR Jr, Morris J. Women's satisfaction with partners' penile implant: inflatable vs noninflatable prosthesis. Urology 1984; 24:552–558.

23. Fallon B, Rosenberg S, Culp DA. Long-term followup in patients with an inflatable penile prosthesis. J Urol 1984; 132:270–271.

24. Comarr AE. Marriage and divorce among patients with spinal cord injury I. J Indian Med Prof 1962; 9:4353–4359.

25. El Ghatit AZ, Hanson RW. Marriage and divorce after spinal cord injury. Arch Phys Med Rehabil 1976; 57:470–472.

26. DeVivo MJ, Fine PR. Spinal cord injury: its short-term impact on marital status. Arch Phys Med Rehabil 1985; 66:501–504.

27. Crewe NM, Krause JS. Marital relationships and spinal cord injury. Arch Phys Med Rehabil 1988; 69:435–438.

28. Wiens A, Brazman R. A rationale and method for the sexual history in family practice. J Fam Pract 1977; 5:213–215.

PART XIII

Therapeutic Modalities

34

Therapeutic Heat and Cold

David C. Weber
G. Keith Stillwell

Therapeutic heat and cold generally are not considered cures but rather are most often valuable adjuncts to other therapies.

HEAT

The two general categories of therapeutic heat are superficial and deep.

Superficial heat does not penetrate more than several centimeters into the tissues. Through vascular activity, the heat is rapidly dissipated. Examples of superficial heat include hot water bottles, infrared heat lamps, electric heating pads, and hydrocollator packs. Although the actual temperature increases do not penetrate deeply with these particular devices, physiologic effects do occur beyond the depth of penetration. The deep-heating modalities, or "diathermies," include microwave, shortwave, and ultrasound. These can penetrate deeper into the tissues. Ultrasound penetrates the deepest. It can penetrate deep enough to heat a hip joint, for instance. Microwave is rarely used in diathermy applications and, therefore, we will not specifically address its indications and contraindications.

The physiologic effects of heat application include an increase in local metabolism, an increase in inflammatory response in the acute setting, and reflex vasodilatation with an increase in capillary flow leading to an increased supply of nutrients, antibodies, and leukocytes. There is increased capillary pressure leading to an increase in edema formation. If the application of heat is sufficient, cardiac output may increase. The pain threshold is elevated and, therefore, analgesia may result. Joint stiffness also may be reduced. Painful muscle spasm may be reflexly reduced. Connective tissue extensibility is increased (Fig. 34–1).

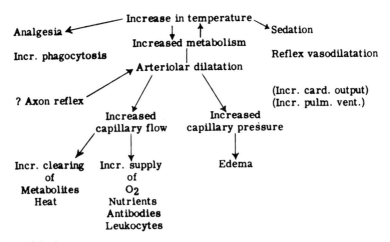

Figure 34-1
Physiologic effects of local heating: local effects that probably are not directly attributable to an increase in local metabolic rate (left) and systemic effects (right). card., cardiac; Incr., increased; pulm. vent., pulmonary ventilation. (From Stillwell GK. The use of physical medicine in office practice with particular emphasis on the aftercare of fractures. J Iowa Med Soc 1963; 53:12–18. By permission of the Society.)

The indications, therefore, for use of local heat include analgesia, increased cutaneous blood flow accelerating suppurative processes, sedation, and, after the acute phase, enhancing the resolution of hemorrhage and edema. Heat often is used primarily for relaxing the musculature in the area of concern before a specific exercise is applied.

Contraindications for the use of heat include impairment in the sensation of heat or pain. Other contraindications include obtundation or inability to provide feedback about the effects of heat (such as in persons who are very young or have an advanced infirmity), impaired cutaneous blood flow, noninflammatory edema, hemorrhagic diathesis (for example, a hemophiliac joint with active bleeding), acute trauma including sprains and bruises, ischemic tissue, local malignancy, and acutely inflamed joints or tissues. Heating a developing fetus should be avoided, as should deep heat in the area of the eyes or gonads.

The usual duration of heat application is from 15 to 30 minutes; an exception is ultrasound, which is typically applied for 5 to 10 minutes depending on the size of the area to be treated. Because the application of heat can be sedating and relaxing, precautions should be taken so that persons who fall asleep during treatment are not harmed by falls or burns. Caution should be maintained not to exceed the cardiorespiratory reserves of elderly or debilitated patients with the application of heat. Depending on the form used, a trial of up to 10 treatments or up to 2 to 3 weeks without therapeutic benefit should be considered an adequate trial of a particular form of heat. If no relief occurs, then a different therapeutic approach could be considered.

Shortwave is a form of diathermy in which the amount of energy that actually enters the patient cannot be accurately known. Therefore, normal sensation and ability to provide feedback are absolutely essential if this method is used. Further, shortwave cannot be used if metal is either imbedded in or in contact with the patient. Thus, it cannot be used in persons with total joint replacements, metal-containing intrauterine devices, or cardiac pacemakers. Also, jewelry must be removed from the patient. Beads of sweat should be absorbed by towels, and contact lenses must be removed. The patient should be on a wooden table during the treatment. Shortwave is, however, particularly helpful for heating large areas such as the back. Shortwave may increase the menstrual flow when applied in the area of the abdomen or low back; therefore, the patient should be advised of this possibility or therapy should be temporarily delayed during the menstrual period.

Ultrasound can be accurately quantified. However, because the area of the applicator head of the ultrasound unit does not heat, the patient must be attentive to changes felt deeper in the tissues. Ultrasound can be used with caution in the presence of metal. However, certain other compounds are often present in the vicinity of the metal for which ultrasound is contraindicated. For example, the methyl methacrylate and high-density polyethylene that may be present with certain total joint arthroplasties are considered by some to be contraindications for the use of ultrasound. Because ultrasound does penetrate deeply into tissues, it should not be used for acute low back pain secondary to a herniated disc. Heating of the edematous nerve root will lead to increasing swelling in an area compromised by compression of the nerve root. Ultrasound should not be used over fluid media such as the eye. Application of ultrasound directly over the spinal cord is not recommended. Laminectomy sites should be avoided because tissue interference will be less before energy induced by the ultrasound reaches the spinal cord. Ultrasound can be particularly beneficial when used simultaneously with gentle prolonged stretching of the tissue being heated. Ultrasound and other forms of diathermy are not recommended over epiphyseal growth centers in children. Ultrasound is to be avoided if a cardiac pacemaker is present in the area to be heated.

Figures 34–2, 34–3, and 34–4 demonstrate a few superficial and deep-heating methods.

Another form of heat application is hydrotherapy. Whirlpool tanks vary in size from small enough for one hand and arm to big enough for the entire body. The Hubbard tank is a butterfly-shaped form of whirlpool for total body submersion. Cautions with the use of hydrotherapy are much the same as those for general heat application. Some additional specific concerns include the need for monitoring vital signs and precautions regarding cardiovascular demands for total body submersion of the ill or elderly. The use of sterile water should be specifically requested when necessary. A "physiologic" salt solution needs to be specifically requested when the extent of the wound is such that the patient's electrolyte balance may be upset with exposure to nonphysiologic fluids. With the use of hydrotherapy in either a whirlpool or a Hubbard tank, the temperatures

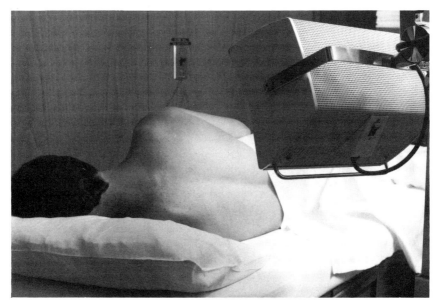

Figure 34–2
Patient receiving radiant heat to upper part of back.

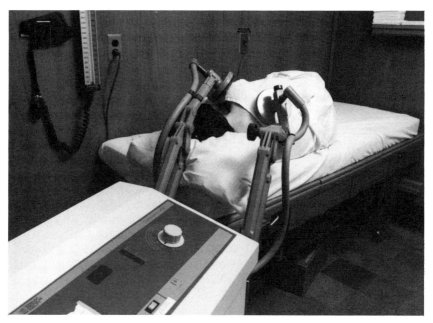

Figure 34–3
Patient receiving shortwave diathermy (drum) to shoulder.

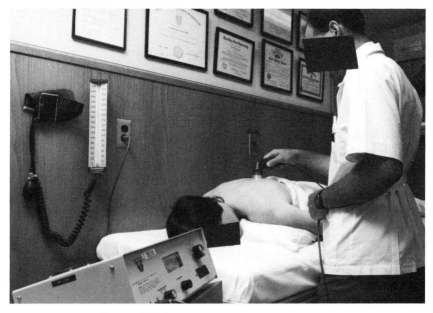

Figure 34–4
Patient receiving ultrasound to paraspinal muscles.

should be specified. Temperatures used range from approximately 90° to 104° F depending on the therapeutic intent and physiologic condition of the patient. Typical whirlpool temperatures could be 100° to 102° F for legs unless circulation is poor, in which case a more neutral temperature, in the range of approximately 95° F, would be more prudent. For the upper extremities, a higher temperature, in the range of 100° to 105° F, may be used unless an operation has been recently performed on the hand or edema is already present, in which case 95° F or less is recommended. The temperature for the Hubbard tank for total body submersion should be kept in the mild range, 98° to 99° F. Other forms of hydrotherapy include walking tanks, in which a patient can walk yet remain partially submerged. Therapeutic swimming pools and fine-water jet streams at room temperatures to assist with debriding and cleansing of wounds are other possibilities. Fluidotherapy is a means of providing relatively high heat in a dry environment. Fluidotherapy units typically have some form of particulate matter such as corn-cob granules that flow in hot air and blow or flow around the area to be heated. Hydrotherapy may be in the form of a contrast bath, in which the immersion of the hand is alternated in hot (110° F) and cold (65° F) water. The extremities are first immersed in the hot water for 10 minutes, then alternating cold water for 1 minute, then hot water for 4 minutes. Treatment is completed with immersion in the hot water. The total duration of treatment is 30 minutes.

Another form of therapeutic heat that is typically used for hands is paraffin with mineral oil baths. This is used for various arthritides and scleroderma problems. The hand is dipped in the heated paraffin and mineral oil mixture and removed after repeated dipping; it is then wrapped in a towel. Dilution of the paraffin with mineral oil (6 parts solid paraffin to 1 part mineral oil) lowers the specific heat of the mixture, such that higher temperatures (126° to 128° F) can be tolerated.

COLD

The physiologic effects of cold include decreased local blood flow secondary to vasoconstriction, slowing and eventually blocking of nerve conduction, reduction in spasticity, reduction in muscle spasms, decrease in local metabolism, decrease in collagen extensibility, decrease in the formation of local edema, decrease in inflammatory response, and decrease in pain sensation. Therefore, indications for the use of cold include reducing extravasation of blood and fluids entering the tissues after acute trauma, analgesia, reduction in spasticity, and reduction of muscle spasm.

Typically, the duration of cold application is 15 to 30 minutes, unless a technique of ice massage is used. For ice massage, ice is placed directly in contact with the patient, and it is applied for only 5 to 7 minutes.

Contraindications to the use of cold include impaired sensation, hypersensitivity with wheal formation, Raynaud's phenomenon, previous frostbite, impaired local circulation or ischemia, cryoglobulinemia, paroxysmal cold hemoglobinuria, and marked cold pressor response. Typically, cold is helpful for reducing edema, pain, and bleeding during the first 12 to 24 hours after an acute trauma. After approximately 48 to 72 hours, however, superficial heat may accelerate resolution of the hemorrhage and edema.

Examples of cold application include ice massage for 5 to 7 minutes, in which ice is placed directly in contact with the area to be treated and moved in a circular motion until the sensation of numbness occurs. Crushed ice can be placed in a container to form an ice pack; it is placed on the area to be treated for 15 to 30 minutes. Dry cold packs from the freezer should be wrapped in toweling and not placed in direct contact with the skin. Evaporation, accomplished by spraying ethyl chloride, can sometimes be helpful. An ice and water slurry may be particularly helpful for an acute sprain.

REFERENCES

1. Lehmann JF, de Lateur BJ. Diathermy and superficial heat, laser, and cold therapy. In: Kottke FJ, Lehmann JF. Krusen's handbook of physical medicine and rehabilitation. 4th ed. Philadelphia: WB Saunders, 1990:283–367.
2. Stillwell GK. Therapeutic heat and cold. In: Sinaki M, ed. Basic clinical rehabilitation medicine. Philadelphia: B.C. Decker, 1987:63–66.

35 | Therapeutic Electricity

Gudni Thorsteinsson

Within the field of physical medicine and rehabilitation, electricity is used for activating muscles and controlling pain. The use of electricity for stimulating specific organs (for example, the heart or urinary bladder) is not discussed in this chapter.

MUSCLE ACTIVATION

Electricity is used to activate muscle through either its nerve supply (innervation intact) or the muscle itself when the nerve supply has been interrupted (denervated muscles).

The amount of electricity (voltage or amperage) needed to stimulate a nerve is much less than that needed to stimulate a muscle directly, and it is also less painful to stimulate a nerve. The effectiveness of electrical stimulation is a function of the rate (frequency) and duration of the stimulus and the magnitude of its change. The minimal duration of an effective stimulus for a nerve is about 0.03 msec and that for a muscle, 1 msec.

Nerve Supply Intact

The indications for electrical stimulation include (1) phrenic nerve stimulation (for example, cases of spinal cord injury above the C-4 segment),[1, 2] (2) electrophysiologic orthosis (for example, in cases of cerebrovascular accidents or spinal cord injury with loss of central motor control),[2-5] (3) spasticity control (for example, in cases of multiple sclerosis, spinal cord injury, or stroke),[2, 3] (4) treatment of scoliosis,[1, 3] (5) neuromuscular reeducation and sensory-motor retraining,[2, 3] (6) fecal incontinence,[3] (7) urinary incontinence,[3] and (8) electroejaculations.[3]

This type of stimulation is used to activate muscles that have lost control from the higher central nervous system but the nerve supply from the spinal cord is intact. For example, phrenic nerve stimulation for respiration is used in cases of spinal cord injury higher than the C-4 level; the diaphragm still has its nerve supply through the phrenic nerve originating below the spinal cord lesion. The same type of electrical stimulation is applied in functional electrical orthosis. The stimulation of muscle with an intact nerve supply may also be used for muscle reeducation. For example, this type is used in cases of disuse atrophy of muscle after trauma, orthopedic procedures, tendon transfers, and tendon repairs. The objective of stimulation is to facilitate and restore mobility, strength, control, endurance, speed, and precision.

The mode of application depends on the condition being treated. The electrode may be implanted, as in the case of phrenic nerve stimulation and some of the electrophysiologic orthoses, or surface electrodes can be used. The intensity, frequency, and duration depend on the condition being treated and differ from one patient to another. They are determined by the function or results one is trying to obtain. For example, rhythmic contractions can be used to obtain different types of function such as breathing, walking, or changes in muscle tones for spasticity control. Surface electrical stimulation of the paraspinal muscles on the apex site of the curve is used to treat scoliosis of 20° to 40° (Cubb); 77% of curves improve or are maintained when treated to bone maturity.[1]

Electrical stimulation is being used for endurance training in patients with spinal cord injury[2, 6] and for strengthening in intact neuromuscular systems.[7]

Denervated Muscle

Denervated muscle can be stimulated by the bipolar method.[3] One electrode is applied over the muscle origin, and the second electrode is at the distal musculotendinous junction. Another method that can be used is the monopolar method, which stimulates the motor points of the muscles. Electrical stimulation has been used to retard denervation atrophy, but recent studies question the benefits.[8] Its effectiveness in such cases depends on the duration, frequency, and intensity used, the electrode placement, and the duration and number of treatment sessions. The therapeutic stimulation should be both isometric and isotonic to obtain maximal results. A rest period of more than 10 minutes is optimal between stimulations.

ANALGESIA[9, 10]

The physiologic basis for the use of electrical stimulation to control pain is the modulation (change) of pain sensation. This occurs at the spinal cord level (dorsal horn) or diencephalon (thalamus). Innocuous stimulation is activated by the use of electrical stimulation, and, at the same time, modulation is achieved by closing the pain gate or overbalancing the scales of modulation in disfavor to the pain. Also, electrical stimulation activates some brainstem reticular nuclei, which activates descending pain control fibers. One type of electrical stimulation also activates the endorphin system, which favors pain control.

Various types of electrical stimulation are used for pain control. One of these is high-frequency transcutaneous electrical nerve stimulation (hi-TENS or traditional TENS). This term is a misnomer because the frequency is less than 200 Hz, but it is used to distinguish it from low-frequency TENS of 1 to 2 Hz. Low-frequency TENS (low-frequency, high-intensity TENS or acupuncture-like TENS) is another type of electrical stimulation used for pain control. High-voltage galvanic stimulation (high-voltage, high-peak current [HVHPC] or Microdyne stimulation) and interferential therapy (medium frequency; 4,000 Hz) are electrical stimulations that have been used recently.

Basically, two types of modulation are being achieved. One activates the thick myelinated fibers (hi-TENS) and causes modulation at the spinal cord, brainstem, and thalamus levels, and the other, which is not as comfortable (low-TENS), involves endorphin activation. Electrical stimulation can be used to control chronic and acute pain. Originally, it was mainly used for chronic pain, but its use for acute pain has gained popularity because the more penetrating stimulation (HVHPC and interferential therapy) also seems to reduce edema, which is so often associated with acute pain that occurs with trauma or postoperatively. Electrical stimulation should not be used with a cardiac pacemaker when it might affect it.

Electrical stimulation has especially been used for neurogenic pain located in the periphery (for example, chronic painful peripheral neuropathy). It has also been used with reasonable results for chronic myofascial pain syndromes, low back pain syndromes, cancer pain, and arthritis. It has not proved successful for controlling central pain.

To control acute pain, electrical stimulation has been used postoperatively and has decreased atelectasis after thoracic operation and decreased ileus associated with abdominal operation. Its application has been shown to decrease the use of narcotics and allowed earlier ambulation when used after orthopedic operation.

Thorough evaluation of patients before prescribing electrical stimulation is important because other conditions such as depression may be present and may need special attention. Electrical stimulation is rarely prescribed alone but is used in combination with other physical therapy measures, such as exercises and training for relaxation, conditioning, and proper posture.

The efficacy of electrical stimulation is usually partial relief (25% to 90%), although complete relief is not uncommon, especially when the stimulation is first introduced. There is a definite placebo effect, but it is not different from that associated with other therapies used to control pain. A definite decline in efficacy occurs over time when treating chronic pain.

The stimulation is applied either over a nerve innervating the area or over the area of pain. Most often the stimulation is used two to three times per day, but sometimes it is used continuously or under certain circumstances when pain is increased, such as while working.[3, 9]

REFERENCES

1. Herbert MA. The treatment of scoliosis using electrical stimulation of muscle. IEEE Eng Med Biol Mag, September, 1983; 43–49.
2. Weber RJ. Functional neuromuscular stimulation. In: DeLisa JA, ed. Rehabilitation medicine: principles and practice. Philadelphia: JB Lippincott, 1988:295–306.
3. Jacobs SR, Jaweed MM, Herbison GJ, Stillwell GK. Electrical stimulation of muscle. In: Stillwell GK, ed. Therapeutic electricity and ultraviolet radiation. 3rd ed. Baltimore: Williams & Wilkins, 1983:124–173.
4. Petrofsky JS, Phillips CA. The use of functional electrical stimulation for rehabilitation of spinal cord injured patients. Central Nervous System Trauma 1984; 1:57–73.
5. Merritt JL. Knee-ankle-foot orthotics. In: Redford JB, ed. State of the Art Reviews, Orthotics. Philadelphia: Hanley & Belfus, 1987:67–82.
6. Phillips CA, Petrofsky JS, Hendershot DM, Stafford D. Functional electrical exercise: a comprehensive approach for physical conditioning of the spinal cord injured patient. Orthopedics 1984; 7:1112–1123.
7. Kramer JF. Muscle strengthening via electrical stimulation. Crit Rev Phys Rehabil Med 1989; 1:97–133.
8. Herbison GJ, Jaweed MM, Ditunno JF Jr. Exercise therapies in peripheral neuropathies. Arch Phys Med Rehabil 1983; 64:201–205.
9. Thorsteinsson G. Electrical stimulation for analgesia. In: Stillwell GK, ed. Therapeutic electricity and ultraviolet radiation. 3rd ed. Baltimore: Williams & Wilkins, 1983:109–123.
10. Basford JR. Physical agents. In: DeLisa JA, ed. Rehabilitation medicine: principles and practice. 2nd ed. Philadelphia: JB Lippincott, 1993:404–424.

36

Biofeedback

Gudni Thorsteinsson

Biofeedback (BFB) is a part of a treatment process in which a biophysical function is recorded and then displayed to the individual. The function can thus be better perceived and gainfully manipulated by the individual.

Various functions can be recorded. In this chapter, some of the many BFB applications are mentioned as they relate to management of the patient in physical medicine and rehabilitation.

The most common function recorded is skeletal muscle activity. Other functions used in BFB are limb motion, skin temperature, brain activity, blood pressure, cardiac function, and respiratory function.[1] The method used to record muscular activity is electromyography. In clinical practice, this is done by surface electrodes. Basmajian,[2] one of the pioneers in BFB applications, gave a vivid account of this method in his book *Muscles Alive*. Other methods used to record functions include electrocardiography, electronic goniometry, and electroencephalography.[1]

Significant advances in the electronic field have made recording function (that is, skin temperature, blood pressure, ventilation), amplification, and display simple, reliable, and economical. The method of display is usually visual or auditory, but it can be by other means. BFB is usually done in combination with other treatments. These could include patient education, relaxation techniques, therapeutic exercises, and medications. This combination therapy has significantly hampered pure, unbiased evaluation of BFB.

BFB is indicated in multiple conditions.[1, 3] In relation to skeletal muscle functions, BFB may be used to decrease muscle activity, such as in tension headaches, tension myalgias, pelvic floor tension myalgias, muscle incoordination, some types of urine bladder dysfunction, and muscle spasticity. It also may be used to increase muscle activity for muscle reeducation, such as in partial paralysis from upper motor neuron disease, lower motor neuron disease, disuse atrophy, or urinary stress incontinence or bowel incontinence.

In these applications of BFB, mainly voluntary function is recorded and modified. BFB is also used to record involuntary function. The manipulation used to improve the function is then originally imaginary, and a trial-and-error type of approach is used to obtain the desired response. Conditions in which this approach is used include temperature elevation in Raynaud's disease and blood pressure elevation in orthostatic hypotension associated with spinal cord injury.

BFB training requires that the patient be motivated and have an ability to learn. It also requires trained physicians and therapists. It is time-consuming. Usually three sessions are needed for the patient to understand the concept, and the treatment may last months. BFB equipment varies according to its point of application in the process and the sophistication of the treatment. Complex multichanneled equipment is used for scanning various functions and to provide printouts, and more simple equipment is available for home treatment.

In the field of physical medicine and rehabilitation, BFB has established itself as a significant addition in the treatment of various conditions.[1, 4]

REFERENCES

1. Basmajian JV. Biofeedback in rehabilitation medicine. In: DeLisa JA, ed. Rehabilitation medicine: principles and practice. Philadelphia: JB Lippincott, 1993:425–439.
2. Basmajian JV. Muscles alive: their functions revealed by electromyography. 4th ed. Baltimore: Williams & Wilkins, 1978.
3. Basmajian JV. Biofeedback in rehabilitation: a review of principles and practices. Arch Phys Med Rehabil 1981; 62:469–475.
4. Brucker BS. Biofeedback in rehabilitation. In: Golden CJ, ed. Current topics in rehabilitation psychology. Orlando, FL, Grune & Stratton, 1984:173–199.

PART XIV

Ambulatory Rehabilitation and Provisional Devices

37

Wheelchair Prescriptions and Types of Wheelchairs

Neil E Miller

In the wheelchair industry, the wheelchair is no longer the "wheelbarrow" that was used 10 to 20 years ago. Today's wheelchair is a sophisticated piece of equipment deserving the same care and fitting of a lower-extremity orthosis. Indeed, the wheelchair of today could be considered a lower-extremity orthosis. No longer can we call the local vendor with a request for an adult-width chair or a narrow adult chair and "call it good." Historically, in the 1970s, a lightweight rigid wheelchair was developed. This chair was designed with wheelchair sports in mind; however, the users soon decided they preferred pushing a 25-lb rigid chair in place of the 50-lb chair for everyday use. From these beginnings mushroomed the lightweight wheelchair industry of today. Manual wheelchairs are not the only type that has undergone significant change. Power, or electric, wheelchairs have become increasingly sophisticated also. The power wheelchair of the 1970s bears only superficial resemblance to the power wheelchair of today. Microswitches and minicomputers are important constituents of the power chairs currently in use. Power tilt or orientation-in-space features, as well as power reclining without shearing, are all common features. The purpose of this chapter is to provide the health practitioner with an overview of the currently available chairs and their prescription.

Two features are common in all chairs, regardless of variety: fit and posture. These two subjects will be addressed before the specifics of various chair models are discussed.

WHEELCHAIR FIT

The areas of wheelchair fit to be considered are back height, armrest height, seat width, seat depth, seat height from the floor, and footrest adjustment.

Back Height

From the top of the chair, back height is best adjusted to approximately 1.5 inches below the inferior angle of the scapula. Another method is to identify this height as approximately 4 inches below the axilla. Either approach is appropriate. Naturally, persons with considerable disability and trunk instability need more back height. Those with the least disability will do well with backs that are considerably lower. A height 1.5 inches below the inferior angle of the scapula allows most chair users adequate freedom of the shoulders and adequate scapular mobility to allow easy propulsion of the chair as well as stability of the chair.

Armrest Height

This feature is relatively easy to measure because most chairs have adjustable armrests. Thus, the final adjustment can be made after the user is in the wheelchair. However, some wheelchairs are still manufactured with armrests of fixed height, and this height should be specified at the time of the wheelchair prescription. This height is measured with the patient seated in a wheelchair on the appropriate cushion, and the arm is relaxed at the patient's side with the elbow bent at 90°. A measurement is then taken from the wheelchair seat to the elbow, and 1 inch is added to this height for the prescription.

Seat Width, Depth, and Height

The widest part of the patient is measured and then 1 to 2 inches is added to the measurement to obtain the appropriate seat width. Some consideration must be given to the stability of this width in each patient. For example, in a child who can be expected to grow rapidly or in a person who has lost a great deal of weight as a result of disability, it may be necessary to order a chair that is slightly wider than the determined measurement. However, it must be remembered that increases in seat width also increase the overall width of the wheelchair.

In conjunction with seat width, seat depth must also be considered. The seat depth must give maximal coverage to the buttocks and thighs without impinging in the popliteal space. Consequently, the seat upholstery should end approximately 2 to 3 inches from the popliteal space. Seats that are too short do not provide enough surface area to support a cushion adequately and, therefore, protect the skin from possible breakdown. If the seat depth is too great, the potential for pressure in the popliteal space and skin breakdown in this area is certainly present.

Seat height is another consideration at the time of prescription. Determination of cushion type must be made at this time (if it has not been made previously) because this will make a difference in the overall seat height. With this in mind, the seat height must give a minimum clearance of 2 inches when the foot plates are properly adjusted.

Footrest Length

For proper footrest adjustment, the feet are well supported on the foot plates and the thighs have good contact with the cushion at all points without increasing the pressure at the distal femur (which occurs when the footrest is too low) or the ischial tuberosities (which occurs when the foot plates are too high). The minimal clearance of foot plates is 2 inches; 3 inches is probably a better adjustment for active users, particularly those who will use their chairs on uneven surfaces.[1-5]

POSTURE

Even with a properly fitted wheelchair, care must be taken to ensure that the user maintains appropriate posture while in the chair and while propelling the wheelchair. For good posture, the buttocks are well back in the wheelchair and weight is evenly distributed on both ischial tuberosities. The pelvis should, therefore, be level. Every effort should be made to maintain the normal curves of the spine, that is, there is some slight lordosis, the head is balanced on the column of the neck without any forward thrusting or severe lordosis of the cervical spine, the arms rest comfortably on the armrest, hand placement on the push rims is in a comfortable natural position, and the feet rest comfortably and firmly on the foot plates.

WHEELCHAIR TYPES

Undoubtedly, the most commonly prescribed wheelchair is a manual wheelchair. During the early 1970s, the wheelchair industry underwent a major transformation. For years, the folding manual wheelchair (Fig. 37–1) was the industry standard. However, users began to demand, or look for, a much lighter-weight wheelchair. These chairs were first manufactured in California as a rigid, nonfolding, but very lightweight wheelchair. Users gave up their folding, but heavy, wheelchairs in favor of these lightweight models. These were followed by folding lightweight chairs (Fig. 37–2). The wheelchair of the 1980s is not only foldable and lightweight but also extremely maneuverable and convenient for the user to lift into an automobile. The heavier folding versions are still available. These chairs are extremely durable and will last a long time. However, users are much more attracted to the features of the lightweight chairs, and these are available in a wide price range as well as a wide range of features and designs.

USERS

Users of manual wheelchairs are as varied as the chairs themselves. In general, those with impaired ability to walk; those with no ability to walk

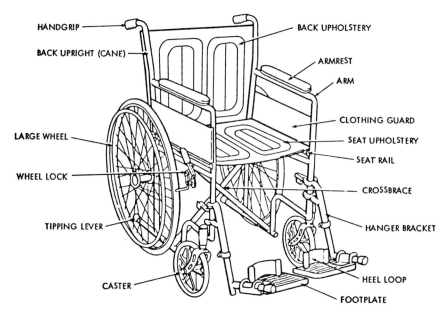

Figure 37–1
Components of folding manual wheelchair. (From The professional wheelchair contact.[7] By permission.)

at all, either because of paralysis or limb loss; or those with greatly impaired endurance levels because of cardiovascular disease are appropriate candidates for a manual wheelchair.

SPECIFICATIONS

Manual wheelchairs come in a wide variety of types and styles as well as weights. The chairs, whether lightweight or conventional, have a standard version. The standard type generally has a back height of 16.5 inches, a seat depth of 16 inches, a seat height of 19 to 20 inches, and a crossframe to allow folding of the chair. Another variety of chair that is frequently used, particularly in a rehabilitation setting, is a low-seat chair. This is often referred to as a hemichair. The seat height from the floor is 2 inches less than the standard type (that is, approximately 17 to 18 inches from the floor). This distance allows the person with some lower-extremity function (for example, a hemiplegic) to propel the wheelchair. Low-seat chairs also have a crossframe and so can be folded.

Lightweight chairs come in two styles: conventional crossframe folding models and rigid chairs that are little more than four wheels with a minimal amount of framework. Rigid chairs should not be dismissed as an everyday wheelchair. Many active users find a rigid chair just as convenient as a folding chair. The use of a rigid chair in a daily setting requires a dif-

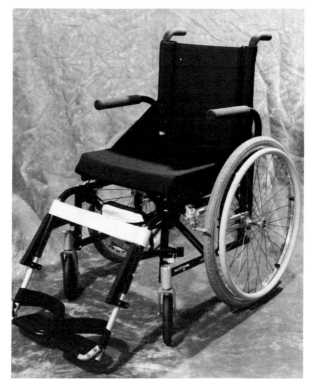

Figure 37–2
Lightweight, daily-use wheelchair.

ferent method for placing the chair into an automobile. The rigid chair can easily be placed into the backseat of most automobiles by removing the quick-release wheels, which are generally available on most chairs, and folding the back down. Choosing a rigid chair over a folding chair is much like choosing a sports car over a conventional car. In many ways, the rigid chair is the high-performance chair, probably due to the fact that all pushing energy is transmitted directly to the wheels and to propelling the chair. With any crossframe-style chair, energy is lost to torque in the crossframe. However, the convenience of transporting a folding chair weighs heavily in favor of crossframe models, and with recent improvements in design, performance of these chairs is approaching that of rigid chairs.

POWER WHEELCHAIRS

Power wheelchairs can be divided into three categories. The first type is the regular or conventional power wheelchair; this has large rear wheels and smaller 8-inch caster wheels. This is the most common configuration of power wheelchairs.

The second category is the power-base wheelchair. This type has the power source, drive mechanisms, and module directly under the seat and covered by a plastic shroud. The power-base chairs have smaller wheels of approximately the same size all around. Usually these wheels are 8 to 10 inches in diameter and 3 inches in width. The seat on a power-base wheelchair is positioned directly above the power base on a pedestal.

The third type of chair is the three-wheeler or scooter. This is made by several companies. The wheels are 6 inches in diameter; there are two wheels in the rear and a third wheel in the front. The chair has a molded fiberglass-type seat that is not readily adjustable, and the chair comes with or without armrests. Forward, reverse, and stop controls are all located on a tiller mechanism positioned above the front wheel.

Conventional

This type is generally operated by a joystick located under either the right or the left hand and attached to the armrest of the chair (Fig. 37−3). Generally, the chairs are based on a 24-volt system, needing charging on a daily basis. These chairs are reliable and give a range of approximately 20 miles during the course of a day. Options available on these chairs are diverse. Recline mechanisms (Fig. 37−4), tilt-in-space mechanisms, and el-

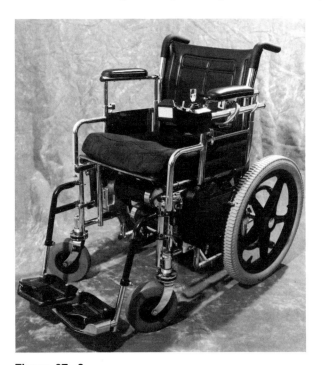

Figure 37−3
Conventional power wheelchair.

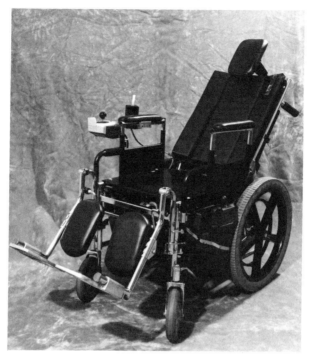

Figure 37–4
Power wheelchair with power recline.

evating leg rests are readily available. If the normal sitting position in a wheelchair is with a trunk-to-thigh angle of roughly 90°, reclining the chair then increases the trunk-to-thigh angle by tipping the seat back away from the seat bottom. The trunk-to-thigh angle may be increased to the point of approximately 170°. Recline mechanisms can be manual and are operated by an attendant through a release mechanism at the rear of the chair. Reclining may also be a power option applied to a reclining-type chair which allows the user to alter the sitting angle. The advantage of this feature is that position can be changed to relieve pressure on the skin and so reduce the possibility of decubitius ulcers. It may facilitate catheterizing a patient in the chair, and it is likely to reduce the need for additional transfers during the day for rest periods. Additionally, it also may be helpful in patients who have hypotension. As the back is lowered, descending during a recline maneuver, the leg rests generally elevate at the same rate that the back descends; the patient thus is in an almost fully recumbent position while still in the chair. One of the major difficulties with using a recliner wheelchair, particularly a power recliner, is shear between the user's back and the seat back during a recline maneuver, and this is even more pronounced during an inclining maneuver (that is, coming back to a fully upright seated position). As the seat back is returned to its normal operating position, the user is pushed forward on the seat of the chair, causing "sacral sitting"; this is a very compromised posture for the remainder of the patient's time in the wheelchair, unless an attendant or another person can assist in repositioning.

Skin care must be of the utmost concern to those prescribing wheelchairs. One of the best features available on power recline chairs is a low-shear or zero-shear system. This system consists of a double-back arrangement that allows the user to adhere to the forward-most back of the chair. Shear is confined between the "front" and "rear" backs of the chair. Reduced shear may also be attained by moving the seat forward as the chair reclines; this approach allows the user's buttocks to slide ahead as the back reclines. On inclining, the seat returns to its normal position and the user stays in correct posture.

Orientation in space, or tilt, is another feature available on power chairs. This feature maintains the roughly 90° position between the trunk and thigh; however, it allows the chair to tilt, bringing the thighs and knees above the trunk and head. This position is useful for maintaining posture in the chair and changing position for skin protection through weight shifting; in some cases, this change facilitates the reduction of spasticity.[6-8]

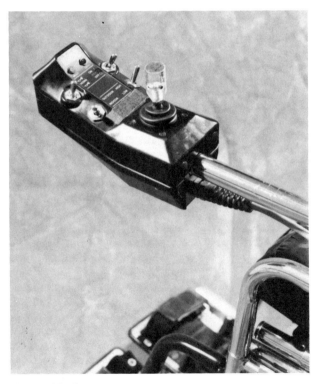

Figure 37–5
Close-up view of controls on a power wheelchair.

Controls are as sophisticated as the other features of power chairs. Many chairs are controlled by a joystick or hand control (Fig. 37–5). This is a small stem attached to the control box; the speed attained is proportional to the amount of pressure placed on it (that is, the harder the stick is pushed, the faster the chair will go). This stick is also directional (forward and reverse, right and left, and all variations in between). Generally, the controls have a high and low range as well as increased power options for carpets, grass, and rough terrain. A control similar to this may be positioned in front of the face for use with the tongue or chin in severely disabled individuals. A third option is a sip-and-puff control (pneumatic control), which drives the chair forward, reverse, right, and left by alterations of air pressure, either positive or negative. These are difficult to learn to use, but after considerable practice, some users can become sophisticated. This system may also be tied into an environmental control system, as can the other controls previously described. By changing the mode on this system, environmental controls (that is, radio, television, stereo, lights, and others) may be operated from this single control. These environmental controls could also include computer use. A most recent adaptation has been a head control system without any apparatus in front of the face; the user is able to direct the chair by head positioning. Two sensors are in the headrest; the further the user moves his or her head from the headrest within a 2-inch range, the faster the chair will go. The various modes of the chair (forward, reverse) must be coded by bumping the head against the headrest. For example, a single bump will turn off the unit, and a series of three bumps will program forward. A different sequence of bumps against the headrest will program an environmental control system.

Power Base

The power-base chair (Fig. 37–6), because of its low center of gravity and wide tires, may allow use outside more readily than the conventional arrangement. However, the power-base chair has some drawbacks; primarily, it is less maneuverable indoors or on carpets, and the large caster wheels have a tendency to wrinkle and roll carpeting, especially small rugs. However, all of the features previously described are available and readily transferred to the power-base chairs. Therefore, users with severe disabilities may also have a chair that is well adapted for outdoor use. This is not to say that conventional chairs are inappropriate for outdoor use, but the low center of gravity and the wider tires of the power-base chair may be more suitable.

Three-Wheeler

The scooter (Fig. 37–7), or three-wheeler, generally is for individuals who are less disabled than users of the other chairs. The cost is somewhat less, and for patients who have difficulty dealing with disability, this type

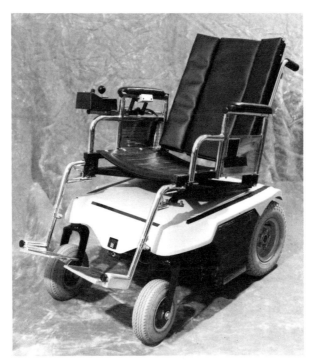

Figure 37–6
Power-base wheelchair.

perhaps suggests that less disability is present and may be more agreeable to people who are in the early stages of, for example, multiple sclerosis. Persons with rheumatoid arthritis or some cardiac conditions may be appropriate users of a scooter-type chair. Features that are available on these chairs include a high-low power seat. A swivel seat feature may be useful for persons who work at a desk. This type of chair is particularly suited for the individual who has some ability to ambulate but cannot do so on a regular or a full-time basis. Transportation of these chairs is perhaps somewhat easier than that of other power chairs. The seat and front tiller mechanism detach from the main base. The largest amount of weight that is necessary to be placed into the trunk of a car is around 50 lb. The user of this chair could generally not place it in an automobile.

Three-wheelers come in two varieties: rear-wheel drive and front-wheel drive. The primary activity of the user should be known at the time of prescription. If the user intends to use the three-wheeler primarily outdoors, a rear-wheel drive type should be prescribed. The disadvantage of this type, however, is that it is somewhat bulkier and heavier. If the primary use is to be indoors, a front-wheel drive type is smaller, lighter weight, and more maneuverable in the tight spaces and confines of a house. The controls and steering of the scooters are the same (that is, on the tiller or on a steering arm above the front wheel).

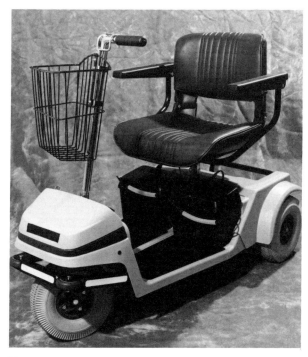

Figure 37–7
Three-wheeler, or scooter-type, chair.

MANUFACTURERS

The description of wheelchair types is not all-inclusive, but it should provide a solid basis for wheelchair prescriptions. Further information about specific wheelchairs and the latest advances is available from a wide variety of manufacturers, as listed below.[6, 7]

Manufacturers of Wheelchairs (All Types)

Active Aid
One Active Aid Road
P.O. Box 259
Redwood Falls, MN 56203-0359

Amigo Mobility International
6693 Dixie Highway
Bridgeport, MI 48722-0402

Everest & Jennings, Inc.
4142 Rider Trail
Earth City, MO 63045

Fortress Scientific
61 Miami Street
Buffalo, NY 14204

Gunnell, Inc.
221 North Water Street
Vassar, MI 48768

Invacare Corporation
899 Cleveland Street
P.O. Box 4028
Elyria, OH 44036-2125

Ortho-Kinetics, Inc.
P.O. Box 436
Waukesha, WI 53187

Permobil of America, Inc.
1403 Massachusetts Avenue
Lexington, MA 02173

Designs, Inc./Quickie
2842 Business Park Avenue
Fresno, CA 93727

Wheel Rings, Inc.
199 Forest Street
Manchester, CT 06040

X-L Manufacturing Co., Inc.
4950-D Cohasset Stage Road
Chiro, CA 45926

Power Recline Systems

Falcon Rehabilitation Products, Inc.
4404 East 60th Avenue
Commerce City, CO 80022

LaBac Systems, Inc.
8955 South Ridgeline Boulevard
Highlands Ranch, CO 80126

REFERENCES

1. Jay PE. Jay Medical seating handbook. Boulder: Jay Medical, Ltd., 1989.
2. Kottke FJ, Lehmann JF. Krusen's handbook of physical medicine and rehabilitation. 4th ed. Philadelphia: WB Saunders, 1990.
3. Measuring the patient. Camarillo, CA: Everest & Jennings, 1979.
4. Pierce DS, Nickel VH, eds. The total care of spinal cord injuries. Boston: Little, Brown, 1977.
5. Guttmann L. Spinal cord injuries: comprehensive management and research. 2nd ed. Oxford: Blackwell Scientific Publications, 1976; 607–613.
6. The perfect fit. Fresno, CA: Quickie Designs, 1987.
7. The professional wheelchair contact. Elyria, OH: Invacare, 1980.
8. Zacharkow D. Wheelchair posture and pressure sores. Springfield, IL: Charles C Thomas, 1984.

38

Ambulatory Aids

David L. Nash
Jeffrey M. Thompson

Practitioners in the field of physical medicine and rehabilitation encounter a wide range of people with physical impairments, many of whom are having some difficulty with ambulation. These gait difficulties may be temporary or permanent. Sometimes a permanent impairment shows improvement with time, such as in a person who has suffered a cerebrovascular accident. In some other conditions the gait impairment will progressively worsen, such as in a person with a progressive neuromuscular disease. This chapter addresses the various conditions that may be associated with gait difficulties and the characteristics of an antalgic gait. Evaluating a patient's needs, the type of gait aid to meet these needs, and the various types of crutch gaits are also discussed, as is applying these principles to write a physical therapy prescription for a gait impairment.

CONDITIONS ASSOCIATED WITH GAIT IMPAIRMENTS

Conditions associated with gait impairments can be classified in many ways. We prefer to divide them into three categories. The first condition is pain, which may be associated with some additional structural lesion in the lower extremity. The second includes conditions that are usually not painful but are associated with impaired balance, coordination, or strength. The third condition is amputation, which is discussed in Chapter 39. Basic biomechanical principles of gait are also reviewed in Chapter 39 (see Fig. 39–1).

Pain With or Without a Structural Lesion

Most patients with temporary needs for a gait aid have pain. Both in emergency rooms and in outpatient clinics, patients present daily with sprains or strains of ligaments or tendons, contusions, lacerations, torn knee cartilage, or tendon or nerve injury. These injuries need proper rest and protection, which can be provided with a gait aid to relieve weight-bearing stresses.

Fracture or Operative Intervention. Fractures or surgical intervention in the lower extremity may be associated with the types of traumatic lesions mentioned above. However, many lower extremity operations are not related to trauma, such as correction of a congenital deformity or treatment of an acquired disease such as osteoarthritis of the hip with a total joint arthroplasty or a focal atherosclerotic obstruction with vascular by-pass. These conditions also usually require a gait aid for protection during healing and to minimize pain from excessive weight bearing.

Inflammatory Diseases. Other conditions requiring protection from painful weight bearing are associated with inflammatory processes. Lower extremity joints may be affected with a systemic connective tissue disease such as rheumatoid arthritis, a crystal-induced arthropathy such as gout, or infection such as septic arthritis. Osteoarthritis can certainly have a painful inflammatory appearance too. Painful inflammatory processes of other soft tissues, such as cellulitis, myositis, or thrombophlebitis, can also warrant the use of a gait aid during the acute phases. Again, the primary goal of a gait aid in these conditions is to facilitate ambulation while protecting painful healing tissue from the stress of weight bearing.

Antalgic Gait. The characteristic gait resulting from weight-bearing pain in one of the lower extremities has several distinguishing features (Table 38–1). The foot is placed flat rather than with the typical heel strike in order to reduce the jarring of impact. Push off may also be avoided to eliminate the associated transmission of forces. The duration of time with weight on the painful leg is shortened relative to the time on the other leg, which results in a shortened swing phase and a prolonged stance phase on the normal side. The normally smooth cadence and rhythm are disrupted. The center of gravity is typically shifted to the painful side, especially with hip disease, to decrease forces at the joint that would be normally in-

TABLE 38–1

Characteristics of an Antalgic Gait

No heel strike
No push off
Reduced stance phase on painful leg
Shortened swing phase of normal leg
Prolonged stance phase on normal leg
Abnormal cadence and rhythm
Center of gravity shifts to painful side during
  weight bearing

creased because of the mechanical properties of the lever arm. When a person stands on one leg with the body weight centered over the pelvis, the pelvis acts as a lever arm and the femoral head in the acetabulum acts as a fulcrum. The hip abductors have to increase the forces at the fulcrum further by contracting to counterbalance the body weight and hold the pelvis level. Shifting one's weight to the painful side reduces these forces.

Impaired Balance, Coordination, or Strength

In this group of disorders, pain is usually not a feature, but unsteadiness of gait places the patient at risk for falls and injuries.

Gait With Spasticity. Spasticity secondary to an upper motor neuron injury occurs most commonly in patients after stroke resulting in hemiplegia, spinal cord injury that leads to quadriparesis or paraparesis, or traumatic brain injury. Spastic cerebral palsy, a perinatally acquired brain injury, certainly fits into this category. The excessive tone and central motor lesion cause difficulties in voluntarily activating and inhibiting muscle groups and result in stiff, jerky styles of gait. Patients with hemiplegia often need to swing their stiff, straight leg out to the side to keep from catching a toe. This type of gait abnormality is referred to as circumduction.

Gait With Weakness. Weakness can result from any number of diseases affecting the motor units. There are many myopathies described that include the muscular dystrophies. The lower motor neuron can be affected in several ways also, for example, by an inflammatory process such as Guillain-Barré syndrome or by inherited idiopathic or acquired peripheral neuropathies, such as occurs with Charcot-Marie-Tooth disease, diabetes, folic acid or vitamin B_{12} deficiency, or environmental toxin exposure. Amyotrophic lateral sclerosis is typified by progressive painless weakness. Also, weakness can be associated with a prolonged illness and bed rest resulting in marked deconditioning.

Gait With Ataxia. Ataxias, disorders of muscular coordination, can be divided into two types. The first is based on impaired cerebellar function that limits, on a central processing basis, the brain's capacity to coordinate muscle activation. Foot placement appears haphazard or drunken and lurching with a wide base. The second type is based on sensory deficits limiting peripheral feedback from the limbs regarding their position in space. Affected patients may have a more noticeable slapping of their feet and become significantly more impaired in the dark because compensatory visual cues are decreased.

Gait With Rigidity. Rigidity most commonly occurs in the gaits of patients with Parkinson's disease who have an extrapyramidal disorder resulting in a gait disturbance characterized by short, shuffling steps, no arm swing, flexed posture, and sometimes difficulty initiating the first step. Their gait may also have a peculiar acceleration referred to as festination.

A combination of the features mentioned above may also be present in some diseases with weakness, upper and lower motor neuron deficits, cerebellar dysfunction, and sensory loss. The most common disease that can include all of these features is multiple sclerosis.

SELECTION OF ASSISTIVE DEVICES

Evaluation of Assets and Impairment of Patient

Before a gait aid can be prescribed, the patient must be evaluated to determine his or her strengths and limitations and any potential complicating factors. The strength and condition of the upper extremities need to be assessed, particularly the shoulder adductors, elbow extensors, and grip strength. Pain or deformity such as in rheumatoid arthritis must be taken into consideration. The strength and condition of the "good leg" are also important to evaluate. Pain or weakness on the less involved side, circulation problems such as claudication, and possibly fragile, vulnerable skin on the weight-bearing surface of the foot affect the choice of gait aids and techniques.

Also pertinent to the assessment is a past history of falls and whether the patient is taking anticoagulants that might warrant extra precautions against falls. A history of cardiac problems, syncope, angina, or orthostatic hypotension should be noted, as should significant pulmonary impairments with marked shortness of breath or general debilitation from prolonged illness and bed rest. The hemoglobin or hematocrit value is also worth noting, especially if the patient has recently undergone an operation.

Ambulatory Aids

The three basic categories of aids are canes, crutches, and walkers (Fig. 38–1).

Canes. A cane is used for conditions with the least degree of gait impairment. It is nearly always used in the hand opposite the impaired leg. In normal gait, the opposing arm and leg swing together in a reciprocal fashion. Using the cane in the hand opposite to the affected limb allows one to simulate this normal gait pattern, and it functionally provides significant weight-bearing relief when used in this manner. A cane is of proper length if, when placed with the tip 6 inches lateral to the forefoot, the elbow is flexed 30°. The cane is used in patients with mild pain or slight instability. After a cemented total hip replacement, one usually advances from crutches to a cane when pain is largely resolved and strength and stability have improved significantly. A cane might be used in cases of femoral trochanteric bursitis to decrease the tension of the hip abductor on the trochanter. Hemiplegia is another common condition for which a cane is

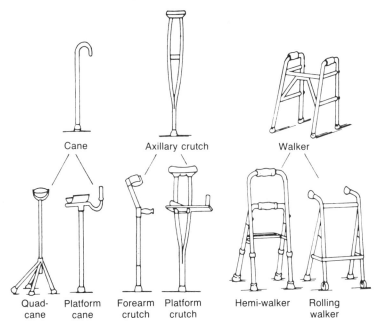

Cane   Axillary crutch   Walker

Quad-   Platform   Forearm   Platform   Hemi-walker   Rolling
cane   cane   crutch   crutch   walker

Figure 38−1
Three basic types of ambulatory aids—canes, crutches, and walkers—and some common modifications.

used. A quadripod cane (Fig. 38−2) is commonly used by hemiplegic patients to broaden the base of support for additional stability.

Crutches. Crutches, in contrast to canes, are most commonly used bilaterally for greater weight-bearing relief. The fitting of crutches is similar to that of a cane; when the hand is resting on the grip and the tip is 6 to 8 inches lateral to the forefoot, the elbow should be flexed 30°. In addition, there should be room for approximately two fingers between the axillary pad and the axilla. Weight should not be placed on the axillary pads because of the potential for complications of neurovascular compression. Axillary crutches are probably the most commonly used gait aid to protect against painful weight bearing on a lower extremity after injury or operation. Crutches may also be used in cases of mild to moderate ataxia or weakness related to a neuromuscular condition. When crutches are expected to be used for a long duration, light-weight aluminum ones are sometimes preferred to the less expensive wooden ones. Also, in patients with chronic conditions who have good shoulder strength, forearm (Lofstrand) crutches may be more convenient because they are shorter and made of aluminum and allow for limited use of the hands while standing.

Walkers. Walkers are most often used for patients with moderate instability. They are often used by elderly and debilitated persons, but they

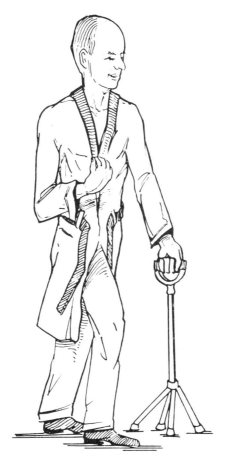

Figure 38–2
Patient using quadripod (quad) cane to broaden base of stability.

are useful for those with ataxia at any age and, in particular, young children with spastic cerebral palsy who are learning to walk. The walker may also be preferred for some persons who are physically capable of using crutches but do not have the motor planning ability required for some crutch gaits.

Several modifications and special features may benefit certain persons. A rolling walker with wheels on the front is beneficial to those with moderately severe ataxia because it eliminates the relatively unstable and unsupported phase of gait that occurs when the walker is lifted up to be advanced. With the wheels, a steady, continuous forward force on the walker keeps it advancing.

The addition of sandbags or ankle weights to the walker may be required to provide additional stability for persons with severe ataxia. Patients who have Parkinson's disease with retropulsive instability may also benefit from these modifications.

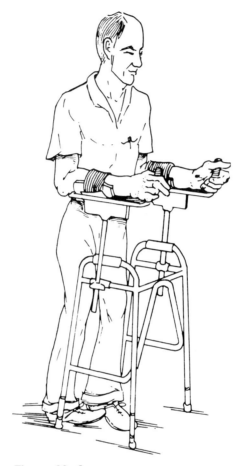

Figure 38–3
Patient using walker with platform attachment.

For patients with rheumatoid arthritis who have severe involvement of the wrists and hands, platform attachments are available both for axillary crutches and walkers (Fig. 38–3). These attachments distribute the weight-bearing pressure across the forearm and decrease the stress to the hands and wrists. The swivel walker that can be advanced one side at a time or the rolling-type walker functions best for patients using platform attachments on a walker.

CRUTCH GAITS

Gaits for Disorders Involving One Leg

The most common crutch gait prescribed and used is called the 3-point gait. In this gait, the two crutches and the involved leg move together as a unit while the "good leg" supports the body weight by itself. When ordering 3-point crutch gait, one also needs to specify the weight-bearing restrictions. For nonweight bearing, the goal is to maintain the normal reciprocal gait pattern with no weight-bearing forces on the affected limb. Touch-only weight bearing has been arbitrarily set at 10 to 30 lb of weight bearing. Some orthopedic surgeons prefer this gait early after total joint arthroplasty. Partial weight bearing allows for up to 40 to 80 lb of weight bearing. When the actual amount of weight is not critical, weight bearing as tolerated is often ordered. It should be noted that it is difficult to reproduce a precise amount of weight bearing consistently. Therefore, these amounts are only approximate and not a precise standard.

The swing gait can be used for one affected lower extremity but it is often discouraged because it does not simulate normal reciprocal motion of the lower extremities. The crutches are advanced together, then the legs are advanced together as a unit. Young patients often prefer this gait because it is conducive to greater speed. The primary indication for its use, however, is for paraplegic patients with long leg braces.

Gaits for Two Affected Limbs

The 4-point (or 4-count) gait is characterized by moving one crutch or limb at a time and always having three points remaining in contact with the floor at any one time. An example of the sequence would be left crutch, right foot, right crutch, left foot. For most people this is a tediously slow gait, but it is tolerated in conditions such as rheumatoid arthritis, with which joints in both legs need protection from weight bearing. Also, some patients with moderately severe ataxia benefit from this gait pattern with its added stability. After starting with the 4-point gait, patients often advance to the quicker 2-point gait, in which one crutch and the opposite foot move together in a more natural reciprocal fashion. This gait is faster than the 4-point gait and has a more natural rhythm, but only one crutch and one leg are in contact with the floor at any one time.

The "walk to" gait is most commonly used with the walker but can be used with crutches. The patient first advances the crutches or walker as a unit and then steps up one foot at a time to the position of the gait aid. This pattern is commonly used by elderly persons who have very limited mobility.

For safety and comfort, axillary and grip pads are standard on most axillary crutches. Also, crutches usually have large rubber tips to prevent slipping. As part of gait training, it is important to instruct patients in the proper technique to be used when encountering curbs or steps or carpeting. For unsteady patients, a safety belt around the waist that the therapist can hold to prevent a sudden fall is the best precaution.

PRESCRIPTION FOR AMBULATORY AIDS

Prescriptions for aids for a gait impairment (Table 38–2) always need to be individualized and may include orders for exercises (including range

TABLE 38–2

Sample Prescriptions for Ambulatory Aids

Clinical Problem	Prescription
Painful soft tissue injury, leg	3-Point axillary crutch gait, nonweight bearing. Instructions for safety on curbs, carpet, and stairs
Rheumatoid arthritis, acute flare or severe chronic deformity with weakness or pain	4-Point platform axillary crutches; advance to 2-point as tolerated
	or
	Platform walker with swivel or rolling mechanism
Multiple sclerosis with marked ataxic gait	"Walk to" or through gait with rolling, weighted walker

of motion, stretching, strengthening, pregait training, balance, coordination, transfers, and gait reeducation). Pregait training may begin on the parallel bars with weight shifting and practicing foot placement in patients with severe gait disorders. Ataxic gaits may be facilitated with weights on the ankles or added to the rolling walker to add stability. Occupational therapy may also be ordered for additional assistance with training and devices for activities of daily living.

39

Prostheses and Orthoses

Rolland P. Erickson
Malcolm C. McPhee

DEFINITIONS

Prosthesis

A prosthesis is an artificial substitute for a missing body part. Although this definition may relate to absent ears, breasts, or dentition, the following discussion pertains only to those devices that are designed to replace a partially or completely absent limb.

Orthosis

An orthosis is a device that, when in contact with the body, improves function. In the greatest sense, this definition could encompass wheelchairs, feeding and grooming aids that improve one's ability to accomplish activities of daily living, crutches, and walkers. However, the following discussion is limited to devices that improve limb function.

INDICATIONS FOR PROSTHESES OR ORTHOSES

Amputation

"Major amputation" is generally defined as proximal to and including complete amputation of the hand or foot. In the United States alone, about 43,000 major amputations are performed every year. The yearly incidence is thus nearly 0.3 amputation per 1,000 persons; the prevalence is about 1 amputation per 250 persons.

Disease. Although etiologic reports vary by region and country, the most common reason for amputation is disease. Peripheral vascular disease manifested as atherosclerosis, thromboangiitis, and diabetes mellitus accounts for 58% to 93% of all amputations and is, as expected, most frequent in elderly populations. The lower extremity is affected most often.

Trauma. Trauma is the second most frequent reason for amputation and is responsible for 29% to 33% of all cases. Like other traumatic conditions, amputations most often affect young adults and certain occupational groups and are most frequent during wartime. Approximately a third involve the upper extremity.

Tumor. Accounting for approximately 5% of the indications for amputation, tumor as an etiologic agent peaks twice. The higher peak occurs during adolescence and is due to osteosarcoma and chondrosarcoma, and a less significant peak occurs during late middle age. Certain medical centers with comprehensive cancer treatment programs have a much greater proportion of amputations due to cancer.

Congenital Limb (Skeletal) Deficiency. In about 5% of persons with absent limbs, the condition has been present since birth. It is more than semantically incorrect to consider such limb loss as a "congenital amputation." Congenital limb deficiencies can be transverse or longitudinal. A transverse deficiency is the absence of all skeletal parts distal to the deficiency along a transverse axis and results in limb loss similar to that of most acquired amputations. Conversely, a longitudinal deficiency extends parallel to the long axis of the limb; an example is absence of the radius, radial carpal bones, and one or more radially situated digit rays. The medical and prosthetic management of transverse deficiencies often parallels that of acquired amputations. However, special surgical, prosthetic, and orthotic interventions are frequently required for the management of longitudinal deficiencies.

In contradistinction to acquired amputations, congenital limb deficiencies occur more frequently in the upper extremity; a transverse deficiency below the elbow is the single most frequent deficiency.

Paralysis

Paralysis as an indication for use of an orthosis cannot be classified as simply as amputations. A myriad of neurogenic lesions involving a single or diffuse portion of the central or peripheral nervous system and also myopathic processes can impact an individual to a degree that orthotic intervention may be required. However, common conditions often requiring one or more orthoses include cerebrovascular accidents with hemiplegia, spinal cord injuries, head injuries, traumatic and entrapment mononeuropathies, Guillain-Barré syndrome, peripheral neuropathies, poliomyelitis, and congenital maladies.

Skeletal Instability

A multitude of conditions with skeletal instability also may benefit from orthotic intervention. Ligamentous injuries to weightbearing joints, monoarthropathies and polyarthropathies with or without inflammation, and fractures of long bones often require one or more orthotic devices to augment or maintain stability. Conditions resulting in painful extremities, although often unassociated with skeletal instability, are included in the discussion.

BIOMECHANICAL PRINCIPLES

Lower Extremity

The human gait cycle (Fig. 39–1) is often addressed using relatively standard terminology. Stance phase is the portion of the gait cycle in which the reference limb is in contact with the floor; it is initiated when the heel first contacts the floor (heel strike). It progresses through full foot-floor contact (midstance) and culminates with heel lift (push off). Swing phase is the portion of the gait cycle in which the reference limb does not contact the floor. It begins with loss of foot-floor contact (toe off), progresses through unencumbered forward movement (swing through), and ends with heel strike.

We walk the way we do, given our anatomic limitations, because it is the most energy-efficient way to transport ourselves physically from one place to another. At first analysis, ambulation may seem to be an easy and automatic activity. Yet, with closer analysis, human gait becomes exceedingly complex.

The body's center of gravity has been calculated to be just anterior to the second sacral vertebra. The energy costs of ambulation would be minimized if we could transport that center of gravity forward in a straight line without vertical or lateral displacement. In that we do not have wheels, this is impossible. Instead, we move ourselves forward by alternating movements of two stick levers (legs), a decidedly inefficient activity because we are constantly raising, lowering, and laterally displacing our center of gravity as it is moved forward. To damp these displacements, our extrapyramidal system uses a complex repertoire of arm, pelvic, hip, knee, ankle, and foot movements and forces constantly practiced and improved on since our first steps as a toddler. Any condition that causes a deviation from our normal gait pattern results in an increased cost of ambulation.

Compared with an able-bodied walker, the average person with a below-knee amputation ambulates with a 41% increase in energy expenditure, and one with an above-knee amputation experiences an 89% increase. In hemiplegics, ambulation consumes 63% more calories.

As energy expenditure rises, the ability for ambulation declines and disability occurs. When coupled with environmental barriers (stairs, lengthy hallways, or rough ground), the disability becomes a handicap.

STANCE PHASE

Heel Strike   **Midstance**   **Push Off**

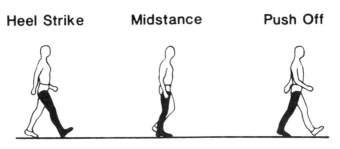

Foot in contact with floor, leg bearing body weight

SWING PHASE

Toe Off   **Swing Through**   **Heel Strike**

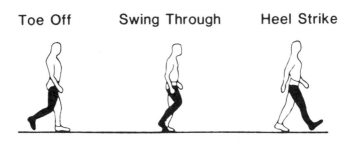

Foot not touching floor, opposite leg bearing body weight

Figure 39–1
Analysis of a single forward step. (From Anderson MH, Bechtol CO, Sollars RE. Clinical prosthetics for physicians and therapists: a handbook of clinical practices related to artificial limbs. Springfield, Illinois: Charles C Thomas, 1959:169. By permission of the publisher.)

   Clearly, it is prudent to design, fabricate, and assess the usefulness of all lower extremity prosthetic and orthotic devices for their ability to approximate normal gait.

Upper Extremity

   Just as ambulation depends on normal lower extremity function, our ability to accomplish the activities of daily living depends on normal upper extremity function. Through complex and coordinated force and movement patterns of the trunk, shoulder, elbow, wrist, and hand, we have the dexterity to thread a needle as well as the strength to lift heavy weights. Any significant disruption in these patterns yields deficits in our ability to feed, dress, groom, toilet, write, work, or recreate.

Upper extremity prosthetic and orthotic devices must be developed and assessed for their ability to approximate normal upper extremity function.

Prosthetic and Orthotic Materials

Materials suitable for prosthetic and orthotic devices have certain desirable characteristics. The material should be lightweight because the intact parts of the impaired limb must not only have the strength to accomplish the activity but also be able to move the device that will perform or assist in the performance of the activity. Newer thermoplastic and metal alloy developments are continually applied to device fabrication to minimize weight. The material should be resistant to fatigue to assist in the repetitious activities of living. The material should be smooth and inert to minimize skin trauma and irritation. For externally powered devices, desirable factors include small size, constant and long-lasting power, and an intimate interface between skin and machine. Every effort should be made to manufacture low-maintenance components. Few prosthetic and orthotic devices accomplish all these goals.

PROSTHETIC PRINCIPLES

Lower Extremity Components

Foot and Ankle. The human foot and ankle absorb decelerating forces during heel strike, provide a stable base of support during midstance, and, in concert with the triceps surae, furnish a rigid lever arm to propel the body up and forward during the later stages of stance phase. Designed to mimic these activities, the standard foot and ankle mechanism for most prostheses is currently the solid ankle-cushion heel. A compressible heel cushions heel strike, and the lack of an articulated ankle provides the lever arm to propel the body forward at the end of stance phase (Fig. 39–2).

Below-Knee Amputation Sockets. A socket is the portion of the prosthesis that incorporates the residual limb. The most frequent design used in below-knee sockets is the patellar-tendon-bearing socket (Fig. 39–3). In that the standard below-knee amputation stump is bony with many pressure-intolerant areas, the patellar-tendon-bearing socket is designed to allow the lion's share of weight bearing at the patellar tendon, just distal to the patella. Edema and skin problems are minimized if the socket is skillfully molded to provide total contact with the stump. Even then, a fabric sock usually separates the stump from direct contact with the prosthesis. The prosthesis is prevented from falling off the stump during swing phase by suspending it either by molding the sides of the prosthesis snugly above the femoral condyles or through a fastening-tape (Velcro) strap. For situa-

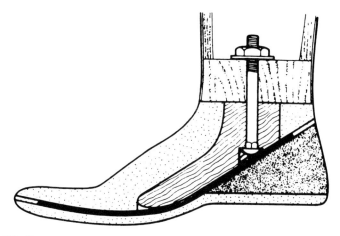

Figure 39−2
Solid ankle-cushion heel. (From Levy SW. Skin problems of the amputee. St. Louis, Missouri: Warren H. Green, 1983:82. By permission of the publisher.)

tions in which the patellar tendon cannot tolerate the weight bearing, or when the knee joint is painful or unstable, significant weight may be redistributed to more proximal tissues via a thigh lacer attached to the prosthesis through lateral and medial knee joints.

   Knee Units.   Prostheses for amputations above the knee require a mechanical knee. The constant friction unit is the most basic type. It consists of a simple bolted articulation in which constant friction can be applied to resist free swing at the knee. Additional security against unexpected knee flexion during stance phase can be provided by the safety knee. When weight is placed on the limb, a friction brake provides resistance against

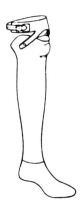

Figure 39−3
Below-knee prosthesis with patellar-tendon-bearing socket. (From Hosmer-Dorrance, Campbell, California. By permission.)

buckling into flexion. Additional stability against knee flexion during stance phase is provided in virtually all knee units by situating the articulation posteriorly. If the wearer is agile and ambulates at multiple speeds, hydraulic mechanisms are often used to provide variable resistance during swing phase.

Above-Knee Amputation Sockets.   The standard above-knee amputation socket is the quadrilateral type (Fig. 39–4). It molds the soft tissues of the stump such that the ischial tuberosity is maintained on a horizontal shelf on the posterior aspect of the socket. Consequently, much of the weight bearing occurs at this point, and the distal pressure-intolerant areas of the stump are thus relieved of significant weight-bearing tasks. Unlike the patellar-tendon-bearing socket, the quadrilateral socket is often used without an intervening sock, and thereby an intimate fit provides suction during swing phase to maintain suspension of the prosthesis on the stump. Modifications to the basic design include the use of a fabric sock and suspensory belt for persons who have difficulty accomplishing the vigorous donning efforts. Recently, flexible thermoplastics have been used in the fabrication of the socket to accommodate dynamic changes of muscle size and stump shape during gait. Another innovation is a socket redesigned to incorporate greater hip adduction, which thereby stretches the hip abductors for more efficiency.

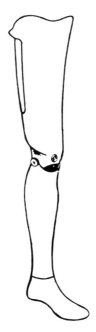

Figure 39–4
Standard above-knee prosthesis. (From Hosmer-Dorrance, Campbell, California. By permission.)

Hip Disarticulation and Hemipelvectomy Prostheses. Although energy inefficient, the Canadian design is used by many people with hip disarticulation and hemipelvectomy (Fig. 39–5). The knee and hip articulations are placed so that simple downward weight bearing stabilizes the joints against buckling. The socket is large and encompasses much of the remaining pelvic soft tissues. Suspension is maintained through a belt that passes above the opposite iliac crest.

Upper Extremity Components

Terminal Devices. In an effort to approximate normal prehension, maintain visual monitoring of manual tasks, and accomplish acceptable cosmesis, many prosthetic hooks and hands have been developed. The terminal device used by many persons with upper extremity amputations is a curved and split hook in which sturdy rubber bands maintain the closed position. It is opened by traction on a cable powered by intact proximal muscles on either side or both sides. Similar mechanisms operate many mechanical hands. Mechanisms to use the cable for closing instead of opening the hook or hand are also available. In recent years, battery-oper-

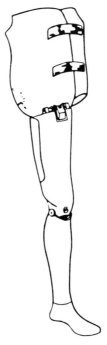

Figure 39–5
Hip disarticulation and hemipelvectomy prosthesis. (From Hosmer-Dorrance, Campbell, California. By permission.)

ated hooks and hands have been developed that are controlled by electromyographic signals from proximal muscles.

Wrist Units. Mechanical wrist units are used to allow operation of the terminal device close to the body and in various degrees of supination and pronation.

Below-Elbow Amputation Sockets. Below-elbow amputation sockets use a double wall to provide both cosmetically acceptable exterior contours and total socket-stump contact. Suspension is provided by either snug capture of the epicondyles or a harnessing system suspended from the involved and uninvolved shoulders (Fig. 39−6).

Elbow Units. For above-elbow amputations, a prosthetic elbow unit is required. This unit must be able to be positioned and maintained in var-

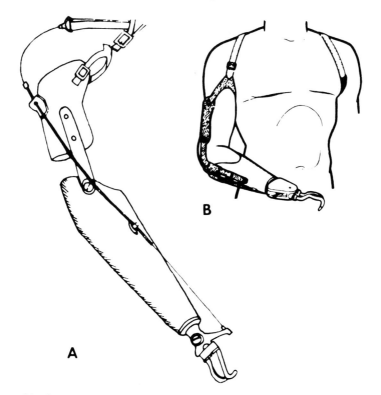

Figure 39−6

A and *B,* Below-elbow prostheses. (*A,* From Below and above elbow harness and control system, Evanston, Illinois: Northwestern University Prosthetic-Orthotic Center, 1966. *B,* From Pursley RJ. Harness patterns for upper-extremity prostheses. In: American Academy of Orthopaedic Surgeons. Orthopaedic appliances atlas. Vol. 2. Artificial limbs. Ann Arbor, Michigan: JW Edwards, 1960:105−128. By permission of the Academy.)

ious angles. Both of these operations are usually accomplished through cable systems similar to the one that operates the terminal device. Expensive
and complex externally powered systems have also been designed to perform these actions.

Above-Elbow Amputation Sockets.   As with below-elbow amputation
sockets, above-elbow amputation sockets are usually double walled, and
suspension is provided through a harnessing system (Fig. 39–7).

Shoulder Disarticulation and Forequarter Prostheses.   Although functional shoulder disarticulation and forequarter prostheses are available, the
lack of proximal muscles for cable operation on the involved side and the
complexity of actions required for the prosthesis to be functional generally
negate effective use. Frequently, affected persons opt for a cosmetic shoulder cap or an endoskeletal system passively positioned by the opposite
hand.

Exoskeletal and Endoskeletal Prosthetic Systems.   Most prostheses are
fabricated with an exoskeleton of laminated plastic. To improve cosmesis

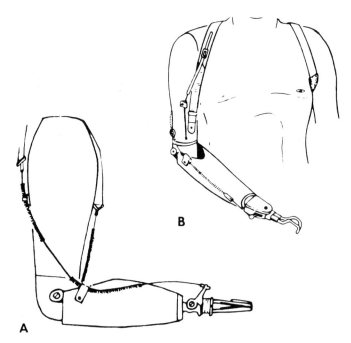

Figure 39–7
A and *B*, Above-elbow prostheses. (*A*, From Below and above elbow harness and control
system, Evanston, Illinois: Northwestern University Prosthetic-Orthotic Center, 1966. *B*,
From Pursley RJ. Harness patterns for upper-extremity prostheses. In: American Academy
of Orthopaedic Surgeons. Orthopaedic appliances atlas. Vol. 2. Artificial limbs. Ann Arbor,
Michigan: JW Edwards, 1960:105–128. By permission of the Academy.)

and minimize weight, endoskeletal component systems have been devised with carefully molded soft surfaces that appear similar to the contralateral limb.

ORTHOTIC PRINCIPLES

Lower Extremity Devices

Ankle-Foot Orthoses. With instability about the ankle, a stable base of support is never achieved during stance phase. With paralytic conditions, not only is stance unstable but footdrop leads to catching of the toe during swing phase. If the triceps surae is involved, no push off is provided.

The conventional (double-upright) orthosis is the prototype ankle-foot orthosis (see Fig. 6–7). A steel stirrup attaches the device to the sole of the shoe. Mechanical ankle joints situated on both the medial and the lateral aspects of the ankle at approximately the height of the anatomic ankle joint connect the stirrup to two metal uprights that pass proximally along the calf. The proximal ends of the uprights are attached to a cuff surrounding the calf. The mechanical ankle joints can be locked or stopped at various angles or fitted with springs that provide resistance to either ankle dorsiflexion or plantar flexion.

With the conventional ankle-foot orthosis, footdrop can be prevented with a stop that prevents plantar flexion during swing phase. Push off is simulated through use of a dorsiflexion stop. With conditions of gross ankle instability, the ankle joints can be rendered immobile. If weight-bearing relief is required, a patellar-tendon-bearing piece is added to redistribute the weight proximally.

With the development of sturdy and resilient thermoplastics, in-shoe ankle-foot orthoses have been designed to incorporate many of the characteristics of the double-bar upright type and yet be lighter weight and provide greater cosmesis (see Fig. 9–9 and 9–10).

Common conditions amenable to the use of an ankle-foot orthosis include hemiparesis, multiple sclerosis, head injury, lumbar radiculopathies, and peroneal neuropathies.

Knee-Ankle-Foot Orthoses. When paralysis or instability occurs at both the knee and the ankle, support must be extended to the proximal thigh, and the knee must be crossed with joints that can be locked. If weight-bearing relief is required at the knee or the ankle, forces can be redistributed even more proximally, incorporating the ischial tuberosity and soft tissues of the proximal thigh.

Upper Extremity Devices

Although upper extremity orthoses vary considerably in design and purpose, there are two basic types. Static orthoses provide structural stability through immobilization to prevent contractures and support joints and muscles weakened by disease or injury. A single joint or several joints may be immobilized with a single device. A burned hand is often immobilized by a static hand orthosis to prevent contractures during healing. A static (resting) wrist-hand orthosis is often used to immobilize and protect joints inflamed by rheumatoid arthritis (see Fig. 24–1). The shoulder can be maintained in abduction for several weeks after a rotator cuff repair to protect the healing tissues.

Functional orthoses improve function through the use of joints, levers, pulleys, and external power sources. The power sources include rubber bands, springs, batteries, and cartridges of compressed gas. Peripheral nerve lesions can be made less disabling by using power sources to simulate the lost motor function. A wrist-hand orthosis that assists wrist and metacarpophalangeal extension through springs or rubber bands may provide added function to a person with radial nerve palsy (see Fig. 24–2). An elbow with posttraumatic instability may be stabilized with a hinged splint. External power may be added to assist elbow flexion or place dynamic stretch to an accompanying flexion contracture.

REHABILITATION

Provision of a prosthesis or an orthosis does not constitute rehabilitation. Rehabilitation is the medical and educational process by which a person, disabled by disease or injury, regains independence in all spheres of life.

Comprehensive rehabilitation is an interdisciplinary team process in which health-care professionals bring together special expertise to maximize a patient's independence.

Because of the large influx of amputees into the health-care system at the end of World War II, Army and Veteran's Administration physicians soon recognized that management of these patients was inadequate and rife with inefficiencies, duplicated services, and patient misconceptions. The team concept was developed and has since succeeded in improved care.

Team Members

Physician. The physician provides the team leadership, directs the amputee clinic, provides the prosthetic prescription, and manages the medical issues. Although most often a physiatrist, the physician may be an orthopedist, a vascular surgeon, or other physician with a special interest and expertise in the management of amputees.

Therapists. For patients with lower extremity amputation, the physical therapist is responsible for muscular reconditioning, gait retraining, and education in stump management and also provides input for the prosthetic prescription. In a like fashion, the occupational therapist often cares for patients with upper extremity amputation. For patients with both upper and lower extremity amputation, the occupational therapist also provides adaptive equipment and retraining for activities of daily living.

Prosthetist.   The prosthetist provides input into the prosthetic prescription, fabricates and fits the prosthesis, and aids in the training for its use.

Nurse.   The hospital-based nurse provides ward care during hospitalization and assists in patient and family education. The public health nurse may be required to monitor the patient after dismissal from the hospital.

Social Worker.   The social worker is responsible for coordinating the financial and vocational issues pertinent to the patient and frequently provides an interface with the patient's family.

Others.   At times, the services of a surgeon, psychologist, psychiatrist, or dermatologist may be required.

The Rehabilitation Process

Preamputation Management.   For situations in which elective amputation is contemplated, the team provides valuable assistance for preparing the patient and family for the procedure and the subsequent rehabilitation. The patient and family learn about the various team members and about the expected duration of hospitalization and prosthetic training and a prosthesis is shown to them.

Phantom sensation should be fully explained. It is a painless awareness of the amputated part that persists for a variable time after amputation. The sensation can be very vivid, includes any sensation felt by an intact limb, and gradually disappears. It is important for the patient to understand that phantom sensation is entirely normal; otherwise, the patient may undergo significant psychologic trauma and yet be too embarrassed to discuss it with anyone.

If additional time is available, a visit with an amputee is arranged, crutch-walking is reviewed, and a reconditioning program is initiated. The physician may counsel the surgeon about the amputation level if potential prosthetic problems are uncovered during the evaluation.

Postoperative Management.   In the hours and days immediately after the amputation, every effort should be made to dissociate the amputee from pain. Appropriate analgesics are very important because evidence suggests that patients with greater surgical pain are more apt to have problems with phantom pain.

Wound management varies according to the circumstances of the amputation and the surgeon's preferences. At first a soft removable dressing is used if the surgeon is concerned about tissue viability and wound healing. If no complications are expected and the medical center has an active amputee team, a rigid cast dressing will often be placed. Attached to the cast is a metal pylon and prosthetic foot. With this immediate postsurgical fitting, wound edema is controlled, stump healing and molding are accelerated, and the patient is able to begin gait retraining on the parallel bars (toe touch only) or upper extremity retraining almost immediately.

Immediate postsurgical fitting is used frequently with below-knee and upper extremity amputations and occasionally with above-knee amputations. Because the stump shrinks and molds as healing occurs, the casts must be changed every 7 to 10 days. The patient is often dismissed after removal of the sutures. Most patients with above-knee amputations are managed with a similar system, except that a removable thermoplastic socket is used. New wound management approaches include rigid, removable systems for below-knee amputations. Application of the dressings (soft or rigid) is discontinued when good wound healing has occurred, and Ace wrapping is used to mold and shrink the stump further. Throughout this period, muscles proximal to the amputated part are strengthened and joint motion is maintained.

Prescription of Prosthesis. When the wound is healed and the edema has cleared (often at 6 to 8 weeks postoperatively), the patient is evaluated by the entire team for prescription of the prosthesis. Each prosthesis must be tailored to the individual needs of the patient. Considerations include medical and cognitive status, stump characteristics, general level of fitness and coordination, financial status, and vocational and avocational interests. The appropriate prescription is completed, and the patient is then examined by the prosthetist to make a mold of the stump. The prosthesis is then fabricated around this mold.

Fitting of Prosthesis and Training in Its Use. Fitting and training are usually accomplished in 1 to 2 weeks on an outpatient basis. Complicating factors, such as cardiopulmonary disease, a marginally healed wound, or a second amputation, may require the patient to be hospitalized. As the patient undergoes training, the prosthetist continues to modify and adjust the prosthesis until it is comfortable and efficient. Fabrication is then completed, and the patient continues retraining until independent use is ensured. Strengthening exercises for endurance are prescribed at the time of dismissal.

Long-Term Management. Many amputees return to their previous employment without difficulty. Whether they have had an upper or lower extremity amputation, many will require modifications to their automobile. Some patients with upper extremity amputation may require modifications in their workplace, and those with occupations requiring bimanual dexterity or heavy physical labor may require vocational assessment and retraining.

The patient returns to the amputee clinic periodically for monitoring and fitting and to address other problems relating to the amputation.

The frequency of prosthetic replacement varies greatly. Light users may not require another prosthesis for many years, whereas a farmer may need a new prosthesis every 2 years. Because the stump often continues to shrink for many years, periodic socket and prosthetic replacement will be required on an ongoing basis.

Complications. The most frequent complication is loss of prosthetic fit due to changes in the size and shape of the stump. Such changes may result in stump irritation, ulceration, infection, or edema and, if not managed with proper prosthetic modification, may require stump modification.

Stump pain and phantom pain are also frequent and must be carefully delineated. Stump pain is most often caused by problems with the prosthetic fit but may also relate to bony overgrowth, adherent scar, or painful neuroma. Phantom pain is defined as a painful phantom sensation; it is not a universal occurrence. Every effort should be made to identify and correct the cause. Although socket modifications, injections for neuroma, and relaxation with biofeedback training may relieve or modify the pain in some patients, many others are resistant to specific treatment. Whenever possible, the single most important management technique is to return the amputee to regular use of a properly fitting prosthesis.

The rehabilitation process is similar when fitting an orthosis and training a patient in its use, although the duration of intervention is usually much shorter.

SUMMARY

The management of amputees serves as an effective model for comprehensive rehabilitation. These patients present with a major disability. Before rehabilitation intervention, such patients cannot ambulate or perform self-care activities and often cannot accomplish vocational tasks. They have a significant loss of body image and are often depressed and anxious about the future. With comprehensive rehabilitation, they can usually be returned to full functional independence at home and work. This can be done without altering the impairment in any way (the patient still has an amputated extremity). Instead, rehabilitation has an impact on the disability (inability to ambulate or to accomplish activities of daily living) by prosthetic fitting and retraining in gait and activities of daily living and on the handicap (inability to drive an automobile or operate machinery) by modifications to the automobile and workplace.

Early intervention must be stressed. Potentially, amputations caused by vascular disease can be prevented by reducing risk factors such as smoking, a high-fat diet, and poor exercise habits. After the onset of peripheral vascular disease, proper management of ischemic ulcers and timely vascular procedures may avoid or delay the time of amputation. After the amputation, early intervention can avoid complications such as contractures, deconditioning, delayed or improper fitting of the prosthesis, and inadequate training that have an adverse impact on acceptance and use of the prosthesis. Several excellent texts have in-depth discussions of prosthetics and orthotics.[1-3]

REFERENCES

1. Banerjee SN, ed. Rehabilitation management of amputees. Baltimore: Williams & Wilkins, 1982.
2. American Academy of Orthopaedic Surgeons. Atlas of limb prosthetics: surgical and prosthetic principles. St. Louis: CV Mosby, 1981.
3. Redford JB, ed. Orthotics etcetera. 3rd ed. Baltimore: Williams & Wilkins, 1986.

PART XV

Spine and Limb Disorders

40 | Painful Disorders of the Spine and Back Pain Syndromes

Bahram Mokri
Mehrsheed Sinaki

EPIDEMIOLOGY AND GENERAL CONSIDERATIONS

Painful diseases of the spine, particularly low back pain, are common clinical problems. In some cases, they can disrupt normal activities enough to require professional medical attention. In the industrialized world, low back pain is second only to headache among the leading causes of pain. It is the leading cause of workers' compensation expenditure, and it is ranked second as a cause of lost work time. One of the most common causes of limitation of activity for persons younger than 45 years is low back pain.[1] It is one of the most costly medical problems in our society for persons aged 30 to 60 years.[1, 2]

Vocational factors that can cause spine pain (particularly low back pain, but also neck pain and dorsal pain) include poor static work postures, strenuous physical work, exertional bending and twisting, heavy lifting, and forceful, repetitive, and strenuous movements of the spine.[3]

Various pathologic conditions can also cause neck pain, dorsal pain, or low back pain. Some of those that are more common are discussed at the end of this chapter and in Chapters 41 and 42.

THE SPINE AS A SUPPORTIVE UNIT OF THE SKELETON

The spine consists of a series of mechanical units and has several functions: (1) it protects a significant part of the central nervous system; (2) it is the major axial mechanical support of the body; (3) the intervertebral disks act like shock absorbers; and (4) the spine functions as a supportive connecting rod for the appendicular skeleton. Each mechanical unit of the spine consists of an anterior and a posterior segment. The anterior segment is composed of two adjacent vertebral bodies and the intervertebral disk. This segment bears weight, and the connecting disk acts like a shock absorber.[4] The posterior segment is formed by the vertebral arches, the transverse and spinous processes, and the inferior and superior articular facets. This portion protects the neural structures and directs movement of the unit in flexion and extension.

Different physical activities generate different forces on the spine. Nachemson showed marked variations in forces in various positions and activities.[5, 6] In the supine position, a force of 100 newtons is exerted on the L-3 disk. While sitting upright without support, an individual generates seven times this force, and when the same person bends forward and rotates while holding a 10-kg weight, the force increases 20-fold.

THE FUNCTION OF MUSCLES ON THE SPINE

Four functional groups of muscles support the spine: the extensors, flexors, lateral flexors, and rotators of the spine.

In normal but not exceptionally athletic individuals, the main supportive muscles of the spine are the extensors and rotators.[7, 8] The center of motion of the vertebral joints is the disk. The movement in the facet joints is a gliding type. The main mass of the back muscles begins in the lumbar region and follows the muscle groups upward. The heavy musculotendinous mass over the upper sacral and the lower lumbar vertebrae is the origin of a large segment of the back musculature known as the *erector spinae*, which extends the vertebral column.

Deep to the erector spinae are the *semispinalis muscles*. The remaining muscles of the back are the *interspinales*, which are between spinous processes and are not present throughout most of the thoracic region.

The main function of the muscles of the back in the erect posture is to resist gravity. On extreme range of motion (such as flexion), regardless of which muscles are used to start the movement, once the vertebral column is bent far enough the muscles of the back that resist this movement must actively contract to prevent falling and to make the movement smooth and controlled.

Some muscles that have no attachment to the vertebral column also play an important role in movements of the spine. The sternocleidomastoid muscles are the main flexors of the neck. They laterally flex and rotate the head. The abdominal muscles are the main flexors and lateral flexors of the trunk and also participate in rotation.

Spinal motion is distributed as follows: flexion occurs mainly at the cervical, upper thoracic, and lumbar levels; extension occurs mainly at the cervical and lumbar levels; lateral mobility in the frontal plane occurs at the cervical level; and rotation in the axial plane is accomplished almost entirely at the cervical and thoracic segments.[9]

RELATIONSHIP BETWEEN VERTEBRAL PAIRS AND SPINAL NERVES

Although in early fetal life the cord fills the entire spinal canal, the final location of the lower end of the spinal cord (sacral cord segments) is at the lower end of L-1 and the upper end of L-2 because of more accelerated growth of bony structures both before and after birth. Therefore, the level of emergence of nerve roots from the spinal canal (especially for the lower levels) is lower than their respective spinal cord segments. The relationship of the spinal nerves (and the related cord segments), their parallel vertebral segments, and the level of exit of the related nerve roots in adults is summarized in Table 40–1.

INTERVERTEBRAL DISKS

The intervertebral disks act as cushions between the vertebral bodies. They are thickest in the lumbar region. Intervertebral disks have two major components: the nucleus pulposus and the annulus fibrosus. The nucleus pulposus is yellowish and elastic and is made of mucoprotein, a meshwork of collagen fibers, and water (the water content is 88% in young individuals and 70% in elderly persons). The annulus fibrosus is a concentrically arranged, thick, tough fibrocartilaginous ring confining the nucleus pulposus. The intervertebral disk is a remnant of the notocord and has a poor blood supply.

Disk Protrusion

As the result of degenerative changes, a portion of the annulus fibrosus may become relatively loose and give way. The result is a localized disk bulge (protrusion). Annular fibers are intact and are not disrupted.[10]

TABLE 40–1
Relationship of Spinal Nerves, Vertebral Segments, and Exit Level of Nerve Roots

Spinal Nerve and Cord Segment	Vertebral Segment	Exit
C-1	C-1	Above C-1
C-8	C-7	Between C7-T1
T-6	T-5	Between T6-T7
T-12	T-8	Between T12-L1
L-2	T-10	Between L1-L2
L-5	T-11	Below L-5
S-3	T-12	Third sacral foramen

From Pansky B. Review of gross anatomy. 2nd ed. New York: Macmillan, 1984:214. By permission of McGraw-Hill.

Disk Herniation

A herniated disk involves disruption of annular fibers at one point through which part of the nucleus pulposus is herniated. Sometimes the herniated nuclear material may burst through the most superficial posterior fibers of the annulus *(extruded disk).* Sometimes an extruded fragment may become sequestrated and lie free in the spinal canal *(sequestrated disk).*[10]

EVALUATION OF THE PATIENT WITH SPINE PAIN

I. Clinical evaluation
   A. History—at the least, the following factors should be determined:
      Mode of onset, whether abrupt or insidious
      Provoking or aggravating factors
      Relieving factors
      Effect of exertion and rest
      Effect of cough, sneeze, or strain on spine pain, especially if these cause pain down any of the limbs
      Presence or absence of nocturnal pain
      Course since the onset—whether the pain has increased, decreased, or fluctuated or has been episodic
      History of back pain
      History of trauma
      Associated limb symptoms (pain, paresthesias, numbness, weakness, cramps, fasciculations)
      Presence or absence of sphincter trouble
      History of back operation (such as laminectomy, fusion)
      Types of medications taken and the effects of these medications on the symptoms
      Presence or absence of litigation or compensation issues
   B. Examination of the back
      1. Inspection: The back is evaluated for deformities, paraspinal spasm, birth marks, list to one side, corkscrew deformity, decrease or increase in lumbar or cervical lordosis, presence of scoliosis, muscular atrophy, or asymmetries
      2. Palpation and percussion: This part of the examination determines whether there are tender or trigger points, local tenderness or pain on percussion, spasm or tightness of the paraspinal muscles
      3. Evaluation of range of motion: Range should be determined in flexion, extension, lateral bending, and rotation. Several techniques and instruments have been used to measure the range of motion of the spine. These have varied from simple and inexpensive methods to expensive and complicated machines. Some of the techniques are described.
         a. Tape measure method: This is used to determine the amount of flexion of the lumbar spine. This test was originally described by Schober.[11] This is a simple and practical method.

A midline mark is made in the line that connects the "dimples of Venus." Then two other marks are made along a vertical line perpendicular to the first line in its midpoint. One mark is 5 cm below and the second mark is 10 cm above the midline mark. Therefore, the distance between these two marks is 15 cm. The patient is then asked to bend forward maximally. The measured distance beyond the original 15 cm gives an estimate of the degree of spinal flexion (see Fig. 3–4). This method provides some indication of spinal flexibility, but it does not provide complete information.[12]

   b. Inclinometers: These were first introduced by Asmussen and Heebøll-Nielsen[13] for measuring spinal motions and were later further developed by Loebl[14] (see Fig. 3–5). There is some variability with this method because it fails to separate hip motion from spine motion. It also varies with the subject's effort.[15]

   There are various electronic and computerized gadgets not only for measurement of range of motion but also for measurement of muscle strength.

C. Neurologic examination[16]
   1. Gait and station: Gait is a complex activity that depends on the integration of several neural mechanisms, but it also can be affected by disturbed posture, disorders of joints, or pain. One should look for antalgic gait, footdrop, spastic or ataxic features, functional features, or hysterical features. The patient should do toe walking, heel walking, and tandem gait. It should be determined whether the patient can stand on either foot or can squat and rise.
   2. Muscle stretch reflexes: An increase, decrease, or absence of muscle stretch reflexes should be recorded. Neither a decrease nor an increase of these reflexes in itself can be interpreted as definitely abnormal. Occasionally, neurologically normal persons may have exaggerated, diminished, or even absent reflexes. Therefore, a patient's reflexes must be compared with other muscle stretch reflexes, particularly of the corresponding opposite side. Reflex asymmetry, however, is most often significant.
   3. Alternate motion rates: These are to be performed rapidly and regularly. They depend on an intact sensory motor system. These can also be affected by pain, diseases of joints, insufficient attempt, poor cooperation, and functional factors.
   4. Muscle bulk: The presence of any muscle atrophy should be determined. Comparison of the circumference of the limbs at different levels is sometimes useful (such as comparison of the circumference of both legs at mid-calf level or mid-thigh level). One should also look for muscle fasciculations.
   5. Muscle strength: It is particularly important to determine whether the muscle weakness is genuine or whether it is functional or a manifestation of giving way as the result of pain or poor effort.

One should determine the exact distribution of the weakness; whether it corresponds to a single root, multiple roots, a peripheral nerve, or plexus; and whether the weakness is of upper motor neuron type. It is equally important to determine whether the patient gives way because of pain or for other reasons.

6. Sensory examination: This is the most difficult and least reliable part of the neurologic examination. It should be done at the end of the examination, when the examiner may have some suspicions about what disorder is affecting the patient. Asking the patient to outline areas of sensory loss will help orient the examiner and save time. The patient should understand the nature of the test. It should be determined whether the reported sensory changes are consistent and reproducible and whether they follow the anatomic dermatomal patterns, although they may be noted in only part of a dermatome.

7. Straight-leg raising and Fabere tests: With the patient in the supine position and the lower limbs extended and relaxed, the symptomatic leg is lifted and gradually elevated until pain in the lower extremity (in sciatic distribution in typical cases) is reported. At this point, the amount of elevation in degrees is recorded. Sometimes elevation of the asymptomatic lower extremity causes pain in the asymptomatic side (the well leg sign), and this is often a reliable sign of root irritation. Fabere test (*f*lexion, *ab*duction, external *r*otation, and *e*xtension) is done to look for any associated hip disease.

8. Spurling test (foraminal compression test): This test is useful in the diagnosis of laterally herniated cervical intervertebral disks. The patient's neck is hyperextended and laterally flexed toward the symptomatic arm. Downward pressure is then applied on top of the head. The test result is considered positive when this maneuver aggravates the pain or paresthesias in the symptomatic upper limb.

II. Diagnostic studies

A. Plain roentgenography: Although the use of plain roentgenography has decreased with the increasing availability and use of computed tomography and magnetic resonance imaging, plain films are still useful as quick and less costly screening. They are helpful for detecting fractures, dislocations, degenerative joint disease, spondylolisthesis, narrowing of intervertebral disk space, and many vertebral bone diseases and tumors. Oblique views are helpful for visualizing the neural foramina. Flexion and extension views are useful for studying subluxations and stability.

B. Radioisotope bone scanning: This remains a valuable test for screening the entire skeleton or a large part of the skeleton. It is useful for the detection of tumors, particularly for a skeletal survey of metastatic tumors. Gallium scanning is used if infection is suspected.

C. Computed tomography (CT) and magnetic resonance imaging (MRI): Both tests are useful for detecting disk disease, herniated or extruded disk, or tumors (vertebral, epidural, meningeal, intradural, or cord). Overall, MRI is superior to CT, especially when it is supplemented with gadolinium-enhanced images. MRI can image the entire lumbar spine in a single scanning session and shows the soft tissues better than CT, and it is an excellent method for detecting epidural, intradural, and some of the intra-axial spinal cord lesions, such as tumor, cyst, or syrinx. However, CT can define bone better. These studies, particularly MRI, may show various degenerative changes, especially in elderly patients. Sometimes these changes may have little relationship to the patient's symptoms. It is essential to interpret the findings in the light of the clinical observations and impressions.

D. Myelography: Although CT and especially MRI have decreased the use of myelography, this test is still used by many surgeons before a final decision is made regarding lumbar surgery. CT-myelography has added to the accuracy of the test by detecting intraspinal lesions. This still remains the most accurate test for the diagnosis of disk herniations and extrusions.

E. Electromyography: This is extensively used for detecting associated neurogenic changes and denervation.

SOME COMMONLY ENCOUNTERED PAINFUL DISORDERS OF THE SPINE

Mechanical Low Back Pain

This is a term commonly used for non-diskogenic back pains provoked by physical activity and relieved by rest. This is a descriptive term, sometimes overused, and does not point to a single or particular etiologic factor. The term, however, is practically useful. This type of pain is often due to stress or strain to the back muscles, tendons, and ligaments and is usually attributed to strenuous daily activities, heavy lifting, or prolonged standing or sitting. Mechanical back pain is a dull aching pain of varying intensity that affects the lower spine and is mostly chronic in nature. It may be localized or may spread to the gluteal areas. The pain often progressively worsens during the day because daily physical activities such as bending, lifting, twisting, prolonged sitting, and standing often aggravate the pain. There is no associated numbness, paresthesia, weakness or neurologic deficit, or cough or sneeze effect on the lower limbs.

Osteoarthritis (Degenerative Joint Disease)

Changes of degenerative joint disease in the spine occur with aging and may begin during the third decade of life.[17] It may be asymptomatic. If symptomatic, the associated pain is centered in the spine and is often increased with movement of the spine. Stiffness and limitation in range of motion of the spine may be present. Pain is relieved by rest. Arthritic changes can compress nerve roots and cause additional radicular pain.

Roentgenograms are diagnostic. In the early stages, roentgenographic findings may be absent. The osteoarthritic and hypertrophic changes are more prominent in the lumbar and cervical spine. Management of pain includes improvement of support of the spinal musculature, improvement of working posture, and provision of proper static and dynamic posture principles such as bending one knee during prolonged standing (placing one foot on a low stool). When there is poor muscle support, application of an elastic support can decrease the strain. Exercises include abdominal and back muscle strengthening exercises (preferably isometric exercises).

Degenerative arthritis of the facet joints results in localized spine pain that sometimes extends to the limb and may mimic radicular pain. Limitation of range of motion, especially with extension, is often needed. Pain is increased with activity and relieved by rest. Operation is rarely required. Most patients can achieve relief of pain to a tolerable level with a carefully adjusted program of weight control, rest, analgesics, or nonsteroidal anti-inflammatory medications.

Back Pain Related to Pregnancy

Enlargement of the uterus during the third trimester in combination with the extra weight added to the abdominal area and pressure over the vena cava leads to night backache.[18] This pain may be managed through reduction of lordosis with nonstrenuous exercises such as pelvic tilt exercises and knee-bent positioning with pillows under the knees or between the knees when lying on the side (Fig. 40–1). During the third trimester of pregnancy, stronger abdominal support is needed to decrease the lordotic posturing. The weight of the uterus and increased intra-abdominal girth add to the strain of the back and abdominal muscles for maintaining normal posture and can result in mechanical back pain. The application of abdominal elastic support with shoulder straps during ambulatory activities during the last 8 weeks of pregnancy can decrease low back pain caused by poor muscle support.

Posttraumatic Compression Fracture

This usually is related to compressive flexion trauma. It can also occur spontaneously in patients with osteoporosis, osteomalacia, multiple myeloma, hyperparathyroidism, hyperthyroidism, and metastatic cancer. The upper lumbar spine or the middle to lower thoracic spine is more commonly affected. The pain usually appears immediately after the fracture and is fairly localized. There may be accompanying paraspinal muscle spasm and limitation of range of motion of the spine. Roentgenography, imaging studies, and bone scanning may be needed to establish the diagnosis.

Pain in the upper back area is helped with back supports that extend cephalad to the lower thoracic spine. The thoracolumbar supports function on the basis of three-point contact. In general, if hyperextension is needed

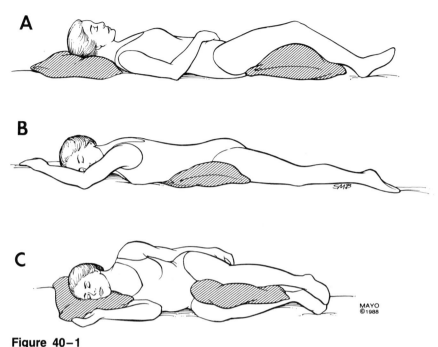

Figure 40–1

Lying posture for pain. *A,* On back, with pillow under the knees. *B,* On abdomen, with use of pillow. *C,* Lying on side, with pillow between knees. (From Sinaki M, Dale DA, Hurley DL. Living with osteoporosis: guidelines for women before and after diagnosis. Toronto: BC Decker, 1988. By permission of Mayo Foundation.)

in cases of thoracic compression fractures, the three points of contact are the base of the sternum, the symphysis pubis, and the lumbar spine, as in the Jewett brace (see Fig. 16–10).

Spondylolysis and Spondylolisthesis: General Considerations and Clinical Manifestations

Spondylolysis is a bony defect in the pars interarticularis. Bilateral spondylolysis of the lumbar spine may lead to forward slipping of vertebral body. Wiltse and associates[19] described five types of spondylolisthesis: (1) dysplastic, (2) isthmic, (3) degenerative, (4) traumatic, and (5) pathologic (Table 40–2). Spondylolisthesis may cause back pain and sometimes, by irritating or compressing the nerve roots, may cause radicular pains or neurologic deficits in the lower limbs. Sometimes the compromise of the spinal canal and its stenosis caused by spondylolisthesis may lead to pseudoclaudication or compromise of the cauda equina and even sphincter dysfunction (see Chapter 41). Range of motion of the back may be limited and lumbar lordosis is exaggerated. The pelvis may be rotated, scoliosis may

TABLE 40–2

Classification of Spondylolisthesis

Type	Criteria
I	Dysplastic—the defect is a congenital dysplasia in the neural arch, which allows subluxation
II	Isthmic—defect in pars interarticularis a. Lytic type, probably a fatigue fracture with hereditary predisposition b. Elongated but intact pars, similar to type IIa, but the fatigue fractures have healed, resulting in an elongated but intact pars c. Acute fracture due to trauma
III	Degenerative—secondary to degenerative changes at the apophyseal joints (this is more frequent at L-4 or L-5 in women older than 40 years)
IV	Traumatic—fracture of posterior elements other than pars
V	Pathologic—due to pathologic changes in posterior elements secondary to malignancy or primary bone diseases

Modified from Wiltse et al.[19]

be noted, and the hamstrings may be tight. Degenerative spondylolisthesis is more common in overweight individuals.

When standing, patients frequently hold their knees in a slightly flexed position. The incidence of spondylolysis is reportedly about 4.5% in preadolescent children, but it increases to 12% in gymnasts. In children, the most common types are of the dysplastic and isthmic types. Strenuous athletic activity in children may produce a fracture of a genetically weak pars interarticularis.

Roentgenographic and Imaging Studies. The defect of pars in spondylolysis is demonstrated as a break in the "Scottie dog's neck" (pars interarticularis) on oblique views of the lumbar spine. Bone scanning may show increased activity on one or both sides.[20]

The overall alignment of the thoracic and lumbosacral spine in the anterior-posterior view is observed. On lateral views of the thoracic and lumbosacral spine, the height of the vertebral interspaces is determined and the evidence for spondylolysis is evaluated. Spondylolisthesis or forward slippage of one vertebra on the other is graded according to Meyerding's classification[21] as grades 1 to 4, depending on the intensity of slippage (Fig. 40–2). Lateral flexion-extension roentgenograms of the lumbosacral spine are obtained to examine the segmental instability. For the evaluation of patients with pseudoclaudication or neurologic deficit, imaging studies (computed tomography, magnetic resonance imaging, myelography) are necessary.

Treatment. In acute cases of spondylolisthesis, a pars defect may actually heal, as in any other fracture. Immobilization for 10 to 12 weeks in a plaster body jacket is the recommended treatment. In chronic cases, in-

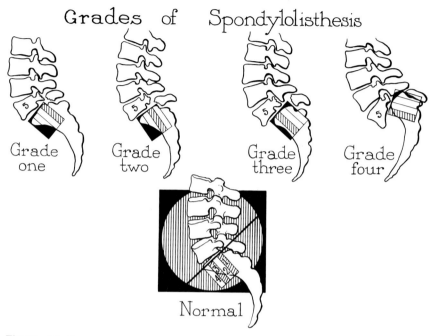

Figure 40–2

Meyerding's classification. The degree of subluxation is divided into four groups: grade 1, slipping on the vertebra less than one-fourth the distance of the lumbosacral angle; grade 2, less than half; grade 3, less than three-fourths; and grade 4, more than three-fourths. (Modified from Meyerding.[21])

structions in back care, abdominal muscle strengthening, and, in persistent cases, application of a brace or corset are recommended. In children, once symptoms resolve, normal activities can be resumed, although a return to vigorous spine-bending athletic events (gymnastics, football) is controversial.

Conservative management of spondylolisthesis is recommended for grades 1 and 2 and in older patients. The physical therapeutic procedures consist of application of heat and massage for reduction of pain and stiffness. Special attention can be given to tightness of hip flexors, hamstrings, and Achilles tendons. A program of stretching exercises is recommended (Fig. 40–3). The objective of an exercise program should be reduction of lumbar lordosis through stretching of the lumbar paraspinal muscles and strengthening of lumbar flexors with isometric exercises[22] (Fig. 40–4 and 16–9 E through H). Strengthening of abdominal muscles is also of great significance in cases of severe weakness of the abdominal muscles and inability for improvement (significant obesity); application of a lumbosacral elastic support can decrease pain until other measures (such as weight loss, improvement of posture) contribute to reduction of pain. In certain cases when spondylolisthesis becomes painful during the advanced

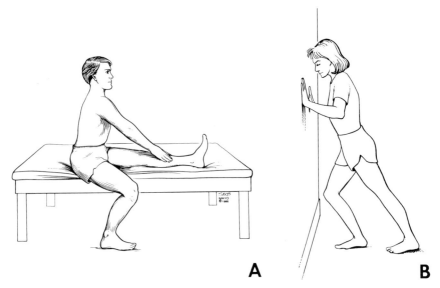

Figure 40−3

A, Hamstring stretches. For a single-leg stretch, the back is kept straight and patient leans forward until a gentle stretch is felt behind the knee. B, Stretches for Achilles tendons. Patient stands at arm's length from wall with palms flat against the wall, slowly bends elbows, and leans toward wall. Involved leg is kept back with knee straight and heel flat on floor. Hold for 5 to 20 minutes as needed or tolerated for each exercise. (By permission of Mayo Foundation.)

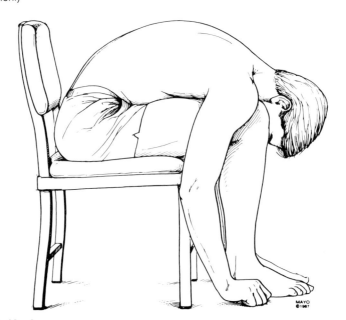

Figure 40−4

Flexion exercise for lumbar spondylolisthesis (developed by M. Sinaki): chest-to-thigh position with pelvis and hip stable. (From Sinaki et al.[22] By permission of Mayo Foundation.)

months of pregnancy, an abdominal pregnancy support may prove helpful. Flexion exercises are also effective for conservative management of spondylolisthesis in children.[23] In some cases, severe osteoporosis occurs with degenerative changes of ligamentous structures and spondylolisthesis. In these instances, a therapeutic exercise program that combines dynamic and static posturing along with isometric spinal flexion exercises and spinal extension exercises without inducing strain on the osteoporotic spine has been shown to be helpful.[24] In severe symptomatic slips and when neurologic symptoms or deficits are present, surgical treatment should be considered.

An understanding of the mechanical factors relevant to spondylolisthesis is necessary to outline an effective conservative treatment program. Patients treated with flexion rather than extension exercises have been shown to have less pain and less need for use of back supports.[22] Patients with severe spondylolisthesis may have cosmetic and postural deformity. Fusion may help to improve these postural deformities.

REFERENCES

1. Kelsey JL, White AA III, Pastides H, Bisbee GE Jr. The impact of musculoskeletal disorders on the population of the United States. J Bone Joint Surg [Am] 1979; 61:959–964.
2. Nachemson AL. The lumbar spine: an orthopaedic challenge. Spine 1976; 1:59–71.
3. Andersson GBJ. Epidemiologic aspects on low-back pain in industry. Spine 1981; 6:53–60.
4. Cailliet R. Low back pain syndrome. 3rd ed. Philadelphia: FA Davis, 1981.
5. Nachemson A. Towards a better understanding of low-back pain: a review of the mechanics of the lumbar disc. Rheumatol Rehabil 1975; 14:129–143.
6. Nachemson AL. Disc pressure measurements. Spine 1981; 6:93–97.
7. Rudins A, Sinaki M, Miller JL, Piper SM, Bergstralh EJ. Significance of back extensors versus back flexors in trunkal support (abstract). Arch Phys Med Rehabil 1991; 72:824.
8. Beimborn DS, Morrissey MC. A review of the literature related to trunk muscle performance. Spine 1988; 13:655–660.
9. Steindler A. Kinesiology of the human body under normal and pathological conditions. 2nd printing. Springfield, IL: Charles C Thomas, 1964.
10. Macnab I, McCulloch J. Backache. 2nd ed. Baltimore: Williams & Wilkins, 1990.
11. Schober P. Ledenwirbelsäule und Kreuzschmerzen. Munchen Med Wschr 1937; 84:336–338.
12. Mayer TG, Mooney V, Gatchel RJ. Contemporary conservative care for painful spinal disorders. Philadelphia: Lea & Febiger, 1991.
13. Asmussen E, Heebøll-Nielsen K. Posture, mobility and strength of the back in boys, 7 to 16 years of age. Acta Orthop Scand 1959; 28:174–189.
14. Loebl WY. Measurement of spinal posture and range of spinal movement. Ann Phys Med 1967; 9:103–110.
15. Mayer TG, Tencer AF, Kristoferson S, Mooney V. Use of noninvasive techniques for quantification of spinal range-of-motion in normal subjects and chronic low-back dysfunction patients. Spine 1984; 9:588–595.

16. Department of Neurology, Mayo Clinic and Mayo Foundation. Clinical examinations in neurology. 6th ed. St. Louis: Mosby Year Book, 1991.
17. Fahrni WH. Conservative treatment of lumbar disc degeneration: our primary responsibility. Orthop Clin North Am 1975 Jan; 6:93–103.
18. Fast A, Weiss L, Parikh S, Hertz G. Night backache in pregnancy: hypothetical pathophysiological mechanisms. Am J Phys Med Rehabil 1989; 68:227–229.
19. Wiltse LL, Newman PH, Macnab I. Classification of spondylolysis and spondylolisthesis. Clin Orthop 1976; 117:23–29.
20. Gelfand MJ, Strife JL, Kereiakes JG. Radionuclide bone imaging in spondylolysis of the lumbar spine in children. Radiology 1981; 140:191–195.
21. Meyerding HW. Spondylolisthesis. Proc Staff Meet Mayo Clin 1934; 9:666–671.
22. Sinaki M, Lutness MP, Ilstrup DM, Chu C-P, Gramse RR. Lumbar spondylolisthesis: retrospective comparison and three-year follow-up of two conservative treatment programs. Arch Phys Med Rehabil 1989; 70:594–598.
23. Plucinski TM, Sinaki M, Currier BL, Rizzo TD. Sports and spondylolisthesis in children. Proceedings of Advances in Idiopathic Low Back Pain. Vienna, Austria. November 27–28, 1992. Blackwell Scientific Press (in press).
24. Sinaki M, Chan C, Plucinski T, Ackerman M. Spondylolisthesis of the osteoporotic spine (abstract). Fourth International Symposium on Osteoporosis & Consensus Development Conference. Hong Kong: Gardner-Caldwell Communications Ltd., March 27–April 2 1993, 106.

41 | Lumbar Disk Syndrome, Lumbosacral Radiculopathies, Lumbar Spondylosis and Stenosis, Spondylolisthesis

Bahram Mokri

Mehrsheed Sinaki

LUMBAR DISK SYNDROME AND LUMBOSACRAL RADICULOPATHIES

Lumbar disk syndrome is one of the common causes of acute, chronic, or recurrent low back pain.[1, 2] Pain may be unilateral, bilateral, or bilateral but more prominent on one side. The cause is usually a flexion injury. Repetitive injury results in degeneration of the posterior longitudinal ligaments and annulus fibrosus. This is more common in men of middle and advanced age, but it also occurs in women and even adolescents, especially if they are involved in strenuous physical activity. Disk herniation may be midline, but it is often to one side.

If irritation or compression of an adjacent nerve root occurs, the pain often radiates into the buttock and to the posterior thigh and lateral calf or lateral or medial malleoli (in the case of L-5 or S-1 radiculopathies) or to the anterior thigh (in the case of L-4 or L-3 radiculopathies). When extrusion of the disk occurs, the low back pain is sometimes decreased or even relieved and the radicular limb symptoms become more prominent. About 5% to 10% of patients with root lesions do not have associated back pain. In these cases, mononeuropathy (such as sciatic, femoral, or obturator nerve) or a lumbosacral plexus lesion has to be ruled out.

The most common levels of lumbar disk protrusion, herniation, or extrusion (in decreasing order of frequency) are S1-L5, L5-L4, L4-L3, and L3-L2. Therefore, the most common lumbosacral radiculopathies related to lumbar disk disease (herniation, extrusion, or degeneration) are S-1, L-5, L-4, and L-3 radiculopathies. Lower lumbar and S-1 radiculopathies are usually secondary to degeneration or herniation of intervertebral disks.[3–5] These are usually unilateral. Midline disk protrusion may cause low back pain but no significant radiculopathy or, if large enough, lateral radiculopathies or even a cauda equina syndrome with bilateral lower lumbosacral radiculopathies and even sphincter trouble. It is unusual for the upper lumbar radiculopathies to be caused by disk disease. Therefore, when evaluating upper lumbar radiculopathy, other etiologic factors, particularly neoplastic disease, should be ruled out.

Examination of the back often shows paraspinal muscle spasms, loss of lumbar lordosis, list of the spine away from the side of root pain, limitation of motions of the lumbar spine with "corkscrew phenomenon" on flexion and straightening, lumbar or sacral tenderness, tenderness at the sciatic notch, positive straight-leg raising test, sometimes "well-leg sign" in cases of S-1 or L-5 radiculopathies (sciatic pain produced in the involved leg when the opposite leg is elevated), and positive Kernig's sign. The chin-chest maneuver may cause low back pain because of upward traction on the cord and lower nerve roots. This may be performed simultaneously with straight-leg raising. Dorsiflexion of the foot may also cause stretching of the sciatic nerve and, therefore, pain. The same phenomenon may be noted when the patient tries to perform heel-walking or tries to bend forward. Cough, strain, or sneeze increases the abdominal pressure and leads to distention of epidural and intervertebral veins, which directly compress and put traction on the nerve roots and, therefore, cause pain in the low back, particularly down the involved lower extremity.

When radiculopathy occurs, several features, including distribution of pain, distribution of weakness, reflex changes, and distribution of the sensory alterations, provide reliable information that enables the clinician to localize the level of disk protrusion or root irritation. Changes in these features as they pertain to each lumbar and sacral nerve root are outlined in Table 41–1.

Laboratory Tests

The value of plain roentgenograms of the spine, imaging studies (computed tomography and magnetic resonance imaging), and myelography[6–9] was discussed in Chapter 40. Overall, magnetic resonance imaging is emerging as a major tool in the diagnosis of herniated and extruded lumbar disks (Fig. 41–1). It is also very useful for demonstrating associated bone disease, vertebral or epidural intraspinal tumors, scar tissue formations, and even some forms of meningeal disease.

Myelography still maintains much of its significance. When coupled with computed tomography (computed tomography-myelography), it is still the most accurate test for documentation of herniated disks, and it is used by many neurosurgeons before proceeding with lumbar disk operation.

Electromyographic examination[10] is very helpful for determining the level of involvement, determining whether root involvement is single or multiple, and differentiating a multiple root from a plexus lesion. After the onset of damage to the root, it usually takes 2 weeks or more for electromyographic evidence of denervation to become detectable by needle electrode examination. Therefore, in the early stages, this test should not be expected to be very helpful.

TABLE 41–1
Clinical Features of Lumbosacral Radiculopathies

Root	Distribution of Pain	Paresthesias and/or Sensory Loss	Weakness	Decreased or Absent Reflexes
L-1	Lower abdomen, groin, or upper anterior medial thigh	Lower abdomen, inguinal region	Iliopsoas (±)	Hypogastric and cremasteric
L-2	Groin, anterior or medial thigh	Anterior and medial thigh	Iliopsoas or adductors of thigh or both	Cremasteric
L-3	Anterior thigh or knee	Anterior thigh and knee	Quadriceps and thigh adductors	Quadriceps
L-4	May extend below the knee, often to inner leg or medial malleolus	Inner leg	Quadriceps and thigh adductors and tibialis anterior (±)	Quadriceps and internal hamstring
L-5	Posterolateral thigh, lateral calf to dorsum of foot	Outer leg and dorsum of foot to great toe	Tibialis anterior, toe extensors, and extensor hallucis longus (therefore impaired heel-walking), hamstrings, perinei, and tibialis posterior, gluteus medius	Internal hamstring; ankle jerk often normal, sometimes decreased but not absent because only L-5 root lesion
S-1	Posterior thigh, calf, and lateral malleolus	Posterior leg, lateral foot, last two toes	Gastrocsoleus and toe flexors (therefore impaired toe-walking), hamstring, gluteus maximus	Ankle jerk and external hamstring
S-2	Posterior thigh and occasionally calf	Variable posterior thigh and saddle area	Intrinsic foot muscles (±), rectal sphincter (±)	Anal
S3-4	Buttock and upper posterior thigh or perianal region	Saddle and perineal area, perianal area	Rectal sphincter	Anal

±, Weakness possibly due to variability of innervation.

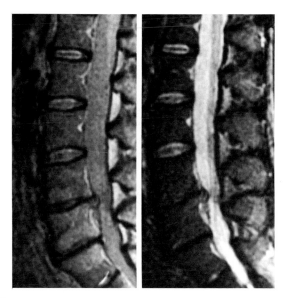

Figure 41–1
Magnetic resonance imaging scan of lumbar spine. T1- *(left)* and T2- *(right)* weighted sagittal images demonstrate extruded L-1 disk.

Treatment

Most patients with back pain related to lumbar disk disease respond to conservative management. Operation is considered when there is definite evidence of radiculopathy or neurologic deficits, especially persistent or progressive neurologic deficits. Progressive neurologic deficits call for early surgical intervention, and large midline disk protrusions with cauda equina syndrome call for urgent treatment and decompression. The success of surgical treatment is greatest when there are bonified objective neurologic deficits. If patients are appropriately selected, about two-thirds will have excellent results, and half of the remaining one-third have improvement to some extent. However, in many patients with lumbar disk syndrome, the major difficulty is low back pain with no evidence of radiculopathy or with only mild or slight root involvement. Most of these patients may respond to conservative management. Lumbar laminectomy and diskectomy for the sole complaint of low back pain often are not justified.[1]

Principles of Conservative Management

Bed Rest. Bed rest for several days with application of cold or heat and a progressive back exercise program, as tolerated, are often recommended. A gradual increase in the level of physical activity is then advised. In patients with significant muscle spasm, a 3- to 4-week course of rest and a subsequent exercise program are required before a return to work. An open-ended off-work program may lead to a longer course of disability.[11, 12]

If pain persists, the use of lumbosacral supports is recommended until the patient's muscular support is improved. This will shorten the duration of bed rest. It is not possible to immobilize a spine unless bed rest is prescribed. Most corsets and braces act on the lumbar spine through increasing intra-abdominal pressure. Through this hydraulic cylinder, the weight of the trunk is supported and the load over the lumbar spine is reduced. If analgesics are indicated, the nonnarcotic type is preferred. If codeine derivatives are used, the prescription course should be limited.

Medications. Analgesics, nonsteroidal anti-inflammatory medications, or muscle relaxants can be used.

Physical Therapy and Rehabilitation Measures. Initially, the objective is to promote muscle relaxation through periods of rest in the supine position (see Fig. 40–3). Later, as the patient's pain permits, gentle flexion exercises or isometric lumbar exercises, or in selected patients mild lumbar extension exercise, can be initiated, and these are gradually advanced to ambulatory activities.

LUMBAR SPINAL STENOSIS

Stenosis of the lumbar spine may involve the central canal at a single level or, often, multiple levels and thus may jeopardize the cauda equina. Sometimes the stenosis may involve the lateral recess or root canal at multiple levels or, often, a single level and, therefore, jeopardize one or more nerve roots. At times, a combination of both may be present. Lumbar spinal stenosis clinically leads to the syndrome of neurogenic claudication or "pseudoclaudication." When the stenosis is limited to the lateral recess or root canal, the lateral recess syndrome of root claudication (a variant of spinal stenosis) is produced. Sometimes the two syndromes coincide. Even then, usually one syndrome dominates the clinical picture.

Pathophysiology

Narrowing of the central spinal canal may be congenital, developmental, or acquired[13, 14] (Table 41–2). Degenerative joint disease is the most common cause and, therefore, the resultant clinical syndromes are often encountered in late middle age or old age.

Degenerative disk disease and narrowing of the intervertebral spaces, spur formation, ligamentous hypertrophy, facet hypertrophy, and overriding all contribute to the decrease in the caliber of the central spinal canal, lateral recess, and root canal. Degenerative disease in the "three-joint complex" (the intervertebral disk and the two facet joints) may render the spine unstable and cause spondylolisthesis with further compromise of the

TABLE 41–2
Different Forms of Spinal Stenosis

I. Primary
  A. Congenital
  B. Developmental (various forms of
     dwarfism)
II. Secondary
  A. Degenerative spondylosis (with or
     without spondylolisthesis)
  B. Late sequelae of fracture
  C. Late sequelae of infection
  D. Systemic bone disease (Paget's
     disease of bone)
III. Mixed
  A. Spinal stenosis due to degenerative
     joint disease in an individual with a
     congenitally narrow spinal canal

From Postacchini.[13] By permission of Springer-
Verlag.

central spinal canal.[15] With advance in the disease process and gradual increase in stenosis, gait endurance is gradually decreased. The caliber of the central spinal canal varies in different individuals; some have congenitally narrow canals. When the spinal degenerative and hypertrophic changes occur in the spine, patients with narrower spinal canals are prone to become symptomatic earlier and more severely.

Clinical Manifestations

Lumbar spinal stenosis clinically manifests as pseudoclaudication (or neurogenic claudication). It is defined as discomfort in the buttocks, thighs, or legs which may be unilateral or bilateral. Symptoms are produced by standing or walking and are relieved within a few minutes by sitting, lying down, or adopting a posture of flexion at the waist. The discomfort is usually pain (in more than 90% of cases), numbness or paresthesias (in more than 60%), or weakness (in more than 40%). Frequently, combinations of these exist. The waist-flexion posture is achieved by such maneuvers as squatting, leaning the back against a wall, or leaning forward on a shopping cart or a church pew.[16]

With flexion, the anteroposterior diameter of the lumbar spinal canal is increased because of separation of the laminae and consequent decrease in the thickness of the ligamenta flava. Meanwhile, the posterior aspect of the annulus is stretched, and the bulge of the disk toward the spinal canal is decreased. Furthermore, with flexion, the caliber of the intervertebral foramina is also increased. The opposite occurs with extension of the lumbar spine (Fig. 41–2).

In spinal stenosis, it is assumed that compression of the roots or cauda

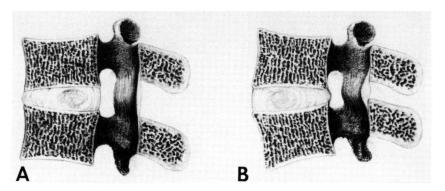

Figure 41-2
Functional changes of the vertebral canal in spinal flexion and extension. *A*, In flexion, the spinal canal lengthens and increases in width in the sagittal plane, due both to separation of the laminae and the consequent decrease in thickness of the ligamenta flava and to the distention of the posterior annulus fibrosus. *B*, Opposite changes occur in extension. (From Postacchini.[13] By permission of Springer-Verlag.)

leads to ischemic changes in these neural structures and, therefore, causes neurologic symptoms. These are reversed when the compression is alleviated and adequate circulation is restored.

Patients frequently prefer to walk in a stooped rather than a straight, erect posture. They may be able to walk uphill easier (waist-flexion posture) than downhill (straight, erect posture). In some patients, pain and discomfort are worsened by lying supine and are relieved by lying on one side, curled in a fetal position.

Symptoms are bilateral in more than two-thirds of patients, although often a marked asymmetry exists with one lower extremity involved much more than the other. Also, in about two-thirds of the patients, low back pain is present. This is typically mechanical in nature and often mild in intensity.

Absence or decrease of ankle jerks is noted in 40% of patients and of knee jerks in about 20% of patients. Weakness can be detected in about one-third of patients. This is usually mild, unilateral, and in the L-5 or S-1 root distribution.

The clinical features of lateral recess syndrome and root claudication are different from those of central canal stenosis.[17] Patients usually report an intense sciatic pain (L-5 or S-1 root irritation) that is provoked by standing or walking and is relieved by sitting, lying down, or flexing the lumbar spine. The pain is typically unilateral. Neurologic deficits, if any, are mild. Results of the straight-leg raising test are usually negative. Back pain is often absent.[18]

Differentiation of Vascular Claudication From Pseudoclaudication

Vascular claudication should be differentiated from neurogenic claudication (pseudoclaudication). Vascular claudication is produced when lower limb muscles are exerted (and, therefore, energy consumption and the requirement for blood and circulation are increased). Walking, climbing stairs, or riding a bicycle (regular or stationary) provokes the pain, which is relieved when exercise is discontinued. Symptoms of pseudoclaudication are produced when the caliber of the spinal canal is decreased by lumbar extension, and they are relieved when the extension posture of the lumbar spine is reversed. Some of the factors useful in differentiating vascular from neurogenic claudication are listed in Table 41–3.

Laboratory Tests

Electromyography. Electromyographic abnormalities are more frequent than the abnormalities detected on neurologic examination. Electromyographic results are abnormal in more than 90% of cases, demonstrating evidence of denervation in the distribution of a single root or multiple roots, usually bilaterally, and sometimes unilaterally with or without paraspinal muscle involvement.[16]

Plain Roentgenography. Most patients have degenerative disk disease, degenerative joint disease, or both with or without spondylolisthesis. In some patients, the lumbar spinal canal may appear congenitally narrow.

Imaging Studies. Myelography shows total or subtotal obstruction to the flow of contrast at one or more levels (Fig. 41–3). Computed tomography and magnetic resonance imaging show stenosis of the central canal, lateral recess, root canal, or a combination of these. Computed tomography myelography is considered an accurate test for evaluation of stenosis in these areas.[6, 9, 19]

Levels of stenosis (in decreasing order of frequency) are L4-L5 (55%), L3-L4 (44%), L2-L3 (26%), L5-S1 (14%), and T12-L1 (3%).

Treatment

The natural history of pseudoclaudication is not entirely clear. It is thought that the symptoms of canal stenosis either remain unchanged or gradually worsen and that symptoms of root claudication either remain unchanged or perhaps gradually improve in some patients but in an unpredictable period. Many patients, however, find that their activities have become markedly limited and seek a solution, including operation. For cases in which progressive neurologic deficits or manifestations of sphincter dysfunction develop, surgical decompression should be seriously considered.[20]

Decompressive operation (decompressive single-level or multilevel laminectomy with or without foraminotomies) provides good results; it alleviates manifestations of pseudoclaudication in a large majority of patients. However, its effect on any associated low back pain is often less satisfactory. When low back pain rather than pseudoclaudication is the

TABLE 41–3
Differentiation of Vascular and Neurogenic Claudication

Factor	Neurogenic Claudication (Pseudoclaudication)	Vascular Claudication	Pitfalls and Remarks
Low back pain	Frequently present	Absent	Sometimes, coincidental degenerative joint disease may be present in patients with vascular claudication
Effect of standing	Provokes symptoms	Does not provoke symptoms	
Direction of radiation of pain in lower limbs	Usually downward	Usually upward	
Sensory symptoms	Present in 66% of patients	Absent	Some patients with vascular claudication may have distal sensory symptoms due to ischemic or diabetic neuropathy
Muscle weakness	Present in more than 40% of patients	Absent	
Reflex changes	Present in about 50% of patients	Absent	In older patients, especially if there is associated neuropathy, reflexes may be decreased or absent
Arterial pulses	Normal	Decreased or absent	In older patients, pulses may be reduced
Arterial bruits	Absent	Frequently present	
Effect of rest while standing	Does not relieve symptoms	Relieves symptoms	
Walking uphill	Symptoms produced later	Symptoms produced earlier	
Walking downhill	Symptoms produced earlier	Symptoms produced later	
Bicycling (stationary or regular)	Does not provoke symptoms	Provokes symptoms	

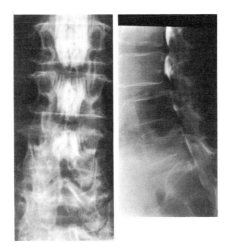

Figure 41–3
Lumbar myelograms. Anteroposterior *(left)* and lateral *(right)* views demonstrate multiple lumbar stenosis.

dominant feature, the expectations for an overall good recovery should be less. Such patients, although they may obtain relief from the symptoms of pseudoclaudication, may still continue to have the low back pain, which was their initial main complaint.

Overall, the more pronounced the degree of spinal canal compromise and neural compression, the better the chance of obtaining a good result from surgical decompression. Patients with long-standing and pronounced neurogenic atrophy and weakness, although they may get relief from the leg pain resulting from the pseudoclaudication, may show only a partial or negligible recovery of the muscle weakness and atrophy.[14]

Conservative Management

Reduction of lumbar lordosis is effective for reducing lumbar stenosis due to postural changes. Therefore, exercises that are aimed at strengthening the abdominal muscles and lumbar flexors are helpful. For patients in whom it is not possible to strengthen the abdominal muscles or those with a protuberant abdomen and extensive weight gain, an elastic abdominal binder is recommended. A program consisting of knee-to-chest exercises, pelvic tilt, and a trial of wall test to decrease lumbar lordosis may be beneficial. Patients should be instructed to avoid exercises that result in hyperextension of the spine.

REFERENCES

1. Simeone FA. Lumbar disc disease. In: Wilkins RH, Rengachary SS, eds. Neurosurgery, vol 3. New York: McGraw-Hill, 1985:2250–2259.

2. Frymoyer JW. Back pain and sciatica. N Engl J Med 1988; 318:291–300.
3. Spangfort EV. The lumbar disc herniation: a computer-aided analysis of 2,504 operations. Acta Orthop Scand Suppl 1972; 142:1–95.
4. Falconer MA, McGeorge M, Begg AC. Observations on the cause and mechanism of symptom-production in sciatica and low-back pain. J Neurol Neurosurg Psychiatry 1948; 11:13–26.
5. Love JG, Walsh MN. Protruded intervertebral disks: report of one hundred cases in which operation was performed. JAMA 1938; 111:396–400.
6. Carrera GF, Williams AL, Haughton VM. Computed tomography in sciatica. Radiology 1980; 137:433–437.
7. Forbes G. Radiologic examination of the spine and myelography. In: Spittell JA Jr, ed. Clinical medicine, vol 11, chapter 31. Philadelphia: JB Lippincott, 1986:1–31.
8. Williams AL, Haughton VM, Syvertsen A. Computed tomography in the diagnosis of herniated nucleus pulposus. Radiology 1980; 135:95–99.
9. Witt I, Vestergaard A, Rosenklint A. A comparative analysis of x-ray findings of the lumbar spine in patients with and without lumbar pain. Spine 1984; 9:298–300.
10. Wilbourn AJ. The value and limitations of electromyographic examination in the diagnosis of lumbosacral radiculopathy. In: Hardy RW Jr, ed. Lumbar disc disease. New York: Raven Press, 1982:65–109.
11. Deyo RA. Conservative therapy for low back pain: distinguishing useful from useless therapy. JAMA 1983; 250:1057–1062.
12. Deyo RA, Diehl AK, Rosenthal M. How many days of bed rest for acute low back pain? A randomized clinical trial. N Engl J Med 1986; 315:1064–1070.
13. Postacchini F. Lumbar spinal stenosis. New York: Springer-Verlag Wien, 1989.
14. Duvoisin RC, Yahr MD. Compressive spinal cord and root syndromes in achondroplastic dwarfs. Neurology 1962; 12:202–207.
15. Yong-Hing K, Kirkaldy-Willis WH. The pathophysiology of degenerative disease of the lumbar spine. Orthop Clin North Am 1983 July; 14:491–504.
16. Hall S, Bartleson JD, Onofrio BM, Baker HL Jr, Okazaki H, O'Duffy JD. Lumbar spinal stenosis: clinical features, diagnostic procedures, and results of surgical treatment in 68 patients. Ann Intern Med 1985; 103:271–275.
17. Ciric I, Mikhael MA, Tarkington JA, Vick NA. The lateral recess syndrome: a variant of spinal stenosis. J Neurosurg 1980; 53:433–443.
18. Fast A. Low back disorders: conservative management. Arch Phys Med Rehabil 1988; 69:880–891.
19. Carrera GF, Haughton VM, Syvertsen A, Williams AL. Computed tomography of the lumbar facet joints. Radiology 1980; 134:145–148.
20. Epstein JA, Epstein NE. Lumbar spondylosis and spinal stenosis. In: Wilkins RH, Rengachary SS, eds. Neurosurgery, vol 3. New York: McGraw-Hill, 1985:2272–2278.

42 | Cervical Disk Syndrome, Cervical Radiculopathies, and Cervical Spondylosis and Stenosis

Bahram Mokri

Mehrsheed Sinaki

CERVICAL DISK SYNDROME AND CERVICAL RADICULOPATHIES

Cervical disk syndrome and cervical radiculopathies are less common than lumbar disk syndromes and lumbar radiculopathies. Lumbar disk herniation occurs 15 times more often than cervical disk herniation. Neck pain resulting from degenerative joint disease and cervical spondylosis is far more common than diskogenic neck pain. Diskogenic neck pains and cervical radiculopathies are often associated with severe aching in the posterior and lateral aspects of the neck. Frequently, there is deep pain near or over the scapula on the involved side. This is thought to be due to irritation of the posterior ramus. Pain may radiate over the shoulder, upper arm, and forearm, but rarely does the pain of cervical radiculopathy extend to the hands or fingers, and it almost never extends to the anterior aspect of the chest. The distribution of the pain may have some localizing value (Table 42–1), but not as much localizing value as the distribution of pain in lumbosacral radiculopathies.

The pain is increased by coughing, sneezing, or straining. The increased intrathoracic pressure causes distension of epidural and intervertebral veins, resulting in traction and compression of the already irritated nerve root.[1] Neck extension or rotation (as occurs when shaving, turning the head, and backing up the car) often causes an increase in pain or may provoke radicular pain or paresthesia by compression or traction of the nerve root. Usually, there is reflex spasm of the neck muscles associated with neck stiffness and a decrease in range of motion. Pain may be worse at night as a result of lengthening of the spinal column. The water content of intervertebral disks is high. Some of this water is lost during the day in the upright position and height is decreased by about 0.5 to 0.75 inch. The

514

TABLE 42–1

Clinical Features of Cervical Radiculopathies

Root	Distribution of Pain	Paresthesias and/or Sensory Loss	Weakness	Decreased or Absent Reflexes
C-5	Upper arm only, not beyond elbow	Often none	*Deltoid* *Supraspinatus and infraspinatus* Brachioradialis Biceps	*Biceps* *Brachioradialis*
C-6	Deep in biceps	Digit 1 or digits 1 and 2	*Biceps* *Brachioradialis* Wrist extensor Supinator Finger flexors	*Biceps* *Brachioradialis*
C-7	Deep in triceps, mid-extensor and mid-flexor aspects of forearm	Digits 1, 2, and 3 or 2 and 3	*Triceps* *Wrist extensors* *Finger extensors* Pectoralis major	*Triceps* Pectoralis
C-8	Posterior arm, medial forearm	Digits 4 and 5	*Interossei* *Intrinsic hand muscles*	*Finger flexor reflex* Triceps

water is reabsorbed and original height is restored at night while lying down. With advance in age, gradually the intervertebral disks dehydrate somewhat. The decrease in height between young adulthood and old age is partly, although not entirely, related to this phenomenon.

The most common levels of cervical disk herniation or extrusion (in decreasing order of frequency) are C6-7, C5-6, C7-T1, and C4-5. Therefore, the most common cervical radiculopathies (in decreasing order of frequency) are C-7 radiculopathy (70%), C-6 radiculopathy (20%), C-8 radiculopathy, and C-5 radiculopathy.[2] A left-sided preponderance has been reported in many series. The disorder occurs more frequently in males. A history of trauma or exertion is not uncommon.

On clinical examination of the neck, evidence of paraspinal muscle spasm is frequent. There is limitation of range of motion of the neck, particularly on extension and lateral flexion. Results of the foraminal compression test of Spurling are often positive. This test is performed by extending the neck and laterally flexing it to the side of the suspected root irritation, and downward pressure is applied to the vertex. This may increase or reproduce the radicular pain or paresthesias.[3] Tenderness of ipsilateral neck and shoulder muscles is frequently noted. Neck traction may cause a decrease in pain. In cervical radiculopathies, often there are changes in muscle stretch reflexes and muscle strength. There are often abnormalities on sensory examination. Furthermore, patients often report paresthesias and numb feelings. The distributions of pain, sensory and motor symptoms and signs, and reflex changes help to localize the level of root irritation. These are summarized in Table 42–1.

Diagnostic Tests

The same diagnostic tests applied in the evaluation of lumbar radiculopathies (see Chapter 41) are used for evaluation of cervical radiculopathies.

Electromyographic evaluation is invaluable for determining which nerve root is involved, whether single or multiple roots are involved, or whether root involvement is bilateral. This test is also helpful for differentiating multiple root from plexus lesions and for identifying incidental or associated compression neuropathies such as carpal tunnel syndrome.

Plain films of the cervical spine may show degenerative changes and osteophyte formation, decreased intervertebral disk space, subluxations, reversal of normal cervical lordosis (Fig. 42–1), deformities (such as swanneck deformity [Fig. 42–2], particularly in patients with a history of multilevel cervical laminectomies), and certain anomalies. They are also helpful for demonstrating fractures, compression fractures, and tumors. Flexion and extension views are useful for identifying cervical instability and any change in the degree of subluxation seen in the standard views. Oblique views (3/4 views) are useful for demonstrating the foramina. If the odontoid process of C-2 is to be studied more clearly, special odontoid views should be obtained.

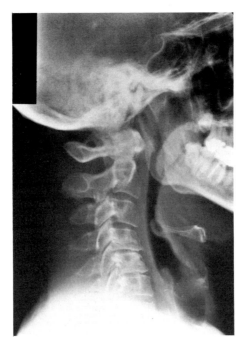

Figure 42–1
Radiograph, lateral view, of cervical spine shows degenerative disk disease with decreased intervertebral disk spaces in lower cervical levels and reversal of normal cervical lordosis.

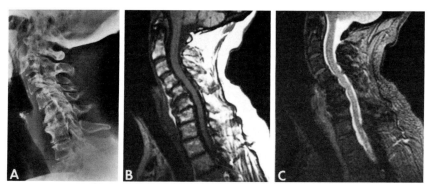

Figure 42–2

A, Radiograph, lateral view, of cervical spine shows degenerative changes of cervical spine, decreased intervertebral disk space, and formation of osteophytes, particularly in middle to lower cervical segments. As a result of these degenerative changes, a "swan-neck" deformity has developed. *B* and *C,* Magnetic resonance imaging scans. On T1- *(B)* and T2- *(C)* weighted images, the related deformity of cervical spinal cord is noted. There is an associated cervical spinal stenosis and segmental compromise of spinal subarachnoid space, particularly anteriorly *(C)*. No intrinsic spinal cord lesion is noted, however.

Magnetic resonance imaging (MRI) is an extremely useful test for demonstrating herniated disk (Fig. 42–3), cervical stenosis (Fig. 42–4) and cord impingement, and particularly the intrinsic cord lesions (tumor, syrinx, even demyelinating plaques). T1-weighted gadolinium-enhanced images may show certain pathologic processes involving the meninges. MRI is a powerful tool for demonstrating tumors involving the vertebral

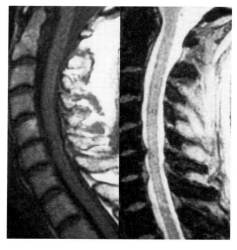

Figure 42–3

Magnetic resonance imaging scans of cervical spine. Sagittal T1- *(left)* and T2- *(right)* weighted images demonstrate extruded C-6 disk.

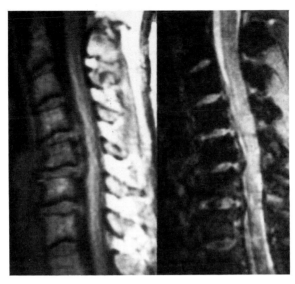

Figure 42-4
Magnetic resonance imaging scan of cervical spine. Sagittal T1- *(left)* and T2- *(right)* weighted images demonstrate multilevel (C-4, C-5, and C-6) disk extrusions causing cervical canal stenosis.

bones and epidural space. Computed tomography (CT) is also capable of showing many of these abnormalities, but often not as accurately as magnetic resonance imaging. However, in the evaluation of certain bony lesions, CT may be more helpful (Fig. 42-5). Myelography, especially when coupled with CT (computed tomography myelography), is the most accurate test for identifying herniated and extruded disks or foraminal stenosis (Figs. 42-6 and 42-7). Despite advances in magnetic resonance imaging, myelography and CT myelography are extensively used by many neurosurgeons before proceeding with operation.

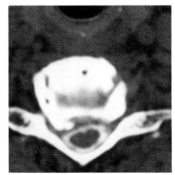

Figure 42-5
Computed tomography myelogram. Note osteophyte at C-6 on the right.

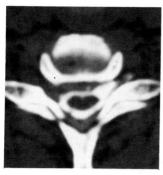

Figure 42–6
Computed tomography myelogram demonstrates extruded C-6 disk on the right with nonfilling of root slope.

Treatment

Most patients with cervical disk syndrome and cervical radiculopathies respond to conservative management. Surgical management is generally reserved for patients with progressive neurologic deficits or intractable pain, particularly when related to compromise of neural structures. Surgical procedures that are usually applied are laminectomy and diskectomy, foraminotomy, anterior diskectomy, and fusion. Symptomatic compromise of the cervical spinal cord often requires early surgical intervention.

Conservative management is basically aimed at relief of symptoms. The principles of conservative management vary according to the severity of the symptoms.

Acute cervical disk syndromes are treated with a supportive collar and analgesics only. Symptomatic measures such as the use of analgesics, nonsteroidal anti-inflammatory medications, or muscle relaxants are helpful at this stage. Foam collars provide warmth to the muscles but do not provide support. At this stage, therapeutic exercise programs can aggravate the pain. Proper positioning during rest and avoidance of aggravating activities are important. Reduction of nuchal myalgia secondary to muscle spasm and overguarding can be managed by supported head positions and relaxation of the neck muscles. If needed, a rigid support to eliminate weight bearing on the cervical spine can be very helpful. Application of cervical

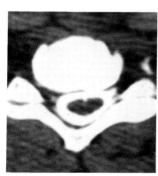

Figure 42–7
Computed tomography myelogram demonstrates foraminal stenosis of C-5 on the right.

traction also contributes to elimination of weight bearing and provides muscle relaxation and reduction of pain. The application of mild heat (such as moist hot packs) is effective for reducing myalgia, but in some instances ice packs are preferred by the patient.

At the subacute stage, muscle overuse, fatigue, and pain may result from the patient's attempt to protect the painful area. In these instances, sedative physical therapy such as hot packs, neck rotation in the supine position, relaxation exercises, and cervical traction may be recommended. The proper position of the cervical spine during traction is with the neck slightly flexed or in the neutral position. This position contributes to foraminal decompression.

After the subacute stage and when it can be tolerated by the patient, isometric strengthening of the nuchal muscles needs to be initiated. The patient should start decreasing the duration of use of the cervical collar to avoid dependence and weakening of the nuchal musculature. Educating the patient in proper spine posture is important.

CERVICAL SPONDYLOSIS AND CERVICAL SPINAL STENOSIS

Cervical spondylosis refers to a condition of progressive degeneration of the cervical spine that begins in the intervertebral disks and is followed by changes in the vertebral bones and spinal ligaments.

The process of disk degeneration may begin in the third decade of life. Loss of water and fragmentation of nuclear material may lead to weakening of the annulus. A sequestered fragment of nucleus pulposus may undergo a frank herniation—the so-called soft disk. This herniation may be midline, ventrolateral, or infraforaminal. Acute forms of cervical radiculopathy are often caused by soft disks. At times, the episode is precipitated by trauma, particularly in the young patient in whom the degenerative process has not yet started or become significant. Midline disk herniation may compress the spinal cord. If herniation does not occur early in the process, disk degeneration continues and leads to disk fibrosis and a decrease in the height of the disk, narrowed intervertebral space, and protrusion of the annulus fibrosus. Generally, these degenerative changes occur more frequently and more prominently in disks below the C3-4 level. The most frequently involved level is C5-6, followed by C6-7. C2-3 is the least commonly affected level.

In the cervical region, the anterior height of the intervertebral disk is greater than its posterior height. This configuration is responsible for normal cervical lordosis. With advance in the process of disk degeneration and loss of height, the normal lordotic curve may be straightened or even, in some cases, reversed. With advanced degeneration, articular cartilages and the vertebral end plates are subjected to more stress, and osteophytic spurs develop around the margins of the vertebral end plates ventrally, dorsally, and laterally. Anterior osteophytes are products of a reactive process in connection with ligamentous stress. Although anterior osteophytes are often larger than posterior osteophytes, they are not closely related to disk degeneration. Posterior osteophytes show a high correlation with disk degeneration. These are most frequently noted in the C5-7 levels. Degeneration of the facets may lead to vertebral subluxation.

Osteophyte formation may lead to foraminal narrowing. The term "hard disk" refers to the presence of osteophytes that originate from the bony confines of the foramina.[4] Anterior osteophytes may become very large and even abut adjacent levels and cause fusion of adjacent vertebral bodies. In advanced spondylosis, mobility of the cervical spine is decreased, particularly on flexion and extension.

With progression of cervical spondylosis and formation of spondylotic ridges anteriorly and hypertrophy of ligamenta flava posteriorly, the anteroposterior diameter of the cervical canal is decreased and cervical stenosis is produced. This, in turn, may compromise the cervical spinal cord (especially in patients who have congenitally narrow cervical spinal canals) and lead to cervical myelopathy.

Clinical Manifestations

Cervical Spondylosis. Radiographic changes of cervical spondylosis may be seen in more than 80% of individuals older than 55 years. There is no direct correlation between these changes and a patient's symptoms. The most common clinical manifestations of cervical spondylosis are neck pain (which is usually not acute or severe), decrease in range of motion of the cervical spine, and muscle contraction-type headaches.

Cervical Spondylosis With Radiculopathy. Radicular symptoms may occur acutely, subacutely, or insidiously. The extent of the nerve root involvement may be variable. A single root or multiple roots may be involved. The involvement may be unilateral or bilateral, and if bilateral it may be symmetric or asymmetric. Sensory symptoms (paresthesias, numbness, dysesthesias) are more common than motor symptoms (muscle weakness and atrophy). The distribution of pain, paresthesias, weakness, and reflex change, similar to that described in cervical disk syndromes (Table 42–1), helps in localizing the one or more nerve roots involved. The clinical picture ordinarily is not affected by whether root compression is due to soft disk (extruded nucleus pulposus) or hard disk (foraminal spur).

Cervical Spondylosis and Stenosis With Myelopathy. Myelopathy associated with cervical spondylosis and stenosis often develops insidiously, but it may occur episodically and sometimes in connection with hyperextension injury. The size and shape of the cervical spinal canal vary considerably in different individuals. The lateral diameter of the canal on average is about 2.5 cm, and the average lateral cord diameter is about 1.3 cm. In cervical spondylosis, the cord is often not compromised laterally but anteroposteriorly. The minimal anteroposterior diameter of the cervical canal is 1.4 cm and at the level of C-5. The spinal cord is somewhat fusiform in the neck, and its maximal girth is at C-5. At this level, the average anteroposterior diameter of the cord is 8 mm. Several factors may interact to produce spondylotic cervical myelopathy, including compressive effect of spondylotic transverse bars on the anterior aspect of the cord, preexisting narrowed canal, changes in canal diameter with motion, vascular changes, cord sensitivity to hypoxia, and shape of the canal.[5, 6]

The course of spondylotic myelopathy is often one of increasing disability over many months. As expected, the symptoms result from involvement of the lower motor neurons and sensory fibers at the segmental level (therefore, these symptoms appear in the upper extremities) and from involvement of long tracts, particularly the pyramidal tracts (therefore, manifested primarily in the lower extremities in the form of spasticity). Patients present with numbness, paresthesias, or dysesthesias of the upper extremities which may be unilateral or bilateral and involve particularly the hands or fingers. Also weakness, atrophy, and sometimes fasciculations or contraction fasciculation of the upper extremities are present. Muscle stretch reflexes at the level of myelopathy are diminished or absent.[7] At the level below the myelopathy, they are exaggerated. Therefore, it is not unusual to encounter patients with absent bicep and brachioradialis reflexes but with exaggerated triceps or finger flexor reflexes. In these cases, when tapping the lower biceps tendon or distal radius to obtain biceps or brachioradialis reflexes, one may observe a triceps muscle contraction or a finger flexion response.

The lower extremities may be involved with a progressive spasticity manifested by clumsiness, spastic gait, and a decrease in alternate-motion rates of the feet. There may be bowel urgency and urinary frequency and urgency and, in severe cases, various degrees of incontinence. Surprisingly, in spondylotic cervical myelopathy, neck pain is not a prominent feature; it may be a mild ache or even absent. Only on questioning do some, but not all, patients report an ache or a decrease in the range of motion of the neck. Sometimes, manifestations of cervical myelopathy appear more rapidly over a few weeks.

When there is absent neck pain and minimal or no sensory symptoms, the patient with cervical spondylosis and myelopathy may display manifestations mimicking those of amyotrophic lateral sclerosis.[8] These patients manifest weakness, atrophy, and sometimes fasciculations in the upper extremities (lower motor neuron manifestations) and spasticity, exaggerated muscle stretch reflexes, and Babinski signs in the lower extremities and even exaggeration of muscle stretch reflexes in some of the lower segments of the upper extremities (such as finger flexors). This combination of upper and lower motor neuron manifestations obviously raises the possibility of amyotrophic lateral sclerosis. In a number of patients suspected of having amyotrophic lateral sclerosis, attempts frequently are made to rule out the possibility of cervical spondylosis and myelopathy.

Diagnostic Tests

The same diagnostic tests and principles described for lumbar radiculopathies and lumbar stenosis (see Chapter 41) and cervical disk syndromes and cervical radiculopathies (earlier in this chapter) apply to cervical spondylosis and cervical spinal stenosis.

On plain radiographs, a congenitally narrow canal may be seen in many patients. Significant spondylosis and subluxations are also frequent.

Computed tomography and especially MRI show the stenosis. MRI is particularly helpful for demonstrating atrophy of the cord or intrinsic cord lesion, which might have been caused by compression of the cord as the result of canal stenosis and compression (Fig. 42–8). Compromise of the spinal subarachnoid space and cord deformity and angulation are also clearly seen with MRI.

Myelography demonstrates various degrees of obstruction to the flow of contrast medium. The degree of obstruction to the flow may vary with the neck in different positions such as flexion or extension and can also be of diagnostic aid.

Electromyography frequently shows active and chronic neurogenic changes in single or often multiple levels which may be unilateral but are often bilateral and frequently asymmetric.

Treatment

Surgical. Cautious clinical judgment must be exercised in selecting patients for operation. Those with progressive neurologic deficits or cord compromise are considered surgical candidates. The problem at hand may vary from single root canal stenosis with compromise of a single root associated with corresponding neurologic deficits to involvement of multiple roots, to cord compression at a single level, to cord compression at multiple levels, and finally to a combination of cord and root compressions. The operative procedure should therefore be designed selectively for the patient. Decompressions of the compromised neural structures with or without fusion may be necessary. Depending on the clinical situation, the experience and preference of the surgeon, and the extent of the disease process, various approaches have been used, including decompressive laminectomies and foraminotomies with a posterior approach, anterior diskectomy, and fusions, if needed. The objectives of surgical treatment are to decompress the involved nerve roots and spinal cord, to remove the offending osteophytes, and provide stability of the spine when needed.[5]

Medical. Many patients with cervical stenosis frequently have little or no pain. Therefore, pain management is frequently a less significant problem than in patients with herniated cervical disk syndromes. When pain is present, the same principles of pain management can be applied here (described earlier in this chapter).

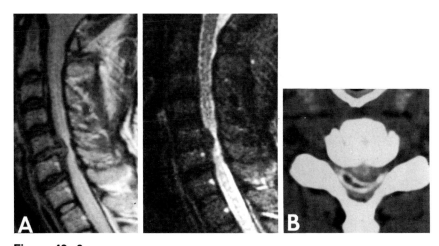

Figure 42–8
A, Magnetic resonance imaging scans of cervical spine. Sagittal T1- *(left)* and T2- *(right)* weighted images demonstrate extruded C-5 disk. Note compression of cervical spinal cord. There was evidence of cervical myelopathy. B, Computed tomography myelogram at level of cord compression, demonstrating marked compression and deformity of cord.

Physical Therapy and Rehabilitative Measures. Postoperative management consists of two categories of physical therapeutic measures. Initial management is to instruct the patient in proper posture, nuchal muscle relaxation techniques, and, if needed, a temporary cervical collar. Isometric muscle strengthening exercises need to be initiated as soon as the patient can tolerate them. Symptoms related to cervical myelopathy such as spasticity, paresthesias, gait disorder, and neurogenic bowel and bladder should be managed accordingly (see Chapters 8, 10, 11, 14, 15, and 38).

REFERENCES

1. Jackson R. The cervical syndrome. 4th ed. Springfield, IL: Charles C Thomas, 1977.
2. Yoss RE, Corbin KB, MacCarty CS, Love JG. Significance of symptoms and signs in localization of involved root in cervical disk protrusion. Neurology 1957; 7:673–683.
3. Department of Neurology, Mayo Clinic and Mayo Foundation. Clinical examinations in neurology. 6th ed. St. Louis: Mosby Year Book, 1991.
4. Lestini WF, Wiesel SW. The pathogenesis of cervical spondylosis. Clin Orthop 1989; 239:69–93.
5. Hoff JT. Cervical disc disease and cervical spondylosis. In: Wilkins RH, Rengachary SS, eds. Neurosurgery, vol 3. New York: McGraw-Hill, 1985:2230–2239.
6. Gooding MR. Pathogenesis of myelopathy in cervical spondylosis. Lancet 1974; 2:1180–1181.
7. Brain WR, Northfield D, Wilkinson M. The neurological manifestations of cervical spondylosis. Brain 1952; 75:187–225.
8. Rowland LP. Surgical treatment of cervical spondylotic myelopathy: time for a controlled trial. Neurology 1992; 42:5–13.

Index